Neuroprotective Effects of Phytochemicals in Neurological Disorders

Neuroprotective Effects of Phytochemicals in Neurological Disorders

Editor: Roy McClen

AMERICAN
MEDICAL PUBLISHERS
www.americanmedicalpublishers.com

AMERICAN
MEDICAL PUBLISHERS
www.americanmedicalpublishers.com

Cataloging-in-Publication Data

Neuroprotective effects of phytochemicals in neurological disorders / edited by Roy McClen.
p. cm.
Includes bibliographical references and index.
ISBN 978-1-63927-747-6
1. Nervous system--Diseases--Chemotherapy. 2. Phytochemicals--Therapeutic use.
3. Nervous system--Diseases. 4. Phytonutrients. 5. Neuroprotective agents. I. McClen, Roy.
RM315 .N48 2023
615.78--dc23

American Medical Publishers,
41 Flatbush Avenue,
1st Floor, New York,
NY 11217, USA

ISBN 978-1-63927-747-6 (Hardback)

Contents

Preface

Every book is a source of knowledge and this one is no exception. The idea that led to the conceptualization of this book was the fact that the world is advancing rapidly; which makes it crucial to document the progress in every field. I am aware that a lot of data is already available, yet, there is a lot more to learn. Hence, I accepted the responsibility of editing this book and contributing my knowledge to the community.

The brain is a complex organ which regulates every action in the human body, including memory, motor skills, respiration, thought, emotion, hunger, touch, vision and temperature. If the brain gets injured, it can have a wide range of consequences, such as changes in sensation, memory and even personality. There are various types of brain disorders, including mental health disorders, brain injuries, neurodegenerative disorders like Parkinson's and Alzheimer's disease, brain tumors and many more. The prognosis for patients suffering from brain disorders is determined by the type and degree of the disorder. Some of the disorders are simple to treat with therapy and medication. However, conditions such as neurodegenerative disorders and some traumatic brain injuries do not have a treatment. Phytochemicals are bioactive compounds which are found in plants, fruits, herbs and vegetables. They are not essential for sustaining cell viability, but have a significant role in providing protection to the neural cells from oxidative stress related with aging, inflammation, and chronic and acute brain diseases related with aging. This book is compiled in such a manner, that it will provide in-depth knowledge about phytochemicals and their effect on the neurological disorders. It presents researches and studies performed by experts across the globe. Those in search of information to further their knowledge will be greatly assisted by this book.

While editing this book, I had multiple visions for it. Then I finally narrowed down to make every chapter a sole standing text explaining a particular topic, so that they can be used independently. However, the umbrella subject sinews them into a common theme. This makes the book a unique platform of knowledge.

I would like to give the major credit of this book to the experts from every corner of the world, who took the time to share their expertise with us. Also, I owe the completion of this book to the never-ending support of my family, who supported me throughout the project.

Editor

1

On the Neuroprotective Role of Astaxanthin: New Perspectives?

Christian Galasso [1], Ida Orefice [1], Paola Pellone [1], Paola Cirino [2], Roberta Miele [1], Adrianna Ianora [1], Christophe Brunet [1,*] and Clementina Sansone [1,*]

1 Department of Marine Biotechnology, Stazione Zoologica Anton Dohrn, Villa Comunale, 80121 Naples, Italy; christian.galasso@szn.it (C.G.); ida.orefice@szn.it (I.O.); paola.pellone@gmail.com (P.P.); robertamiele90@libero.it (R.M.); adrianna.ianora@szn.it (A.I.)

2 Department of Research Infrastructures for Marine Biological Resources, Stazione Zoologica Anton Dohrn, Villa Comunale, 80121 Naples, Italy; paola.cirino@szn.it

* Correspondence: christophe.brunet@szn.it (C.B.); clementina.sansone@szn.it (C.S.)

Abstract: Astaxanthin is a carotenoid with powerful antioxidant and anti-inflammatory activity produced by several freshwater and marine microorganisms, including bacteria, yeast, fungi, and microalgae. Due to its deep red-orange color it confers a reddish hue to the flesh of salmon, shrimps, lobsters, and crayfish that feed on astaxanthin-producing organisms, which helps protect their immune system and increase their fertility. From the nutritional point of view, astaxanthin is considered one of the strongest antioxidants in nature, due to its high scavenging potential of free radicals in the human body. Recently, astaxanthin is also receiving attention for its effect on the prevention or co-treatment of neurological pathologies, including Alzheimer and Parkinson diseases. In this review, we focus on the neuroprotective properties of astaxanthin and explore the underlying mechanisms to counteract neurological diseases, mainly based on its capability to cross the blood-brain barrier and its oxidative, anti-inflammatory, and anti-apoptotic properties.

Keywords: astaxanthin; neuroinflammation; neuroprotective effect; neuroactive carotenoids; neurodegenerative diseases

---

1. Introduction

Carotenoids have gained scientific and commercial interest during the last decades, due to their huge chemical diversity (about 750 carotenoids have been characterized) and their strong beneficial effects on human health and wellbeing. These bioactive compounds exert antioxidant, repairing, antiproliferative, antiaging and anti-inflammatory effects and can be used either as skin photo-protection to inhibit adverse effects of solar UV radiation or as nutraceutical and cosmeceutical ingredients to prevent oxidative stress-related diseases and chronic inflammation [1–3].

Astaxanthin is one of the most successful carotenoids on the market (Figure 1), since many studies in recent years have demonstrated its inhibitory role against oxidative stress and inflammation, dangerous processes at the basis of many chronic diseases. Moreover, astaxanthin exerts a strong protective effect on human brain; its unique chemical structure allows it to readily cross the blood-brain barrier (BBB) [4]. Thus, the brain is considered the most important target organ of astaxanthin.

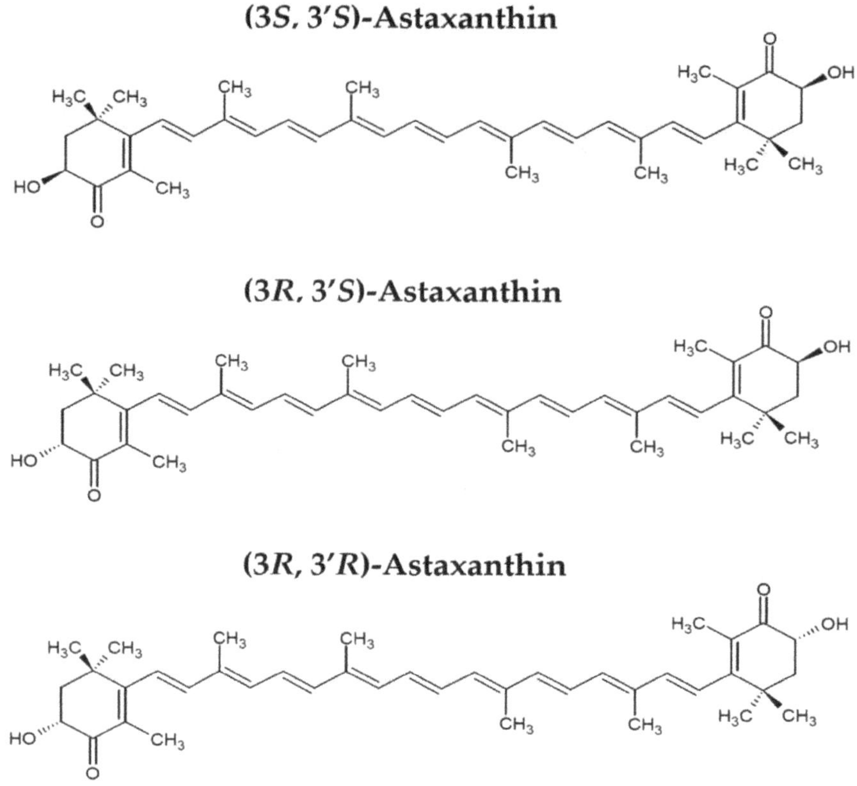

Figure 1. Stereoisomers of astaxanthin.

Astaxanthin is present especially in the marine environment and is produced mainly by microorganisms such as bacteria, microalgae, and yeast; it can also be found in marine invertebrates and vertebrates [5–7]. The most important producers of astaxanthin are the marine bacterium *Agrobacterium aurantiacum*, the green microalgae *Haematococcus pluvialis* and *Chlorella zofingiensis*, and the red yeast *Xanthophyllomyces dendrorhous* (called also *Phaffia rhodozyma*). Animals cannot synthesize astaxanthin but can obtain it through the diet [8]. Astaxanthin is thus present in salmon, trout, shrimp, lobster, and fish eggs which confers a reddish-orange hue to these organisms. Nevertheless, the majority of astaxanthin-based products on the market are derived from its synthetic production, since its natural production is still not well standardized for industrial scale. Unfortunately, synthetic astaxanthin is significantly more inferior than algal-based astaxanthin in terms of anti-inflammatory and antioxidant properties [9].

Given that oxidative damage and increased neuro-inflammation are critically related with the pathogenesis of late-onset massive neuronal loss in neurodegenerative diseases, the neuroprotective effect of natural compounds, such as astaxanthin, has been of specific interest as co-treatments and prevention for these diseases [10]. The most common neurodegenerative diseases include Alzheimer Disease (AD), Parkinson Disease (PD), Huntington's disease (HD), and amyotrophic lateral sclerosis (ALS) [11,12]. Although different neurodegenerative diseases can have several causative factors, they have some common characteristics such as an increase in ROS levels in neuronal cells caused by mitochondrial insults and the release of redox metals interacting with oxygen [13], resulting in neuronal cell death [14]. This can lead to an increase in protein aggregates that inflame and activate microglia cells [15]. Once neuroinflammation is chronically activated, cytokines and chemokines are released, producing an increment of oxidative stress, with dangerous detrimental effects on neurons [16].

The aim of this review is to report the most recent scientific findings on the protective and curative role of astaxanthin on human brain against neuroinflammation, oxidative stress and, more in general, on the beneficial effects for patients with neurodegenerative disorders (Table 1).

Table 1. In vitro and in vivo studies of biological roles of astaxanthin.

Model	Effect	Concentration	Target	Disease	Reference
Mice	Anti-inflammatory	25 mg/Kg/day	NF-κB, TNF-α	Cognitive impairment	[17]
SH-SY5Y cells	Anti-apoptotic	1 to 20 μM	6-OHDA, Casp3, Casp9, PARP	Not specific disease	[18]
PC12 cells	Antioxidant	5, 10, 20 μM	NOX2, NFR2, HO-1 Sp1/NR1	Not specific disease	[19,20]
Rats	Cell regeneration	20 mg/Kg/day	GFAP, MAP-2, BDNF, GAP-43 SOD, GSH,	Not specific disease	[21]
Rats	Neuroprotective	25 mg/kg	Not investigated	Cognitive disorders	[22]
Human	Antioxidant	6 or 12 mg/d	PLOOH	Dementia	[23]
Rats	Anti-inflammatory	1, 10 or 100 mg/Kg	TNF-α, PGE2, IL-1β	AD	[24]
BV-2 cells	Anti-inflammatory	50 μM	p-IKKα, p-IκBα, NF-κB p65, IL-6, MAPK	AD	[25]
Mice	Antioxidant	2 mg/kg	SOD, GSH, MDA, APOP	AD	[26]
PC12 cells	Antioxidant	0.1 μM	Bax, IL-1β, TNFα, NF-κB	AD	[27]
Primary hippocampal neurons	Antioxidant	0.1 μM	NFATc4, RyR2	AD	[28]
Neural Progenitor Cells (NPCs)	Pro-proliferative	5 and 10 ng/mL	PI3K, MEK, CDK2	AD	[29,30]
Mice	Neuroprotective	3 mg/kg	TH, IBA-1	PD	[4]
SH-SY5Y cells	Antioxidant	100 nM	PARP, CYTc	PD	[31]
Motor neurons	Antioxidant	100 nM	SOD1	ALS	[32]
SH-SY5Y cells and Rats	Neuroprotective	10 to 50 μM (cells) 30 mg/kg (rats)	iNOS, HSPs	IR	[33]
Mice	Neuroprotective	20 mg/kg	GHS, SOD, Cyt C, Casp3	IR	[34]
Rats	Neuroprotective	10 mg/Kg	SOD, MVA, Nef2, HO-1, NQO1	IR	[35]

2. Brain Processes Involved in Neurodegeneration and Protective Effects of Carotenoids

The human Central Nervous System (CNS) contains 100 billion neuronal cells and an equal number of glia cells, such as microglia, astrocytes, and oligodendrocytes [36]. The CNS includes all nerves in the brain and spinal cord and is isolated from the other compartments of the human body through the blood-brain barrier (BBB). This barrier is fundamental to control and restrict the penetration of molecules (e.g., neurotoxins) and cells (e.g., immune cells or infectious agents) from peripheral parts of the body into the CNS. Tight junctions between cells forming the vascular endothelium at the CNS level confer to BBB its selective property.

CNS is able to activate the innate immune system in response to several forms of injuries, including trauma, infections, stroke and neurotoxins. A variety of cell types belonging to CNS, such as astrocytes, microglia, vascular cells, neutrophils, and macrophages, are involved in neuroinflammation [37]. Neuroinflammation is a local response of the CNS during several processes, such as neurodegeneration, trauma, and autoimmune disorders, that leads to innate immune cells mobilization and activation. Glia cells release cytokines, reactive oxygen species (ROS) and reactive nitrogen species (RNS), which could be harmful for neurons and oligodendrocytes when neuroinflammation is not a transient event. There is growing evidence suggesting that a long-standing chronic neuroinflammatory response can lead to neuronal damage, producing neurodegeneration via sustained accumulation of neurotoxic pro-inflammatory mediators [10]. The release of pro-inflammatory mediators, together with pro-oxidant agents, results in morphological and functional changes of intracellular organelles and contributes to the insurgence and progression of neurodegenerative pathologies. An example are mitochondria, intracellular targets of oxidative injuries, where chronic inflammation could produce mitochondrial dysfunction [38–40].

The CNS is considered highly vulnerable to oxidative stress and inflammation due to its low cell renewal potential and high cellular metabolism, since this organ requires about 25% of total body energy. This energy is fundamental for neuronal connection, axonal transport, and myelination, while mitochondrial activity produces a high amount of ROS. ROS are involved in several signal transduction pathways, such as survival, growth, proliferation and defense mechanisms against microbial infection. An unbalance between ROS production and endogenous mechanisms for detoxification of reactive oxygen intermediates leads to dysregulation of the above-mentioned mechanisms and consequent neurotoxicity and neurodegeneration [41,42].

In normal conditions and young brains, mitochondrial dysfunction is regulated and deleted by autophagy, a clearance mechanism able to remove intracellular components. In particular, mitophagy is a specific autophagic process, which is activated when damaged or superfluous mitochondria need to be removed. This signal leads to formation of autophagosomes with consequent degradation of unnecessary mitochondria. The efficiency of these clearance mechanisms diminishes with increasing age, with the accumulation of toxic molecules and damaged organelles [43–45]. Aging is considered the major risk factor for the insurgence and development of many neurodegenerative diseases, as also confirmed by studies describing the autophagy reduction in aging CNS cells [46–48]. For example, mitochondrial complex I (NADH dehydrogenase) dysfunction is strictly correlated to the idiopathic Parkinson's disease phenotype; similarly, injury of complex II (succinate dehydrogenase) yields the Huntington's disease phenotype. mtDNA mutations either inherited or caused by oxidative damage have been shown to contribute to Alzheimer's disease pathology [37]. Loss of cognitive function is a common symptom in neurodegenerative diseases and there are few commercially available drugs that are able to reduce the occurrence of neuroinflammation.

Research on molecules with anti-neuroinflammatory effects and with protective properties against oxidative stress in neuronal cell models shows interesting results about some carotenoids [49,50]. Recently, it was demonstrated that astaxanthin attenuates cognitive disorders in *in vivo* and *in vitro* models for neurodegenerative diseases [4,51–53]. The first study in measuring carotenoids within brain compartments was carried out by Craft et al. [54]. This study quantified carotenoid content in five elderly brains and found a seeming preference for xanthophylls in the human brain.

In the last decade, some natural carotenoids, in particular those belonging to the xanthophyll family, such as lutein, crucin, crocetin, have been shown to have anti-neuroinflammatory and antioxidant effects [50,55]. The marine derived xanthophylls, such as fucoxanthin and astaxanthin, have anti-inflammatory effects and antioxidant activity on different cell lines [56,57]. Furthermore, astaxanthin has also been found to reduce hippocampal and retinal inflammation in streptozotocin-induced diabetic rats, alleviating cognitive deficits, retinal oxidative stress, and depression [17,58,59], while fucoxanthin exerts anti-inflammatory effects against various stimuli through Akt, NF-κB, and mitogen-activated protein kinase pathways [60].

The most common mechanism of action for marine xanthophylls is the suppression of inflammation pathways through the radical scavenging activity against oxygen-reactive species [5,61]. In particular, astaxanthin exerts protective effects in liver cells after induction of an inflammatory injury [62,63] and protects neuronal cells from oxidative stress [18,64], through the activation of specific pathways, such as HO-1/NOX2 axis [19] and Sp1/NR1 signaling [20]. Recent studies have demonstrated the beneficial effects of carotenoids for the treatment of neurodegenerative diseases, while a number of epidemiological studies have linked the consumption of a carotenoid rich diet with a decreased risk of neurodegenerative diseases in humans [65–68].

Extensive studies suggest that carotenoids may inhibit neurodegenerative diseases through a variety of molecular mechanisms [68,69]. For example, fucoxanthin treatment reduced Aβ-induced damage in a cultured cell model through several mechanisms including downregulation of apoptotic factors, inhibition of inflammatory cytokine-mediating action, and simultaneous reduction of ROS [70]. High levels of carotenoids within the brain, such as lutein and zeaxanthin, can enhance cognitive function in elderly people, exerting neuroprotection with a reduction of neuronal mortality [71]. In addition, high carotenoid concentrations in other body compartments provide protection against neurological pathologies. In particular, Dias and collaborators [72] found lower concentrations of carotenoids (lutein, lycopene and zeaxanthin) in dementia patients with respect to control subjects.

Many studies confirm that astaxanthin delays or ameliorates the cognitive impairment associated with normal aging or alleviates the pathophysiology of various neurodegenerative diseases [73,74].

It is known that astaxanthin can cross the blood-brain barrier, a crucial feature for the treatment of neurodegenerative diseases with antioxidant compounds [75]. A recent study demonstrated that dietary astaxanthin accumulated in the hippocampus and cerebral cortex of rat brains after single and repeated ingestion. The accumulation of dietary astaxanthin in the cerebral cortex may affect maintenance and improvement of cognitive functions [76].

Astaxanthin pre-treatment promotes nerve cell regeneration, increasing gene expression of glial fibrillary acidic protein (GFAP), microtubule associated protein 2 (MAP-2), brain derived neurotrophic factor (BDNF) and growth-associated protein 43 (GAP-43) [21]. These proteins are involved in brain recovery. For example, GFAP is important in the repairing process after CNS injury, being involved in cell communication and functioning of the BBB [77]. MAP-2 is responsible of microtubule growth and neuronal regeneration; BDNF is involved in neuronal survival, growth, and differentiation of new neurons [78], while up-regulation of GAP-43 3 activates a protein kinase pathway, promoting neurite formation, regeneration, and plasticity [79].

3. Astaxanthin against Cognitive Disorders

Cognitive disorders are a group of mental health diseases that cause several effects on mental abilities, such as learning, problem solving, memory and perception. The most important cognitive disorders are delirium, dementia, and amnesia. Delirium is an acute confusional state characterized by inactivation, disorganized thinking, and confusion of space and time. Dementia is a progressive deterioration of the brain, memory impairment, confusion, and loss of concentration. Amnesia is a memory disorder characterized by loss of short-term memory that interferes with daily life.

Among cognitive disorders, chemobrain, a cognitive impairment caused by chemotherapeutic agents, is receiving increasing attention. These chemical agents could produce in cancer patients a strong reduction in the quality life, since they induce memory impairment, slow processing speed, and inability to concentrate. These cognitive dysfunctions seem to be linked to a reduction of neuronal integrity at the hippocampus and frontal system levels [80]. Recently, El-Agamy and collaborators [22] investigated the potential effect of astaxanthin as a protective compound able to drastically contrast the decline of cognitive functions induced by doxorubicin (DOX). Astaxanthin showed neuroprotection and memory-enhancing effects and was able to switch off inflammation and oxidative stress, mitigating the increase of acetylcholinesterase activity and suppressing several pro-apoptotic stimuli [22].

Astaxanthin also produces beneficial effects in other body compartments and cells, with direct repercussion on brain health. In particular, the positive influence of a diet rich in polar carotenoids, such as astaxanthin, on an abnormal accumulation of phospholipid hydroperoxides (PLOOH) in the erythrocytes of patients affected by dementia [23] has been described. PLOOH are the primary oxidation products of phospholipids and their accumulation in erythrocytes induce a reduction in oxygen transport to the brain, facilitating the progression of dementia [81–83]. Nakagawa and collaborators [23] described lower PLOOH levels in the erythrocytes and blood cells of patients treated with astaxanthin with respect to the control (placebo group), demonstrating that this bioactive molecule is responsible for the improvement of erythrocyte antioxidant status, which may contribute to the prevention of dementia.

Some marine food products are recommended by many medical authorities worldwide [84]. In particular, fish oil usually contains tocopherols, saturated fats, monounsaturated fats (mostly palmitoleic and oleic acids), and polyunsaturated fatty acids (PUFA, such as eicosapentaenoic acid, EPA, and docosahexaenoic acid, DHA). A balanced proportion between EPA and DHA (3:2, regularly found in natural fish oil) seems to be a key factor for beneficial effects, such as the slowing down of cognitive decline and reduced depression, whereas many other PUFAs (for instance the pro-inflammatory arachidonic acid) could be responsible for massive ROS production with consequent activation of immune cells [85]. The combination of astaxanthin and fish oil enhances the positive effect on brain health by reducing harmful effects due to PUFAs [86]. In particular, a Wistar rat fed with 1 mg/kg of astaxanthin and 1 mg/kg of fish oil presented lipid protection status at the anterior forebrain level. Moreover, Trolox equivalent antioxidant capacity (TAEC) and Ferric Reducing Antioxidant Power (FRAP) assessed in brain homogenates was found to increase in rats fed with a mix of astaxanthin and fish oil, with respect to only fish oil. A similar investigation was performed by Nolan et al. [87], who studied the beneficial effects of a mixture of xanthophyll carotenoids and fish oil (containing EPA and DHA) on the human brain. This particular functional food, probably due to its strong antioxidant potential, was able to reduce the progression of neurodegeneration, acting on memory, sight, and mood. The reduction of ROS production linked to marine functional foods, such as fish oil, represents a valid mechanism to prevent cognitive dysfunctions.

4. Astaxanthin against Alzheimer Disease (AD)

Alzheimer's disease (AD) is one of the most severe chronic neurodegenerative disorders, characterized by memory impairment and cognitive dysfunction, due to neuronal loss mainly in the neocortex and hippocampus. The incidence of AD has increased dramatically in the last decades. From few cases at the beginning of the 20th century, in 2017 AD was reported to affect one out of five persons aged 65 and over worldwide [88]. This incidence increases drastically up to 40% over the age of 85. AD is the most common form of dementia, first described in 1906 by Alois Alzheimer. Nowadays there are many unknown aspects regarding the physiopathology of AD. Various theories have tried to explain the molecular mechanisms responsible for the initiation and progression of AD. Not one of these hypotheses alone is able to fully explain this complex neurodegenerative disease. Abnormal formation and aggregation in the brain of amyloid beta plaques are considered initial causes of AD [89]. Many studies have already demonstrated that the formation of these plaques is caused by an imbalance between synthesis and clearance of amyloid beta [90]. Accumulation of amyloid beta induces oxidative stress and inflammation at the neurofibrillary tangle level, inducing neuronal death stimuli in the brain of patients with AD [91,92]. Moreover, some studies have described the presence of high numbers of damaged mitochondria in the neurons of AD patients, probably due to mutations in mitochondrial DNA [93]. Oxidative stress at the expense of mitochondria occurs during the early stages of AD, suggesting a predominant role of oxidative stress for the progression of this disease [94]. For this reason, natural compounds with antioxidant and anti-inflammatory properties are recommended for preventing or reducing the progression of this specific neurodegeneration. In particular, astaxanthin is able to act against oxidative injuries, through various mechanisms, by quenching of singlet oxygen, scavenging of radicals, inhibiting lipid peroxidation, and regulating gene expression related to oxidative stress [5,95].

Astaxanthin exhibited strong anti-inflammatory effect, suppressing the expression of inflammatory mediators, such as TNF-α, PGE_2 and IL-1β and blocking the production of nitric oxide (NO) and the NF-κB-dependent signaling pathway [24,25,96].

Similar anti-inflammatory effects of astaxanthin were described in other studies, using different experimental models. In particular, astaxanthin (50 μM) drastically reduced the release of inflammatory mediators in activated microglial cells (BV-2 cell line), through the modulation of factors involved in the NF-κB cascade (e.g., p-IKKα, p-IκBα, and p-NF-κB p65, IL-6 and MAPK) [97].

These findings validate the astaxanthin administration as an adjuvant therapy for AD, since this carotenoid is able to attenuate microglial activation and the consequent release of pro-inflammatory cytokines. This effect has positive repercussions on neuronal integrity, especially in elderly people, which tend to show increased inflammation in the brain [98].

Endogenous antioxidant enzymes lower their activity and efficiency with age. Results from recent studies support the beneficial effect of astaxanthin on activation of antioxidant mechanisms, increasing the levels or stimulating the activity of endogenous enzymes, such as superoxide dismutase (SOD) and catalase [26,99]. A recent study [27] investigated in mice the effect of astaxanthin on antioxidant enzymes expressed in major brain structures. Catalase and SOD were found highly expressed, together with a reduction in the level of glutathione, when mice were supplemented with 2 mg/Kg of astaxanthin for 1 month. Al-Amin and collaborators [27] also showed a reduction of malondialdehyde (MDA) and advanced protein oxidation product (APOP) levels in some brain areas, such as the frontal cortex, hippocampus, cerebellum and striatum, which showed a decrease in lipid peroxidation levels.

PC12 are neuronal cells from rats used as an artificial nervous system tissue model to study neurodegeneration and, in particular, AD. These cells were protected from neurotoxicity induced by 30 μM of beta-amyloid peptide, when treated with 0.1 μM of astaxanthin. This protective effect was due to caspase 3, Bax, IL-1β and TNFα, NF-κB inactivation, and suppression of ROS production [28]. Other studies have demonstrated the protective effect of astaxanthin on amyloid beta-induced generation of ROS and calcium dysregulation in primary hippocampal neurons [100] and the significant decrease of oxidative stress levels and cell death in PC12 cells injured with n-methyl-4-phenylpyridinium iodide (MPP+) [19].

Recent studies [4,101] have reported on the direct relationship between the healthy effects of astaxanthin on human brain and promotion of neurogenesis and plasticity, two processes that significantly decrease with age [29] and lead to cognitive decline among elderly people. Although the molecular process has not been completely elucidated, astaxanthin promotes neurogenesis and improves behavioral performance in hippocampal-dependent tasks; this could represent the predominant mechanism induced by astaxanthin, acting on cognitive functions and neurodegeneration caused by AD [4]. Neural stem cells exhibit higher proliferation rates and colony-forming capacity in a time- and dose dependent manner when treated with astaxanthin [30]. This result was corroborated by the upregulation of cyclin-dependent kinase 2 (CDK2), genes involved in proliferation control. Together with these pro-proliferative effects, astaxanthin showed protective properties in neural progenitor cells (NPC), significantly reducing apoptotic machinery in NPCs exposed to pro-oxidant agents [102].

5. Astaxanthin against Parkinson Disease (PD)

Parkinson's disease (PD) affects 0.1–0.2% of the global population and this percentage drastically increases with age, reaching 1% incidence in persons aged 60 years and over [103]. Considering the prevalence of neurodegenerative diseases, PD is the second most common disorder. PD has been better characterized in recent years as a multisystem neurodegenerative disorder [104], with motor and non-motor features. In particular, the loss of dopaminergic neurons leads to motor symptoms, such as bradykinesia, rest tremor and rigidity, while degeneration of non-dopaminergic pathways is mainly responsible for the alteration of posture, balance and gait. Oxidative stress and inflammation at the CNS level contributes to insurgence and progression of PD. Unfortunately, there are few treatments that are able to reduce symptoms and to prevent or restore the loss of neurons in the CNS. As for other neurodegenerative diseases, carotenoids, in particular astaxanthin, can represent a valid co-adjuvant treatment for the prevention and/or delay of disease progression. Indeed, astaxanthin reduced neurotoxicity in PD mice [31], when animals were fed with astaxanthin derived from *Haematococcus pluvialis*, for four weeks. Grimmig and collaborators [4] demonstrated that astaxanthin possesses anti-inflammatory effects, attenuating microglia activation in substantia nigra and striatum. SH-SY5Y are human neuroblastoma cell line used to assess the potential antioxidant effect of pure compounds. Astaxanthin is a powerful antioxidant, contrasting the activation of ROS-mediated apoptosis in a dose dependent manner [105] in SH-SY5Y cells. This positive effect of astaxanthin is due to suppression of apoptosis, inhibition of mitochondrial abnormalities and the creation of intracellular ROS [18,105].

6. Astaxanthin against Amyotrophic Lateral Sclerosis (ALS)

Amyotrophic lateral sclerosis (ALS) is a lethal motor neuron disorder characterized by a progressive loss of the upper and lower motor neurons at the spinal or bulbar levels. There are two forms of ALS, sporadic- and familiar-type. The first type does not have a genetically inherited component. The mean age of onset varies from 50 to 65 years, while only in 5% of cases the age of onset is less than 30 years. However, ALS incident is most pronounced in people 80 years or older [106]. 5–10% of ALS cases have a genetic cause. Indeed, in some geographic areas, such as parts of Japan, Guam, Kii Peninsula of Japan and South West New Guinea, the incidence of this disease is 50–100 times higher than in other parts of the world [106].

The most common cause of ALS corresponds to a mutation of the gene encoding Cu/Zn superoxide dismutase 1 (SOD1). SOD1 is a dimeric ubiquitous enzyme mainly localized in the cytosol that catalyses the dismutation of superoxide radical into hydrogen peroxide (H_2O_2) and molecular oxygen (O_2); it plays a pivotal role in the cellular homeostasis of ROS [107–109]. Mutant SOD1 has a structural instability that causes a misfolds in the mutated enzyme, which can lead to aggregation in the motor neurons within the CNS. More than 110 mutations of the SOD1 gene have been described and many of these mutants retain their enzymatic activity, suggesting the possibility of a toxic functional gain of these forms of mutated SOD1 in ALS [32,109,110]. One of the proposed mechanisms of neuronal death in ALS is the free radical accumulation resulting from oxidative stress. This may lead to oxidative damage of lipid, proteins, and nucleic acids, causing cell death. Free radicals are normally neutralized by antioxidant enzymes and nutrient derived antioxidants, such as vitamin C, vitamin E, and astaxanthin. The effect of different antioxidants in the treatment of people with ALS has been evaluated.

Isonaka and co-authors [111] investigated the use of antioxidants in cultured rat spinal neurons treated with the SOD1 inhibitor diethyldithiocarbamate (DDC). Results demonstrated that the use of DDC induced an increase of endogenous oxidative stress, inhibiting thus neurite growth. Antioxidants, such as L-ascorbic acid, L-histidine, α-tocopherol, β-carotene and astaxanthin may rescue the motor neurons injured by SOD1 inhibition. It is important to note that astaxanthin is the most powerful carotenoid for this specific effect. In fact, low concentrations of astaxanthin (100 nM) are needed to obtain a comparable effect of other antioxidant molecules (1 mM) [111].

7. Astaxanthin against Cerebral Ischemia/Reperfusion (IR)

Cerebral ischemia triggers an almost immediate loss of oxygen and glucose to the cerebral tissue and ultimately causes irreversible neuronal injuries in the ischemic core within few minutes from the onset. Cerebral ischemia/reperfusion (IR) injury is the tissue damage caused when blood supply begins to the brain after a period of ischemia. The lack of oxygen for a certain period in specific brain regions, creates a pathological microenvironment, in which the following restoration of blood circulation induces activation of inflammatory process and production of oxidative damage, rather than re-establishment of normal condition and cerebral functions. IR injury can lead to progressive learning and memory impairment as well as the loss of pyramidal neurons, which result in the progression of vascular cognitive impairment.

Ischemia induces an imbalance of endogenous pro-oxidants and antioxidants, and the overproduction of toxic free radicals. Abnormal levels of malondialdehyde (MVA), an important indicator of lipid peroxidation, as well as glutathione (GSH), and superoxide dismutase (SOD), both important as free radical scavengers, have been found in the brain tissue after cerebral IR [112,113]. In addition, the destruction of the normal structure of neurons consequently enhances oxidative stress damage and leads to neuronal apoptosis [114]. In particular, it has been demonstrated that loss of hippocampal pyramidal neurons after cerebral IR contributes to learning and memory dysfunction [33,115].

Recent studies have investigated the effect of astaxanthin supplementation to prevent the risk of ischemia on brain recovery after a cerebral IR injury.

For instance, Lee et al. [34] described *in vitro* and *in vivo* antioxidant and neuroprotective effects of astaxanthin. Oxygen Glucose Deprivation (OGD) was induced in neuronal cells (SH-SY5Y cell line) and such damaged cells were recovered in the presence of astaxanthin. The latter was able to recover cells from OGD injury in a dose dependent manner. Moreover, astaxanthin was able to reduce iNOS (inducible Nitric Oxide Synthase), HO-1 (Heme oxygenase-1, HSP32), and HSP70 (heat shock protein 70) protein levels, after OGD injury [34]. The same study highlighted the neuroprotective effect of astaxanthin on global cerebral ischemia in rats.

Xue and co-authors [35] evaluated the efficacy of AST treatment after repeated cerebral IR injury in a mouse model. These researchers demonstrated that astaxanthin improved learning and decreased memory impairment and neuronal damage. Astaxanthin treatment increased the number of pyramidal neurons of the hippocampus and restored normal neuron morphology. In addition, astaxanthin induced a strong antioxidant activity and an inhibitory effect on neuronal apoptosis in IR mice. Moreover, astaxanthin treatment reduced oxidative stress, restoring GHS levels and SOD activity, and significantly suppressed the concentration of MDA. Xue and co-authors [35] also highlighted a decrease in protein expression of cytochrome C (Cyt C) and caspase-3 (cleaved Caspase-3), both involved in the occurrence and development of apoptosis.

Pan and co-authors [116] demonstrated that astaxanthin was able to protect against brain injuries induced by transient cerebral ischemia in adult rats. The protective effect was proportional to the administered dose. Results of this study demonstrated that pre-treatment with astaxanthin lowered oxidative stress induced by ischemia, increasing the gene expression levels of SOD and decreasing those of MVA, that indicated a minor lipid peroxidation. In addition, astaxanthin increased gene expression of the nuclear factor erythroid 2-related factor 2 (Nef2), Heme oxygenase-1 (HO-1) and NAD(P)H quinone oxidoreductase 1 (NQO1), activating the Nrf2- antioxidant response element (ARE) signaling pathway.

Astaxanthin pre-treatment reduced the rate of cell death, increasing the gene expression of anti-apoptotic factor B-cell lymphoma 2 (Bcl-2), and reducing the gene expression of pro-apoptotic factor Bcl2-associated X (Bax). These two proteins are active mediators of apoptosis; in particular, Bcl-2 suppresses abnormal Ca^{2+} release from the endoplasmic reticulum (ER) and prevents ER Ca^{2+} depletion [117–120], while Bax is a homologous protein of Bcl-2 that promotes apoptosis. The balance between Bcl-2 and Bax plays an important role on ER Ca^{2+} homeostasis and in determining the fate of the cells during transient cerebral ischemia [121,122]. In conclusion, use of astaxanthin exerts protective and anti-apoptotic effects against IR injuries.

8. Conclusions

There is a growing body of evidence regarding the benefits of several molecules in a healthy diet that can help to prevent some age-related diseases. There is large public and scientific interest about natural nutritional supplements able to reduce the risk of age-related disease insurgence and to avoid the exacerbation of degenerative processes leading to death.

In the last decade the high demand by consumers for nutraceutical products containing bioactive compounds is directing research towards the discovery and development of renewable natural sources of bioactive molecules. In this framework, the marine environment represents a new and unexploited source for the identification or production of bioactive compounds. The global market for marine biotechnological products and processes is predicted to reach 4.8 billion USD by 2020, rising to 6.4 billion USD by 2025. In Europe, marine biotechnology was identified by the EU Blue Growth Strategy (2012) as an activity of high potential for the bioeconomy [123]. In this context, 1.20 billion USD was the estimated value for the global carotenoid market in 2016, which is expected to reach 1.53 billion USD by 2021, at a compound annual growth rate (CAGR) of 3.78% from 2016 to 2021 [124]. Such an economic growth related to these compounds is a direct result of the increased number of health conscious customers and a growing trend for natural products industries.

Among carotenoids that have beneficial effects on human health astaxanthin is one of the most successful compounds on the market. Its large scale cultivation mainly from the green microalga *H. pluvialis* is still considered more expensive [125,126]. The synthetic production of astaxanthin is still predominant in the market. This synthetic version of the carotenoid is wrongly thought as "a natural equivalent". Actually, this production process leads to a mixture of astaxanthin isomers, which conferee important molecular and biological differences with respect to the natural carotenoid. In detail, natural astaxanthin (3S, 3′S) is more than 90% esterified, while the synthetic version is all free form, or unesterified. This chemical feature of the natural astaxanthin allows interactions with fatty acids to one or both ends of the compounds, with consequent high bioavailability [9].

Researchers are trying to improve the growth rate and astaxanthin yield of *H. pluvialis* by modulating several culture conditions [127]. In addition, preliminary studies have demonstrated the possibility of the natural astaxanthin production through sea urchin *Arbacia lixula* aquaculture without sacrifice them, since the natural carotenoid is accumulated in eggs [8]. For this reason, it is important to find a new and efficient process for the natural production of astaxanthin. Although the economic advantage of the synthetic way can obtain only racemic chemical formulation with a decrease of biological activity at 50%; this aspect encourages research to lower the cost and enhance the efficiency in the production of the natural compound.

Author Contributions: All authors have equally contributed to the manuscript.

Acknowledgments: The authors thank reviewers for their helpful suggestions. C.S. thanks her dad for inspiration.

References

1. Nichols, J.A.; Katiyar, S.K. Skin photoprotection by natural polyphenols: Anti-inflammatory, anti-oxidant and DNA repair mechanisms. *Arch. Dermatol. Res.* **2010**, *302*, 71–83. [CrossRef] [PubMed]
2. Berthon, J.Y.; Nachat-Kappes, R.; Bey, M.; Cadoret, J.P.; Renimel, I.; Filaire, E. Marine algae as attractive source to skin care. *Free Radic. Res.* **2017**, *51*, 555–567. [CrossRef] [PubMed]
3. Gonzalez, S.; Gilaberte, Y.; Philips, N.; Juarranz, A. Current trends in photoprotection—A new generation of oral photoprotectors. *Open Dermatol. J.* **2011**, *5*, 6–14. [CrossRef]
4. Grimmig, B.; Kim, S.H.; Nash, K.; Bickford, P.C.; Douglas Shytle, R. Neuroprotective mechanisms of astaxanthin: A potential therapeutic role in preserving cognitive function in age and neurodegeneration. *GeroScience* **2017**, *39*, 19–32. [CrossRef] [PubMed]
5. Galasso, C.; Corinaldesi, C.; Sansone, C. Carotenoids from marine organisms: Biological functions and industrial applications. *Antioxidants* **2017**, *6*, 96. [CrossRef] [PubMed]
6. Yuan, J.P.; Peng, J.; Yin, K.; Wang, J.H. Potential health-promoting effects of astaxanthin: A high-value carotenoid mostly from microalgae. *Mol. Nutr. Food Res.* **2011**, *55*, 150–165. [CrossRef] [PubMed]
7. Cirino, P.; Brunet, C.; Ciaravolo, M.; Galasso, C.; Musco, L.; Vega Fernández, T.; Sansone, C.; Toscano, A. The sea urchin *Arbacia lixula*: A novel natural source of astaxanthin. *Mar. Drugs* **2017**, *15*, 187. [CrossRef] [PubMed]
8. Galasso, C.; Orefice, I.; Toscano, A.; Vega Fernández, T.; Musco, L.; Brunet, C.; Sansone, C.; Cirino, P. Food modulation controls astaxanthin accumulation in eggs of the sea urchin *Arbacia lixula*. *Mar. Drugs* **2018**, *16*, 186. [CrossRef] [PubMed]
9. Capelli, B.; Bagchi, D.; Cysewski, G.R. Synthetic astaxanthin is significantly inferior to algal-based astaxanthin as an antioxidant and may not be suitable as a human nutraceutical supplement. *Nutrfoods* **2013**, *12*, 145–152. [CrossRef]
10. Cho, K.S.; Shin, M.; Kim, S.; Lee, S.B. Recent advances in studies on the therapeutic potential of dietary carotenoids in neurodegenerative diseases. *Oxid. Med. Cell. Longev.* **2018**, 4120458. [CrossRef] [PubMed]
11. Barnham, K.J.; Masters, C.L.; Bush, A.I. Neurodegenerative diseases and oxidative stress. *Nat. Rev. Drug Discov.* **2004**, *3*, 205–214. [CrossRef] [PubMed]
12. Hardy, J.; Selkoe, D.J. The amyloid hypothesis of Alzheimer's disease: Progress and problems on the road to therapeutics. *Science* **2002**, *297*, 353–356. [CrossRef] [PubMed]
13. Lin, M.T.; Beal, M.F. Mitochondrial dysfunction and oxidative stress in neurodegenerative diseases. *Nature* **2006**, *443*, 787–795. [CrossRef] [PubMed]

14. Uttara, B.; Singh, A.V.; Zamboni, P.; Mahajan, R.T. Oxidative stress and neurodegenerative diseases: A review of upstream and downstream antioxidant therapeutic options. *Curr. Neuropharmacol.* **2009**, *7*, 65–74. [CrossRef] [PubMed]
15. Wyss-Coray, T.; Mucke, L. Inflammation in neurodegenerative disease—A double-edged sword. *Neuron* **2002**, *35*, 419–432. [CrossRef]
16. Prakash, A.; Kumar, A. Implicating the role of lycopene in restoration of mitochondrial enzymes and BDNF levels in β-amyloid induced Alzheimer's disease. *Eur. J. Pharmacol.* **2014**, *741*, 104–111. [CrossRef] [PubMed]
17. Zhou, X.; Zhang, F.; Hu, X.; Chen, J.; Wen, X.; Sun, Y.; Liu, Y.; Tang, R.; Zheng, K.; Song, Y. Inhibition of inflammation by astaxanthin alleviates cognition deficits in diabetic mice. *Physiol. Behav.* **2015**, *151*, 412z420. [CrossRef] [PubMed]
18. Ikeda, Y.; Tsuji, S.; Satoh, A.; Ishikura, M.; Shirasawa, T.; Shimizu, T. Protective effects of astaxanthin on 6-hydroxydopamine-induced apoptosis in human neuroblastoma SH-SY5Y cells. *J. Neurochem.* **2008**, *107*, 1730–1740. [CrossRef] [PubMed]
19. Ye, Q.; Huang, B.; Zhang, X.; Zhu, Y.; Chen, X. Astaxanthin protects against MPP+-induced oxidative stress in PC12 cells via the HO-1/NOX2 axis. *BMC Neurosci.* **2012**, *13*, 156. [CrossRef] [PubMed]
20. Ye, Q.; Zhang, X.; Huang, B.; Zhu, Y.; Chen, X. Astaxanthin suppresses MPP^+-induced oxidative damage in PC12 cells through a Sp1/NR1 signaling pathway. *Mar. Drugs* **2013**, *11*, 1019–1034. [CrossRef] [PubMed]
21. Wu, W.; Wang, X.; Xiang, Q.; Meng, X.; Peng, Y.; Du, N.; Liu, Z.; Sun, Q.; Wang, C.; Liu, X. Astaxanthin alleviates brain aging in rats by attenuating oxidative stress and increasing BDNF levels. *Food Funct.* **2014**, *5*, 158–166. [CrossRef] [PubMed]
22. El-Agamy, S.A.; Abdel-Aziz, A.K.; Wahdan, S.; Esmat, A.; Azab, S. Astaxanthin ameliorates doxorubicin-induced cognitive impairment (chemobrain) in experimental rat model: impact on oxidative, inflammatory, and apoptotic machineries. *Mol. Neurobiol.* **2018**, *55*, 5727–5740. [CrossRef] [PubMed]
23. Nakagawa, K.; Kiko, T.; Miyazawa, T.; Kimura, G.C.F.; Satoh, A.; Miyazawa, T. Antioxidant effect of astaxanthin on phospholipid peroxidation in human erythrocytes. *Br. J. Nutr.* **2011**, *105*, 1563–1571. [CrossRef] [PubMed]
24. Ohgami, K.; Shiratori, K.; Kotake, S.; Nishida, T.; Mizuki, N.; Yazawa, K.; Ohno, S. Effects of astaxanthin on lipopolysaccharide-induced inflammation in vitro and in vivo. *Investig. Ophthalmol. Vis. Sci.* **2003**, *44*, 2694–2701. [CrossRef] [PubMed]
25. Solomonov, Y.; Hadad, N.; Levy, R. The combined anti-inflammatory effect of astaxanthin, Lyc-O-Mato and Carnosic acid *in vitro* and *in vivo* in a mouse model of peritonitis. *J. Nutr. Food Sci.* **2018**, *8*, 1. [CrossRef]
26. Haider, S.; Saleem, S.; Perveen, T.; Tabassum, S.; Batool, Z.; Sadir, S.; Liaquat, L.; Madiha, S. Age-related learning and memory deficits in rats: role of altered brain neurotransmitters, acetylcholinesterase activity and changes in antioxidant defense system. *Age* **2014**, *36*, 1291–1302. [CrossRef] [PubMed]
27. Al-Amin, M.M.; Akhter, S.; Hasan, A.T.; Alam, T.; Hasan, S.N.; Saifullah, A.; Shohel, M. The antioxidant effect of astaxanthin is higher in young mice than aged: A region specific study on brain. *Metab. Brain. Dis.* **2015**, *30*, 1237–1246. [CrossRef] [PubMed]
28. Chang, C.H.; Chen, C.Y.; Chiou, J.Y.; Peng, R.Y.; Peng, C.H. Astaxanthin secured apoptotic death of PC12 cells induced by β-amyloid peptide 25–35: Its molecular action targets. *J. Med. Food* **2010**, *13*, 548–556. [CrossRef] [PubMed]
29. Shetty, G.A.; Hattiangady, B.; Shetty, A.K. Neural stem cell- and neurogenesis-related gene expression profiles in the young and aged dentate gyrus. *Age* **2013**, *35*, 2165–2176. [CrossRef] [PubMed]
30. Kim, J.H.; Nam, S.W.; Kim, B.W.; Choi, W.; Lee, J.H.; Kim, W.J.; Choi, Y.H. Astaxanthin improves stem cell potency via an increase in the proliferation of neural progenitor cells. *Int. J. Mol. Sci.* **2010**, *11*, 5109–5119. [CrossRef] [PubMed]
31. Grimmig, B.; Daly, L.; Subbarayan, M.; Hudson, C.; Williamson, R.; Nash, K.; Bickford, P.C. Astaxanthin attenuates neurotoxicity in a mouse model of Parkinson's disease. *Oncotarget* **2018**, *9*, 10388–10401. [CrossRef] [PubMed]
32. Dion, P.A.; Daoud, H.; Rouleau, G.A. Genetics of motor neuron disorders: new insights into pathogenic mechanisms. *Nat. Rev. Genet.* **2009**, *10*, 769–782. [CrossRef] [PubMed]
33. Kim, H.A.; Miller, A.A.; Drummond, G.R.; Thrift, A.G.; Arumugam, T.V.; Phan, T.G.; Srikanth, V.K.; Sobey, C.G. Vascular cognitive impairment and Alzheimer's disease: Role of cerebral hypoperfusion and oxidative stress. *Naunyn-Schmiedeberg's Arch. Pharmacol.* **2012**, *385*, 953–959. [CrossRef] [PubMed]

34. Lee, D.H.; Lee, Y.J.; Kwon, K.H. Neuroprotective effects of astaxanthin in oxygen-glucose deprivation in SH-SY5Y cells and global cerebral ischemia in rat. *J. Clin. Biochem. Nutr.* **2010**, *47*, 121–129. [CrossRef] [PubMed]
35. Xue, Y.; Qu, Z.; Fu, J.; Zhen, J.; Wang, W.; Cai, Y.; Wang, W. The protective effect of astaxanthin on learning and memory deficits and oxidative stress in a mouse model of repeated cerebral ischemia/reperfusion. *Brain Res. Bull.* **2017**, *131*, 221–228. [CrossRef] [PubMed]
36. Azevedo, F.A.; Carvalho, L.R.; Grinberg, L.T.; Farfel, J.M.; Ferretti, R.E.; Leite, R.E.; Jacob Filho, W.; Lent, R.; Herculano-Houzel, S. Equal numbers of neuronal and nonneuronal cells make the human brain an isometrically scaled-up primate brain. *J. Comp. Neurol.* **2009**, *513*, 532–541. [CrossRef] [PubMed]
37. Masgrau, R.; Guaza, C.; Ransohoff, R.M.; Galea, E. Should we stop saying "glia" and "neuroinflammation"? *Trends Mol. Med.* **2017**, *23*, 486–500. [CrossRef] [PubMed]
38. Sadeghian, M.; Mastrolia, V.; Rezaei Haddad, A.; Mosley, A.; Mullali, G.; Schiza, D.; Sajic, M.; Hargreaves, I.; Heales, S.; Duchen, M.R.; et al. Mitochondrial dysfunction is an important cause of neurological deficits in an inflammatory model of multiple sclerosis. *Sci. Rep.* **2016**, *6*, 33249. [CrossRef] [PubMed]
39. Urrutia, P.J.; Mena, N.P.; Núñez, M.T. The interplay between iron accumulation, mitochondrial dysfunction, and inflammation during the execution step of neurodegenerative disorders. *Front. Pharmacol.* **2014**, *5*, 38. [CrossRef] [PubMed]
40. Campbell, G.; Mahad, D.J. Mitochondrial dysfunction and axon degeneration in progressive multiple sclerosis. *FEBS Lett.* **2018**, *592*, 1113–1121. [CrossRef] [PubMed]
41. Beckhauser, T.F.; Francis-Oliveira, J.; De Pasquale, R. Reactive oxygen species: Physiological and physiopathological effects on synaptic plasticity. *J. Exp. Neurosci.* **2016**, *10*, 23–48. [CrossRef] [PubMed]
42. Liu, Z.; Zhou, T.; Ziegler, A.C.; Dimitrion, P.; Zuo, L. Oxidative stress in neurodegenerative diseases: From molecular mechanisms to clinical applications. *Oxid. Med. Cell. Longev.* **2017**, 2525967. [CrossRef] [PubMed]
43. Mecocci, P.; MacGarvey, U.; Kaufman, A.E.; Koontz, D.; Shoffner, J.M.; Wallace, D.C.; Beal, M.F. Oxidative damage to mitochondrial DNA shows marked age-dependent increases in human brain. *Ann. Neurol.* **1993**, *34*, 609–616. [CrossRef] [PubMed]
44. Montine, T.J.; Neely, M.D.; Quinn, J.F.; Beal, M.F.; Markesbery, W.R.; Roberts, L.J.; Morrow, J.D. Lipid peroxidation in aging brain and Alzheimer's disease. *Free Radic. Biol. Med.* **2002**, *33*, 620–626. [CrossRef]
45. Sun, N.; Youle, R.J.; Finkel, T. The Mitochondrial Basis of Aging. *Mol. Cell* **2016**, *61*, 654–666. [CrossRef] [PubMed]
46. Hubbard, V.M.; Valdor, R.; Macian, F.; Cuervo, A.M. Selective autophagy in the maintenance of cellular homeostasis in aging organisms. *Biogerontology* **2012**, *13*, 21–35. [CrossRef] [PubMed]
47. Reevel, A.; Simcox, E.; Turnbull, D. Ageing and Parkinson's disease: Why is advancing age the biggest risk factor? *Ageing Res. Rev.* **2014**, *14*, 19–30. [CrossRef] [PubMed]
48. Metaxakis, A.; Ploumi, C.; Tavernarakis, N. Autophagy in age-associated neurodegeneration. *Cells* **2018**, *7*, 37. [CrossRef] [PubMed]
49. Nicholls, D.G. Oxidative stress and energy crises in neuronal dysfunction. *Ann. N. Y. Acad. Sci.* **2008**, *1147*, 53–60. [CrossRef] [PubMed]
50. McGeer, P.L.; McGeer, E.G.; Yasojima, K. Alzheimer disease and neuroinflammation. *J. Neural Transm. Suppl.* **2000**, *59*, 53–57. [PubMed]
51. Che, H.; Li, Q.; Zhang, T.; Wang, D.; Yang, L.; Xu, J.; Yanagita, T.; Xue, C.; Chang, Y.; Wang, Y. The effects of astaxanthin and docosahexaenoic acid-acylated astaxanthin on Alzheimer's disease in APP/PS1 double transgenic mice. *J. Agric. Food Chem.* **2018**, *66*, 4948–4957. [CrossRef] [PubMed]
52. Katagiri, M.; Satoh, A.; Tsuji, S.; Shirasawa, T. Effects of astaxanthin-rich *Haematococcus pluvialis* extract on cognitive function: A randomised, double-blind, placebo-controlled study. *J. Clin. Biochem. Nutr.* **2012**, *51*, 102–107. [CrossRef] [PubMed]
53. Wu, H.; Niu, H.; Shao, A.; Wu, C.; Dixon, B.J.; Zhang, J.; Yang, S.; Wang, Y. Astaxanthin as a potential neuroprotective agent for neurological diseases. *Mar Drugs* **2015**, *13*, 5750–5766. [CrossRef] [PubMed]
54. Craft, N.E.; Haitema, T.B.; Garnett, K.M.; Fitch, K.A.; Dorey, C.K. Carotenoid, tocopherol, and retinol concentrations in elderly human brain. *J. Nutr. Health Aging* **2004**, *8*, 156–162. [PubMed]
55. Sasaki, M.; Ozawa, Y.; Kurihara, T.; Noda, K.; Imamura, Y.; Kobayashi, S.; Ishida, S.; Tsubota, K. Neuroprotective effect of an antioxidant, lutein, during retinal inflammation. *Investig. Ophthalmol. Vis. Sci.* **2009**, *50*, 1433–1439. [CrossRef] [PubMed]

56. Franceschelli, S.; Pesce, M.; Ferrone, A.; De Lutiis, M.A.; Patruno, A.; Grilli, A.; Felaco, M.; Speranza, L. Astaxanthin treatment confers protection against oxidative stress in U937 cells stimulated with lipopolysaccharide reducing O_2^- production. *PLoS One* **2014**, *9*, e88359. [CrossRef] [PubMed]
57. Zhang, X.S.; Zhang, X.; Wu, Q.; Li, W.; Wang, C.X.; Xie, G.B.; Zhou, X.M.; Shi, J.X.; Zhou, M.L. Astaxanthin offers neuroprotection and reduces neuroinflammation in experimental subarachnoid haemorrhage. *J. Surg. Res.* **2014**, *192*, 206–213. [CrossRef] [PubMed]
58. Yeh, P.T.; Huang, H.W.; Yang, C.M.; Yang, W.S.; Yang, C.H. Astaxanthin inhibits expression of retinal oxidative stress and inflammatory mediators in streptozotocin induced diabetic rats. *PLoS One* **2016**, *11*, e0146438. [CrossRef] [PubMed]
59. Zhou, X.Y.; Zhang, F.; Hu, X.T.; Chen, J.; Tang, R.X.; Zheng, K.Y.; Song, Y.J. Depression can be prevented by astaxanthin through inhibition of hippocampal inflammation in diabetic mice. *Brain Res.* **2017**, *1657*, 262–268. [CrossRef] [PubMed]
60. Zhao, D.; Kwon, S.H.; Chun, Y.S.; Gu, M.Y.; Yang, H.O. Anti-neuroinflammatory effects of fucoxanthin via inhibition of Akt/NF-κB and MAPKs/AP-1 pathways and activation of PKA/CREB pathway in lipopolysaccharide-activated BV-2 microglial cells. *Neurochem. Res.* **2017**, *42*, 667–677. [CrossRef] [PubMed]
61. Sansone, C.; Galasso, C.; Orefice, I.; Nuzzo, G.; Luongo, E.; Cutignano, A.; Romano, G.; Brunet, C.; Fontana, A.; Esposito, F.; et al. The green microalga *Tetraselmis suecica* reduces oxidative stress and induces repairing mechanisms in human cells. *Sci. Rep.* **2017**, *7*, 41215. [CrossRef] [PubMed]
62. Shen, M.; Chen, K.; Lu, J.; Cheng, P.; Xu, L.; Dai, W.; Wang, F.; He, L.; Zhang, Y.; Chengfen, W.; et al. Protective effect of astaxanthin on liver fibrosis through modulation of TGF-β1 expression and autophagy. *Mediators Inflamm.* **2014**, 954502. [CrossRef] [PubMed]
63. Li, J.; Wang, F.; Xia, Y.; Dai, W.; Chen, K.; Li, S.; Liu, T.; Zheng, Y.; Wang, J.; Lu, W.; et al. Astaxanthin pretreatment attenuates hepatic ischemia reperfusion-induced apoptosis and autophagy via the ROS/MAPK pathway in mice. *Mar. Drugs* **2015**, *13*, 3368–3387. [CrossRef] [PubMed]
64. Lee, D.H.; Kim, C.S.; Lee, Y.J. Astaxanthin protects against MPTP/MPP+-induced mitochondrial dysfunction and ROS production *in vivo* and *in vitro*. *Food Chem. Toxicol.* **2011**, *49*, 271–280. [CrossRef] [PubMed]
65. Dai, Q.; Borenstein, A.R.; Wu, Y.; Jackson, J.C.; Larson, E.B. Fruit and vegetable juices and Alzheimer's disease: The Kame Project. *Am. J. Med.* **2006**, *119*, 751–759. [CrossRef] [PubMed]
66. Li, F.J.; Shen, L.; Ji, H.F. Dietary intakes of vitamin E, vitamin C, and β-carotene and risk of Alzheimer's disease: A meta-analysis. *J. Alzheimers Dis.* **2012**, *31*, 253–258. [CrossRef] [PubMed]
67. Kesse-Guyot, E.; Andreeva, V.A.; Ducros, V.; Jeandel, C.; Julia, C.; Hercberg, S.; Galan, P. Carotenoid-rich dietary patterns during midlife and subsequent cognitive function. *Br. J. Nutr.* **2014**, *111*, 915–923. [CrossRef] [PubMed]
68. Mohammadzadeh Honarvar, N.; Saedisomeolia, A.; Abdolahi, M.; Shayeganrad, A.; Taheri Sangsari, G.; Hassanzadeh Rad, B.; Muench, G. Molecular anti-inflammatory mechanisms of retinoids and carotenoids in Alzheimer's disease: A review of current evidence. *J. Mol. Neurosci.* **2017**, *61*, 289–304. [CrossRef] [PubMed]
69. Fiedor, J.; Burda, K. Potential role of carotenoids as antioxidants in human health and disease. *Nutrients* **2014**, *6*, 466–488. [CrossRef] [PubMed]
70. Xiang, S.; Liu, F.; Lin, J.; Chen, H.; Huang, C.; Chen, L.; Zhou, Y.; Ye, L.; Zhang, K.; Jin, J.; et al. Fucoxanthin inhibits β-amyloid assembly and attenuates β-amyloid oligomer-induced cognitive impairments. *J. Agric. Food Chem.* **2017**, *65*, 4092–4102. [CrossRef] [PubMed]
71. Johnson, E.J.; Vishwanathan, R.; Schalch, W.; Poon, L.; Wittwer, J.; Johnson, M.A.; Hausman, D.; Davey, A.; Green, R.; Gearing, M.; et al. Brain levels of lutein (L) and zeaxanthin (Z) are related to cognitive function in centenarians. *FASEB J.* **2011**, *25*.
72. Dias, I.H.; Polidori, M.C.; Li, L.; Weber, D.; Stahl, W.; Nelles, G.; Grune, T.; Griffiths, H.R. Plasma levels of HDL and carotenoids are lower in dementia patients with vascular comorbidities. *J. Alzheimers Dis.* **2014**, *40*, 399–408. [CrossRef] [PubMed]
73. Wen, X.; Huang, A.; Hu, J.; Zhong, Z.; Liu, Y.; Li, Z.; Pan, X.; Liu, Z. Neuroprotective effect of astaxanthin against glutamate-induced cytotoxicity in HT22 cells: Involvement of the Akt/GSK-3β pathway. *Neuroscience* **2015**, *303*, 558–568. [CrossRef] [PubMed]
74. Xu, L.; Zhu, J.; Yin, W.; Ding, X. Astaxanthin improves cognitive deficits from oxidative stress, nitric oxide synthase and inflammation through upregulation of PI3K/Akt in diabetes rat. *Int. J. Clin. Exp. Pathol.* **2015**, *8*, 6083–6094. [PubMed]

75. Petri, D.; Lundebye, A.K. Tissue distribution of astaxanthin in rats following exposure to graded levels in the feed. *Comp. Biochem. Physiol. C Toxicol Pharmacol.* **2007**, *145*, 202–209. [CrossRef] [PubMed]
76. Manabe, Y.; Komatsu, T.; Seki, S.; Sugawara, T. Dietary astaxanthin can accumulate in the brain of rats. *Biosci. Biotechnol. Biochem.* **2018**. [CrossRef] [PubMed]
77. Cullen, D.K.; Simon, C.M.; LaPlaca, M.C. Strain rate-dependent induction of reactive astrogliosis and cell death in three-dimensional neuronal-astrocytic co-cultures. *Brain Res.* **2007**, *1158*, 103–115. [CrossRef] [PubMed]
78. Ahmed, S.; Reynolds, B.A.; Weiss, S. BDNF enhances the differentiation but not the survival of CNS stem cell-derived neuronal precursors. *J. Neurosci.* **1995**, *15*, 5765–5778. [CrossRef] [PubMed]
79. Benowitz, L.I.; Routtenberg, A. GAP-43: An intrinsic determinant of neuronal development and plasticity. *Trends Neurosci.* **1997**, *20*, 84–91. [CrossRef]
80. Correa, D.D.; Ahles, T.A. Neurocognitive changes in cancer survivors. *Cancer J.* **2008**, *14*, 396–400. [CrossRef] [PubMed]
81. Ajmani, R.S.; Metter, E.J.; Jaykumar, R.; Ingram, D.K.; Spangler, E.L.; Abugo, O.O.; Rifkind, J.M. Hemodynamic changes during aging associated with cerebral blood flow and impaired cognitive function. *Neurobiol. Aging* **2000**, *21*, 257–269. [CrossRef]
82. Mohanty, J.G.; Eckley, D.M.; Williamson, J.D.; Launer, L.J.; Rifkind, J.M. Do red blood cell-b-amyloid interactions alter oxygen delivery in Alzheimer's disease? *Adv. Exp. Med. Biol.* **2008**, *614*, 29–35. [PubMed]
83. Leijenaara, J.F.; van Maurik, I.S.; Kuijer, J.P.A.; van der Flier, W.M.; Scheltens, P.; Barkhof, F.; Prins, N.D. Lower cerebral blood flow in subjects with Alzheimer's dementia, mild cognitive impairment, and subjective cognitive decline using two-dimensional phase-contrast magnetic resonance imaging. *Alzheimers Dement.* **2017**, *9*, 76–83. [CrossRef] [PubMed]
84. Cunnane, S.C.; Plourde, M.; Pifferi, F.; Bégin, M.; Féart, C.; Barberger-Gateau, P. Fish, docosahexaenoic acid and Alzheimer's disease. *Prog. Lipid Res.* **2009**, *48*, 239–256. [CrossRef] [PubMed]
85. Gorjão, R.; Azevedo-Martins, A.K.; Rodrigues, H.G.; Abdulkader, F.; Arcisio-Miranda, M.; Procopio, J.; Curi, R. Comparative effects of DHA and EPA on cell function. *Pharmacol. Ther.* **2009**, *122*, 56–64. [CrossRef] [PubMed]
86. Mattei, R.; Polotow, T.G.; Vardaris, C.V.; Guerra, B.A.; Leite, J.R.; Otton, R.; Barros, M.P. Astaxanthin limits fish oil-related oxidative insult in the anterior forebrain of Wistar rats: Putative anxiolytic effects? *Pharmacol. Biochem. Behav.* **2011**, *99*, 349–355. [CrossRef] [PubMed]
87. Nolan, J.M.; Mulcahy, R.; Power, R.; Moran, R.; Howard, A.N. Nutritional intervention to prevent Alzheimer's Disease: potential benefits of xanthophyll carotenoids and Omega-3 Fatty acids combined. *J. Alzheimers Dis.* **2018**, *64*, 367–378. [CrossRef] [PubMed]
88. Karlawisha, J.; Jack, C.R.; Rocca, W.A.; Snyder, H.M.; Carillo, M.C. Alzheimer's disease: The next frontier—Special report 2017. *Alzheimers Dement.* **2017**, *13*, 374–380. [CrossRef] [PubMed]
89. Irvine, G.B.; El-Agnaf, O.M.; Shankar, G.M.; Walsh, D.M. Protein aggregation in the brain: The molecular basis for Alzheimer's and Parkinson's diseases. *Mol. Med.* **2008**, *14*, 451–464. [CrossRef] [PubMed]
90. Wildsmith, K.R.; Holley, M.; Savage, J.C.; Skerrett, R.; Landreth, G.E. Evidence for impaired amyloid β clearance in Alzheimer's disease. *Alzheimers Res. Ther.* **2013**, *5*, 33. [CrossRef] [PubMed]
91. Manczak, M.; Anekonda, T.S.; Henson, E.; Park, B.S.; Quinn, J.; Reddy, P.H. Mitochondria are a direct site of Aβ accumulation in Alzheimer's disease neurons: Implications for free radical generation and oxidative damage in disease progression. *Hum. Mol. Genet.* **2006**, *15*, 1437–1449. [CrossRef] [PubMed]
92. Hanzel, C.E.; Pichet-Binette, A.; Pimentel, L.S.; Iulita, M.F.; Allard, S.; Ducatenzeiler, A.; Do Carmo, S.; Cuello, A.C. Neuronal driven pre-plaque inflammation in a transgenic rat model of Alzheimer's disease. *Neurobiol. Aging* **2014**, *35*, 2249–2262. [CrossRef] [PubMed]
93. De la Monte, S.M.; Wands, J.R. Molecular indices of oxidative stress and mitochondrial dysfunction occur early and often progress with severity of Alzheimer's disease. *J. Alzheimers Dis.* **2006**, *9*, 167–181. [CrossRef] [PubMed]
94. Nunomura, A.; Perry, G.; Aliev, G.; Hirai, K.; Takeda, A.; Balraj, E.K.; Jones, P.K.; Ghanbari, H.; Wataya, T.; Shimohama, S.; et al. Oxidative damage is the earliest event in Alzheimer disease. *J. Neuropathol. Exp. Neurol.* **2001**, *60*, 759–767. [CrossRef] [PubMed]

95. Dose, J.; Matsugo, S.; Yokokawa, H.; Koshida, Y.; Okazaki, S.; Seidel, U.; Eggersdorfer, M.; Rimbach, G.; Esatbeyoglu, T. Free radical scavenging and cellular antioxidant properties of astaxanthin. *Int. J. Mol. Sci.* **2016**, *17*, 103. [CrossRef] [PubMed]
96. Suzuki, Y.; Ohgami, K.; Shiratori, K.; Jin, X.H.; Ilieva, I.; Koyama, Y.; Yazawa, K.; Yoshida, K.; Kase, S.; Ohno, S. Suppressive effects of astaxanthin against rat endotoxin-induced uveitis by inhibiting the NF-κB signaling pathway. *Exp. Eye Res.* **2006**, *82*, 275–281. [CrossRef] [PubMed]
97. Kim, Y.H.; Koh, H.K.; Kim, D.S. Down-regulation of IL-6 production by astaxanthin via ERK-, MSK-, and NF-κB-mediated signals in activated microglia. *Int. Immunopharmacol.* **2010**, *10*, 1560–1572. [CrossRef] [PubMed]
98. Satoh, A.; Tsuji, S.; Okada, Y.; Murakami, N.; Urami, M.; Nakagawa, K.; Ishikura, M.; Katagiri, M.; Koga, Y.; Shirasawa, T. Preliminary clinical evaluation of toxicity and efficacy of a new astaxanthin-rich *Haematococcus pluvialis* extract. *J. Clin. Biochem. Nutr.* **2009**, *44*, 280–284. [CrossRef] [PubMed]
99. Puertas, M.C.; Martinez-Martos, J.M.; Cobo, M.P.; Carrera, M.P.; Mayas, M.D.; Ramirez-Exposito, M.J. Plasma oxidative stress parameters in men and women with early stage Alzheimer type dementia. *Exp. Gerontol.* **2012**, *47*, 625–630. [CrossRef] [PubMed]
100. Lobos, P.; Bruna, B.; Cordova, A.; Barattini, P.; Galáz, J.L.; Adasme, T.; Hidalgo, C.; Muñoz, P.; Paula-Lima, A. Astaxanthin protects primary hippocampal neurons against noxious effects of Aβ-oligomers. *Neural Plast.* **2016**, 3456783. [CrossRef] [PubMed]
101. Yook, J.S.; Okamoto, M.; Rakwal, R.; Shibato, J.; Lee, M.C.; Matsui, T.; Chang, H.; Cho, J.Y.; Soya, H. Astaxanthin supplementation enhances adult hippocampal neurogenesis and spatial memory in mice. *Mol. Nutr. Food Res.* **2016**, *60*, 589–599. [CrossRef] [PubMed]
102. Kim, J.H.; Choi, W.; Lee, J.H.; Jeon, S.J.; Choi, Y.H.; Kim, B.W.; Chang, H.I.; Nam, S.W. Astaxanthin inhibits H_2O_2-mediated apoptotic cell death in mouse neural progenitor cells via modulation of P38 and MEK signaling pathways. *J. Microbiol. Biotechnol.* **2009**, *19*, 1355–1363. [CrossRef] [PubMed]
103. Tysnes, O.B.; Storstein, A. Epidemiology of Parkinson's disease. *J. Neural. Transm.* **2017**, *124*, 901–905. [CrossRef] [PubMed]
104. Archibald, N.; Miller, N.; Rochester, L. Neurorehabilitation in Parkinson disease. *Handb. Clin. Neurol.* **2013**, *110*, 435–442. [CrossRef] [PubMed]
105. Liu, X.; Shibata, T.; Hisaka, S.; Osawa, T. Astaxanthin inhibits reactive oxygen species-mediated cellular toxicity in dopaminergic SH-SY5Y cells via mitochondria-targeted protective mechanism. *Brain Res.* **2008**, *1254*, 18–27. [CrossRef] [PubMed]
106. Zarei, S.; Carr, K.; Reiley, L.; Diaz, K.; Guerra, O.; Altamirano, P.F.; Pagani, W.; Lodin, D.; Orozco, G.; Chinea, A. A comprehensive review of amyotrophic lateral sclerosis. *Surg. Neurol. Int.* **2015**, *6*, 171. [CrossRef] [PubMed]
107. Fridovich, I. Superoxide radical and superoxide dismutases. *Annu. Rev. Biochem.* **1995**, *64*, 97–112. [CrossRef] [PubMed]
108. Russo, M.; Cocco, S.; Secondo, A.; Adornetto, A.; Bassi, A.; Nunziata, A.; Polichetti, G.; De Felice, B.; Damiano, S.; Serù, R.; et al. Cigarette smoke condensate causes a decrease of the gene expression of Cu-Zn superoxide dismutase, Mn superoxide dismutase, glutathione peroxidase, catalase, and free radical-induced cell injury in SH-SY5Y human neuroblastoma cells. *Neurotox. Res.* **2011**, *19*, 49–54. [CrossRef] [PubMed]
109. Damiano, S.; Sasso, A.; Accetta, R.; Monda, M.; De Luca, B.; Pavone, L.M.; Belfiore, A.; Santillo, M.; Mondola, P. Effect of mutated Cu, Zn superoxide dismutase ($SOD1^{G93A}$) on modulation of transductional pathway mediated by M1 muscarinic receptor in SK-N-BE and NSC-34 cells. *Front. Physiol.* **2018**, *9*, 611. [CrossRef] [PubMed]
110. Strong, M.J.; Kesavapany, S.; Pant, H.C. The pathobiology of amyotrophic lateral sclerosis: A proteinopathy? *J. Neuropathol. Exp. Neurol.* **2005**, *64*, 649–664. [CrossRef] [PubMed]
111. Isonaka, R.; Hiruma, H.; Katakura, T.; Kawakami, T. Inhibition of superoxide dismutase selectively suppresses growth of rat spinal motor neurons: comparison with phosphorylated neurofilament-containing spinal neurons. *Brain Res.* **2011**, *1425*, 13–19. [CrossRef] [PubMed]
112. Zhang, R.; Liu, C.; Liu, X.; Guo, Y. Protective effect of *Spatholobus suberectus* onbrain tissues in cerebral ischemia. *Am. J. Transl. Res.* **2016**, *8*, 3963–3969. [PubMed]
113. Vani, J.R.; Mohammadi, M.T.; Foroshani, M.S.; Jafari, M. Polyhydroxylated fullerene nanoparticles attenuate brain infarction and oxidative stress in rat model of ischemic stroke. *EXCLI J.* **2016**, *15*, 378–390. [PubMed]

114. Park, E.; Choi, S.K.; Kang, S.W.; Pak, Y.K.; Lee, G.J.; Chung, J.H.; Park, H.K. Cerebral ischemia-induced mitochondrial changes in a global ischemic rat model by AFM. *Biomed. Pharmacother.* **2015**, *71*, 15–20. [CrossRef] [PubMed]
115. Bennett, S.; Grant, M.M.; Aldred, S. Oxidative stress in vascular dementia and Alzheimer's disease: A common pathology. *J. Alzheimers Dis.* **2009**, *17*, 245–257. [CrossRef] [PubMed]
116. Pan, L.; Zhou, Y.; Li, X.F.; Wan, Q.J.; Yu, L.H. Preventive treatment of astaxanthin provides neuroprotection through suppression of reactive oxygen species and activation of antioxidant defense pathway after stroke in rats. *Brain Res Bull.* **2017**, *130*, 211–220. [CrossRef] [PubMed]
117. Lam, M.; Distelhorst, C.W. Evidence that Bcl-2 represses apoptosis by regulating endoplasmic reticulum-associated Ca^{2+} fluxes. *Proc. Natl. Acad. Sci. USA* **1994**, *91*, 6569–6573. [CrossRef] [PubMed]
118. Distelhorst, C.W.; Lam, M.; McCormick, T.S. Bcl-2 inhibits hydrogen peroxide-induced ER Ca^{2+} pool depletion. *Oncogene* **1996**, *12*, 2051–2055. [PubMed]
119. He, H.; Lam, M.; Mccormick, T.S.; Distelhorst, C.W. Maintenance of calcium homeostasis in the endoplasmic reticulum by Bcl-2. *J. Cell Biol.* **1997**, *138*, 1219–1228. [CrossRef] [PubMed]
120. Wei, H.; Wei, W.; Bredesen, D.E.; Perry, D.C. Bcl-2 protects against apoptosis in neuronal cell line caused by thapsigargin-induced depletion of intracellular calcium stores. *J. Neurochem.* **1998**, *70*, 2305–2314. [CrossRef] [PubMed]
121. Antonsson, B.; Conti, F.; Ciavatta, A.; Montessuit, S.; Lewis, S.; Martinou, I.; Bernasconi, L.; Bernard, A.; Mermod, J.J.; Mazzei, G.; Maundrell, K. Inhibition of Bax channel-forming activity by Bcl-2. *Science* **1997**, *277*, 370–372. [CrossRef] [PubMed]
122. Antonsson, B.; Montessuit, S.; Lauper, S.; Eskes, R.; Martinou, J.C. Bax oligomerization is required for channel-forming activity in liposomes and totrigger cytochrome c release from mitochondria. *Biochem. J.* **2000**, *345*, 271–278. [CrossRef] [PubMed]
123. European Marine Board and Marine Biotechnology (ERANET). Marine Biotechnology: Advancing Innovation in Europe's Bioeconomy. In *EMB Policy Brief*; European Marine Board: Oostende, Belgium, 2017; ISBN 978-94-92043-35-1.
124. Markets and Markets Website—New Market Reports. Available online: http://www.marketsandmarkets.com/search.asp?Search=carotenoid&x=0&y=0 (accessed on 24 April 2015).
125. Raja, R.; Hemaiswarya, S.; Kumar, N.A.; Sridhar, S.; Rengasamy, R. A perspective on the biotechnological potential of microalgae. *Crit. Rev. Microbiol.* **2008**, *34*, 77–88. [CrossRef] [PubMed]
126. Misawa, N. Pathway engineering of plants toward astaxanthin production. *Plant Biotechnol.* **2009**, *26*, 93–99. [CrossRef]
127. Cheng, J.; Li, K.; Yang, Z.; Zhou, J.; Cen, K. Enhancing the growth rate and astaxanthin yield of *Haematococcus pluvialis* by nuclear irradiation and high concentration of carbon dioxide stress. *Bioresour. Technol.* **2016**, *204*, 49–54. [CrossRef] [PubMed]

2

Carotenoids as Novel Therapeutic Molecules Against Neurodegenerative Disorders: Chemistry and Molecular Docking Analysis

Johant Lakey-Beitia [1,†], Jagadeesh Kumar D. [2,†], Muralidhar L. Hegde [3,4,5] and K.S. Rao [6,*]

1 Center for Biodiversity and Drug Discovery, Instituto de Investigaciones Científicas y Servicios de Alta Tecnología (INDICASAT AIP), Clayton, City of Knowledge 0843-01103, Panama; jolivel.l@gmail.com
2 Department of Biotechnology, Sir M. Visvesvaraya Institute of Technology, Bangalore 562157, India; jk4research@gmail.com
3 Department of Radiation Oncology, Houston Methodist Research Institute, Houston, TX 77030, USA; mlhegde@houstonmethodist.org
4 Center for Neuroregeneration, Department of Neurosurgery, Houston Methodist, Houston, Texas 77030, USA
5 Weill Medical College of Cornell University, New York, NY 10065, USA
6 Center for Neuroscience, Instituto de Investigaciones Científicas y Servicios de Alta Tecnología (INDICASAT AIP), Clayton, City of Knowledge 0843-01103, Panama
* Correspondence: kjr5n2009@gmail.com
† These authors contribute equally to this work.

Abstract: Alzheimer's disease (AD) is the most devastating neurodegenerative disorder that affects the aging population worldwide. Endogenous and exogenous factors are involved in triggering this complex and multifactorial disease, whose hallmark is Amyloid-β (Aβ), formed by cleavage of amyloid precursor protein by β- and γ-secretase. While there is no definitive cure for AD to date, many neuroprotective natural products, such as polyphenol and carotenoid compounds, have shown promising preventive activity, as well as helping in slowing down disease progression. In this article, we focus on the chemistry as well as structure of carotenoid compounds and their neuroprotective activity against Aβ aggregation using molecular docking analysis. In addition to examining the most prevalent anti-amyloidogenic carotenoid lutein, we studied cryptocapsin, astaxanthin, fucoxanthin, and the apocarotenoid bixin. Our computational structure-based drug design analysis and molecular docking simulation revealed important interactions between carotenoids and Aβ via hydrogen bonding and van der Waals interactions, and shows that carotenoids are powerful anti-amyloidogenic molecules with a potential role in preventing AD, especially since most of them can cross the blood-brain barrier and are considered nutraceutical compounds. Our studies thus illuminate mechanistic insights on how carotenoids inhibit Aβ aggregation. The potential role of carotenoids as novel therapeutic molecules in treating AD and other neurodegenerative disorders are discussed.

Keywords: Alzheimer's disease; Amyloid-β aggregation; carotenoid; apocarotenoid; biosynthesis; molecular docking analysis; structure-activity relationship

1. Introduction

The onset of neurodegenerative disease is a consequence of abnormal conformational/structural changes in proteins [1]. Alterations in the biochemical homeostasis of the nervous system due to metal deposition, oxidative stress, disturbances in cholinesterase, and amyloid and tau plaque formation are highly associated with the initiation and progress of neurodegenerative disease [2–11]. In addition, the accumulation of misfolded amyloidogenic proteins in the central nervous system (CNS) has been linked to progressive neurological impairment [5]. AD, Parkinson's disease (PD), Huntington's disease (HD), and amyotrophic lateral sclerosis (ALS) are the most devastating neurodegenerative diseases, and all of these conditions affect normal behavior [7,8,12]. AD is the most prevalent worldwide with more than 45 million aging people suffering from this condition today and the number of cases expected to triple by 2050 [2]. According to the Aβ hypothesis, Aβ peptide is considered the main trigger of AD pathogenesis due to reduced Aβ clearance [13,14]. In the human brain, Aβ fibrils are considered the hallmark of AD and are found in the hippocampus and neocortical regions [13]. Drug discovery for AD faces two major challenges, namely the lack of an animal model which represents all events that occur in a patient with AD and the absence of a reliable biomarker that enables monitoring of disease progression [15–18].

Natural products, such as polyphenols, carotenoids, and other compounds, play an important role in the prevention of neurodegenerative diseases [19–23]. Polyphenols, such as resveratrol, epigallocatechin gallate (EGCG), and curcumin, constitute a large family of compounds that have demonstrated neuroprotective activity [6]. The biggest challenges with these compounds are their stability and bioavailability. However, structural modification of polyphenols has been demonstrated to improve their biological activity [24].

Carotenoids are another type of natural product reported to play a role in the prevention of brain disorders [25,26]. These molecules are natural products distributed widely in plants, animals, and microorganisms [27], and more than 750 carotenoids exist in nature. These compounds are responsible for the yellow, orange, and red color in various plants and animals (birds, reptiles, fish), and the color is indicative of the type of carotenoid [28–33]. Carotenoids are secondary metabolites produced by enzymatic reactions, and these reactions generate different carotenoids with biological importance [34,35]. Carotenoids play a variety of important functions in plants, animals, and in the human brain. In plants, carotenoids are synthetized de novo where most are enriched with a small quantity of its biosynthetic precursor [36]. The biosynthesis of carotenoids is mediated by different enzymes and occurs in the plastids. They have functions such as light harvesting in the photosynthetic membranes and protection of the photosynthetic apparatus against photo-oxidation [34,37]. Carotenoids also act as precursors of the phytohormone abscisic acid (ABA) [38] and are involved in the process of pollination as attractors of pollinators and seed dispersal agents [34]. Some animals can synthetize carotenoids, but most depend on dietary intake. In humans, these compounds have several therapeutic properties, including antioxidation, prevention of neuro-inflammation, anti-cancer, anti-diabetes, prevention of cardiovascular disease, and potentially the prevention and treatment of neurodegenerative disorders [39–43]. The antioxidant property of carotenoids is the main therapeutic characteristic of this compound where the conjugate polyene chain plays a crucial role in the reduction of free radicals [43–46]. This paper is focused on the chemistry of carotenoids and, through molecular docking analysis, proposes plausible mechanisms by which they may inhibit Aβ aggregation.

2. Chemistry of Carotenoid Compounds

Carotenoids belong to a class of terpenoid compounds with a characteristic conjugated polyene chain composed of eight C_5 isoprenoid units (Figure 1). The trans-carotenoid isomer is most predominant in nature [47–51]. The large polyene chain enables light absorption in the range of 450–550 nm of the visible spectrum [52]. The *cis*- and trans-carotenoid isomers have varying melting points, with *cis*-isomers having a lower value than trans-carotenoids due to the decreased tendency of *cis*-isomers to crystallize [28,53]. Meanwhile, *cis*-carotenoids can absorb light at a shorter wavelength, with a lower absorption coefficient [54]. The soluble property of carotenoids is based on their hydrophobic chemical structure, which makes them insoluble in water and dimethylsulfoxide, but favors their solubility in organic solvents such as ethyl ether, chloroform, acetone, ethyl acetate, and ethanol [55]. Most carotenoids are lipophilic with the ability to cross the blood-brain barrier [56].

Carotenoids are considered "molecular rivets" since the width of this type of compound is the same as that of the phospholipid bilayer which confers stability and rigidity to the phospholipid membrane [57,58].

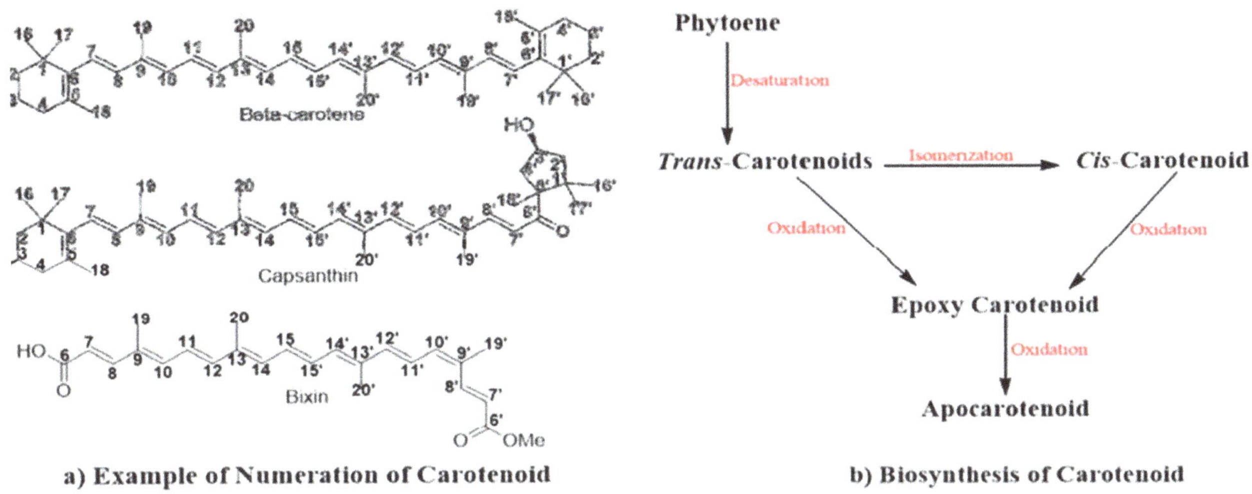

Figure 1. Numeration and biosynthesis of carotenoids: (**a**) Beta-carotene, capsanthin, and bixin are examples of how carotenoids and apocarotenoid can be numerated; (**b**) the biosynthesis of carotenoids starts with phytoenes that produce trans- and *cis*-carotenoids that can produce an epoxy carotenoid and finally an apocarotenoid.

Carotenoids are classified into two groups, namely carotenes and xanthophylls, both of which can be acyclic or cyclic compounds [59–61]. Carotenes have carbon and hydrogen atoms. The most common acyclic carotene is lycopene, which is found in tomato, red-fleshed papaya, and guava [55]. The most common cyclic carotene is β-carotene, which is found mainly in carrot, apricot, and mango [55]. Other cyclic carotenes are β-zeacarotene, α-zeacarotene, γ-carotene, δ-carotene, and α-carotene. Xanthophylls contain carbon, hydrogen, and oxygen atoms in their structure forming hydroxyl, epoxide, and keto groups [59,60]. Xanthophylls are formed from enzymatic reactions involving hydroxylases, epoxidases, or synthases. Carotenols are xanthophylls that possess a hydroxyl group (e.g., β-cryptoxanthin, zeaxanthin, and lutein), while epoxycarotenoids are xanthophylls with an epoxide group (e.g., antheraxanthin, violaxanthin, neoxanthin, β-carotene-5, 6-epoxide, β-carotene-5, 6, 5′,6′-diepoxide, and β-Cryptoxanthin-5,6-epoxide) (Figure 2). Ketocarotenoids, such as astaxanthin, fucoxanthin, capsanthin, and capsorubin, are xanthophylls with a keto group [62].

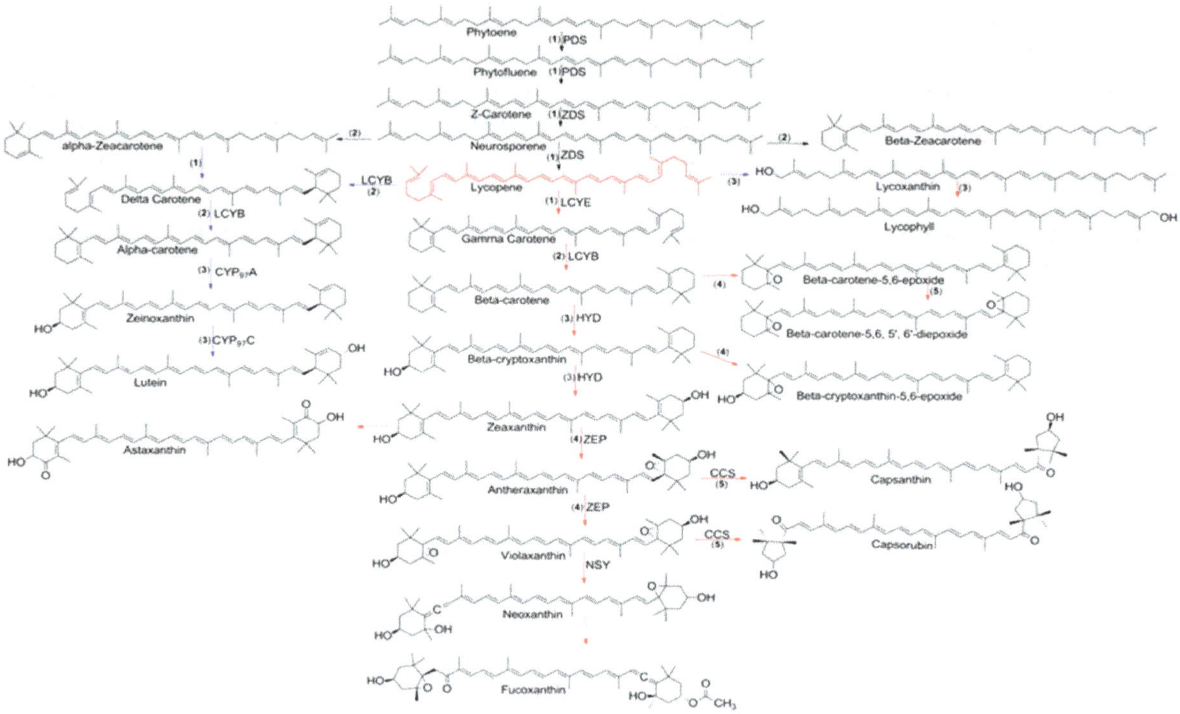

Figure 2. Biosynthesis of carotenoids and their five crucial reactions: desaturation (**1**), cyclization (**2**), hydroxylation (**3**), epoxidation (**4**), and epoxide-furanoxide rearrangement (**5**).

3. Biosynthesis of Carotenoids

Carotenoid synthesis can begin with the mechanism (1–4′) head-to-tail condensation of three isopentenyl diphosphates (IPP) and one dimethylallyl diphosphate (DMAPP) to produce the isoprenoid compound known as geranylgeranyl diphosphate (GGPP) [63]. The olefinic double bond of IPP nucleophilically attacks the carbocation produced through release of the allylic diphosphate group [63]. This reaction is catalyzed by GGPP synthase (GGPPS), and this enzyme has a mechanism of cyclic condensation: ionization-condensation-elimination [48,63]. GGPP is the precursor of different types of compounds such as carotenoids, plastoquinones, tocopherols, chlorophyll side chains, and phytohormones [63]. The head-to-head coupling of two GGPP catalyzed by phytoene synthase (PSY) produces a dimerized compound known as phytoene [34,64]. A phytoene compound is characterized by the presence of three conjugated double bonds in a chain.

The production of carotenoids starts with phytoene synthesis, and this process is considered the rate-controlling reaction in the pathway [63]. The biosynthesis of phytoene is the first committed step in the desaturation process which leads to the formation of the conjugate double bond that is characteristic of carotenoids (Figure 2). The enzyme phytoene desaturase (PDS) introduces two conjugated double bonds into the long chain, forming a phytofluene compound. Then, the desaturation reaction gives rise to another two conjugated double bonds, producing ζ-carotene. The poly-cis-carotenoid compound generated in this biosynthetic process is converted into trans-carotenoid by carotene isomerase (CRTISO) or ζ-carotene isomerase (ZISO). The neurosporene compound is biosynthesized by ζ-carotene desaturase (ZDS), which introduces two conjugate double bonds into the chain [64]. This desaturase enzyme continues the enzymatic process to form the lycopene compound by introducing two conjugate double bonds. The cyclization of lycopene was proposed by Porter and Lincoln, who hypothesized that cyclization can occur on one or both sides of the carotenoid to generate different type of compounds [63]. Two different rings, such as β- or ε-ionone rings, are generated from lycopene cyclization. Usually, the main modification of the carotenoid occurs on the end, and only a few modifications occur in the long chain of the carotenoid. The enzyme responsible for lycopene cyclization is lycopene cyclase (LCY), which is found in plants and cyanobacteria. The type of carotenoid is determined by the LCY subtype, namely β–ionone (LCYB) rings, ε-ionone (LCYE) rings, or bifunctional β/ε-ionone

(LCYB/E) rings. An unsubstituted β-ionone ring is considered a source of vitamin A, a molecule important for human health. In the presence of LCYB, lycopene is transformed into γ-carotene. Meanwhile, lycopene in the presence of LCYE is transformed into δ-carotene. Both compounds contain a six-member-ring at the end of the chain. LCYB can transform γ-carotene into β-carotene, a compound with two six-member rings at the end of the chain. A similar transformation occurs with δ-carotene, which is transformed into α-carotene. The addition of hydroxyl and keto groups to carotenoids can be achieved through two different classes of enzymes, ferredoxin-dependent nonheme diiron enzymes (HYD) and enzymes to belonging to the cytochrome P450 family [63]. The first is a type of β-hydroxylase that is responsible for β-cryptoxanthin and zeaxanthin formation. Cytochrome P450 has a novel ε-hydroxylase that is responsible for hydroxylation of the ε-ionone ring to form zeinoxanthin. The enzyme capsanthin-capsorubin synthase converts epoxycarotenoids into κ-cyclic carotenoids such as capsanthin and capsorubin [65]. Epoxidation reactions also occur in carotenoids through epoxidases such as zeaxanthin epoxidase (ZEP), which is responsible for antheraxanthin and violaxanthin formation.

Apocarotenoids have a structure similar to carotenoids but without C_{40} atoms (Figure 3). An apocarotenoid is considered a product of oxidative cleavage of carotenoids, and the most well-known apocarotenoids are Apo-12′-capsorubinal and bixin [66,67].

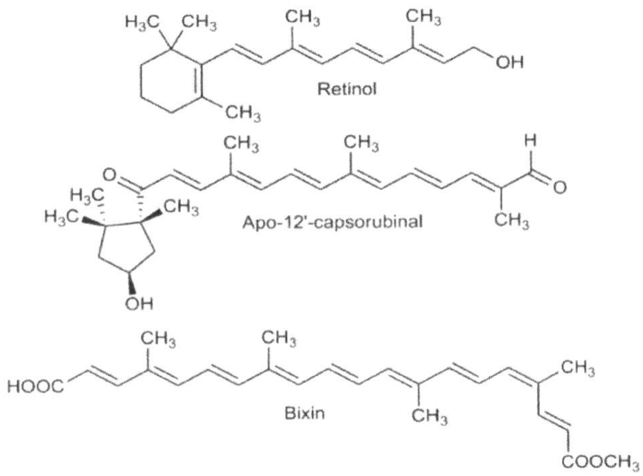

Figure 3. Examples of structures of some of the apocarotenoids.

The five important reactions involved in carotenoid biosynthesis are desaturation (1), cyclization (2), hydroxylation (3), epoxidation (4), and epoxide-furanoxide rearrangement (5) (Figure 2) [55]. The desaturation reaction (Figure 4) is essential for the formation of conjugate double bonds in the chain of the carotenoid. Formation of the lycopene compound starts with desaturation of phytoene, which contains three conjugated double bonds, and then proceeds with the formation of phytofluene, which contains five conjugated double bonds, ζ-carotene, which possesses seven conjugated double bonds, neurosporene with nine conjugated double bonds, and finally lycopene, which contains 11 conjugated double bonds [55,68]. Because the flavin cofactor can accept one or two electrons, four mechanisms have been reported to demonstrate how phytoene desaturation proceeds, namely through single electron transfer, the formation of hydride from substrate, transfer to flavin adenine dinucleotide (FAD), hydrogen atom transfer, and nucleophilic attack [68]. The cyclization reaction (Figure 4) is important in ring formation of the carotenoid. Lycopene is the important carotenoid which starts the cyclization process [69]. The reaction mechanism consists of attacking the alkene in the C_2 position of the lycopene to generate an acid-producing carbocation in the lycopene, which is stabilized by deprotonation of hydrogen in C_4, C_{18}, or C_6 to yield a β-end-group, γ-end-group, or ε- end-group (Figure 3). Two types of rings can be formed, such as the β-ionone ring, at the end-group of both sides (e.g., β-carotene) [69]. The ε-ring can be formed at one side of the compound such as in α-carotene [69].

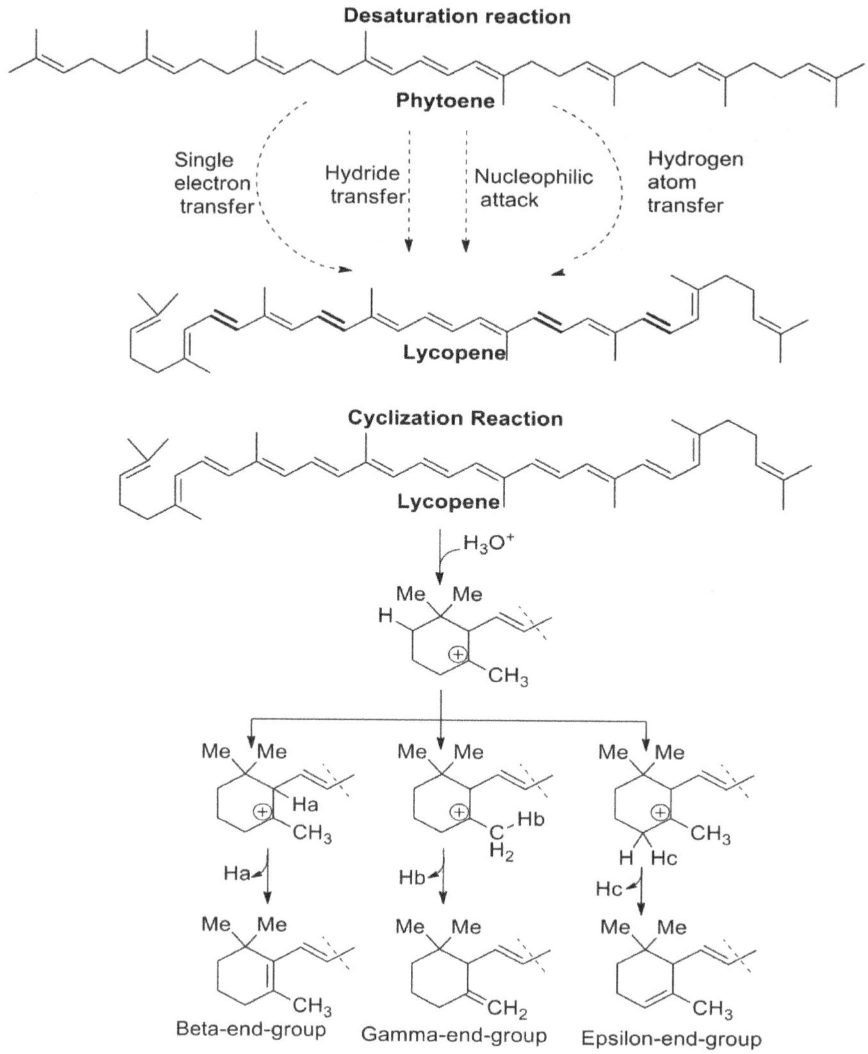

Figure 4. Desaturation and cyclization reaction.

The hydroxylation reaction (Figure 5) is quite common in β- or ε-ionone rings in carotenoids. The addition of this group to the ring causes a loss in vitamin A properties [63]. Xanthophyll functions in preventing damage caused by photo-oxidation. The hydroxylation reaction is carried out by two classes of enzymes, namely ferredoxin-dependent nonheme diiron enzymes (HYD) and enzymes of the cytochrome P450 family [70,71]. A plausible mechanism of carotenoid hydroxylation by HYD has been proposed based on studies of alkane mono-oxygenase and L-*p*-amino phenylalanine hydroxylase, where the first step consists of binding of one oxygen molecule to an iron cluster to form the peroxodiferric intermediate. This step is followed by hydrogen abstraction of the carotenoid by a potent oxidant (Q), resulting in the formation of a carotenoid radical that interacts with the iron complex to hydroxylate the carotenoid [70–72]. The epoxidation reaction (Figure 5) of carotenoids can lead to structural modification of the β-ionone ring at the 5,6-position (e.g., antheraxanthin is epoxidized at one site by zeaxanthin epoxidase (ZEP) [38,69]. However, the epoxidation reaction is a reversible reaction in the presence of violaxanthin de-epoxidase (VDE), forming the xanthophyll cycle which plays an important role in the regulation of photosynthetic energy conversion [73]. In the epoxide-furanoide rearrangement reaction (Figure 5), the epoxide carotenoid can undergo epoxide-furanoxide rearrangement in the presence of acid to produce a different type of end-group. The type of end-group is determined by the carbocation position and hydrogen abstraction by a base (B^-), such as the *k*-end-group, γ-end-group, or ε-end-group, which is produced when the carbocation is in the C_5 position. Meanwhile, the epoxide-furanoxy rearrangement known as 5,8-epoxide carotenoid occurs when the carbocation is in the C_6 position [69]. Capsanthin-capsorubin synthase (CCS) is the enzyme responsible for *k*-end-group formation, where pinacol rearrangement occurs to form a new family of carotenoids [67].

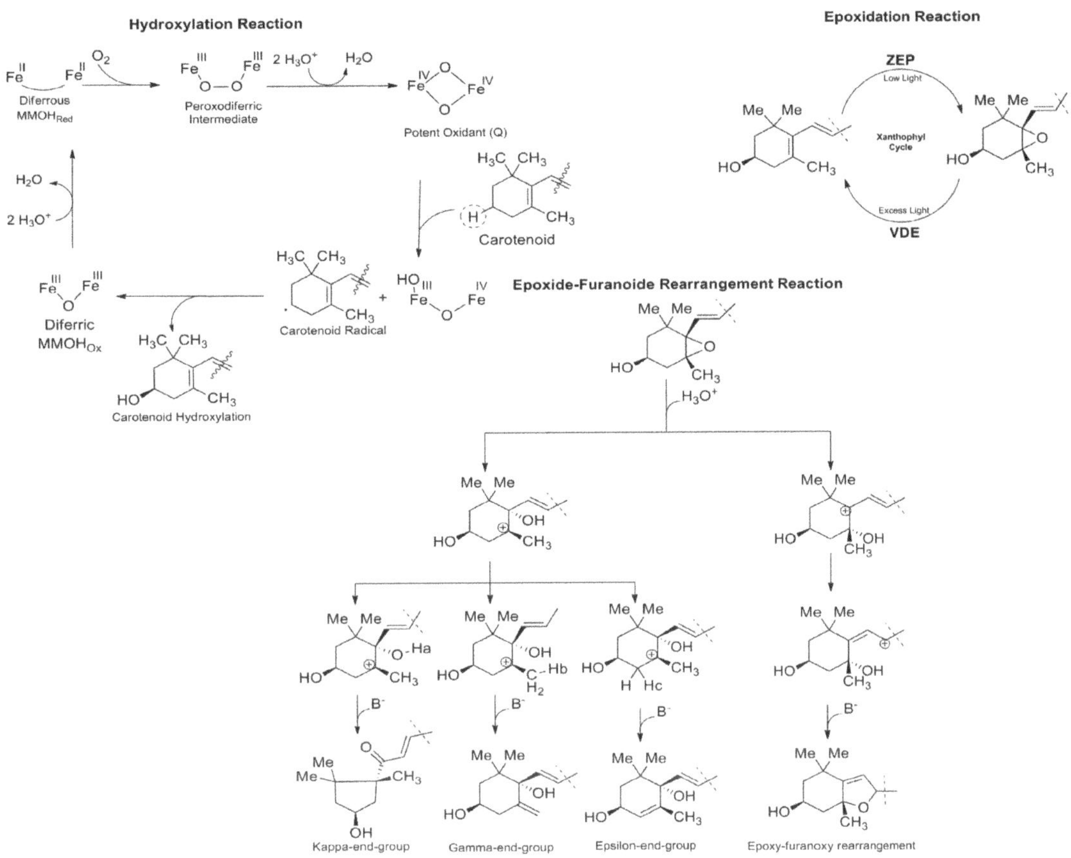

Figure 5. Hydroxylation, epoxidation, and epoxide-furanoide rearrangement reactions.

4. Types of Carotenoid Derivatives

The synthesis of carotenoid derivatives with hydrophilic properties are a good alternative for incorporating this type of molecule with multiple therapeutic properties in aqueous medium [74,75]. Carotenoids have an important nutritional value since most of them are a source of vitamin A, antioxidant molecules with anti-carcinogenic properties, and the ability to prevent cardiovascular disease [41,45]. Synthesizing hydrophilic carotenoid derivatives is important due to their use as therapeutic molecules that improve the biological activity of carotenoids. Another reason to produce synthetic carotenoid derivatives is their increased water solubility. This property allows carotenoids to be widely used in the food industry as natural dyes. Several types of carotenoid derivatives have been synthetized, including reduced carotenoids, carotenoid epoxides, carotenoid esters, carotenoid glycosides, and PEGylated carotenoids (Figure 6) [75]. Below, we briefly describe the types of carotenoid derivatives synthesized with hydrophilic properties.

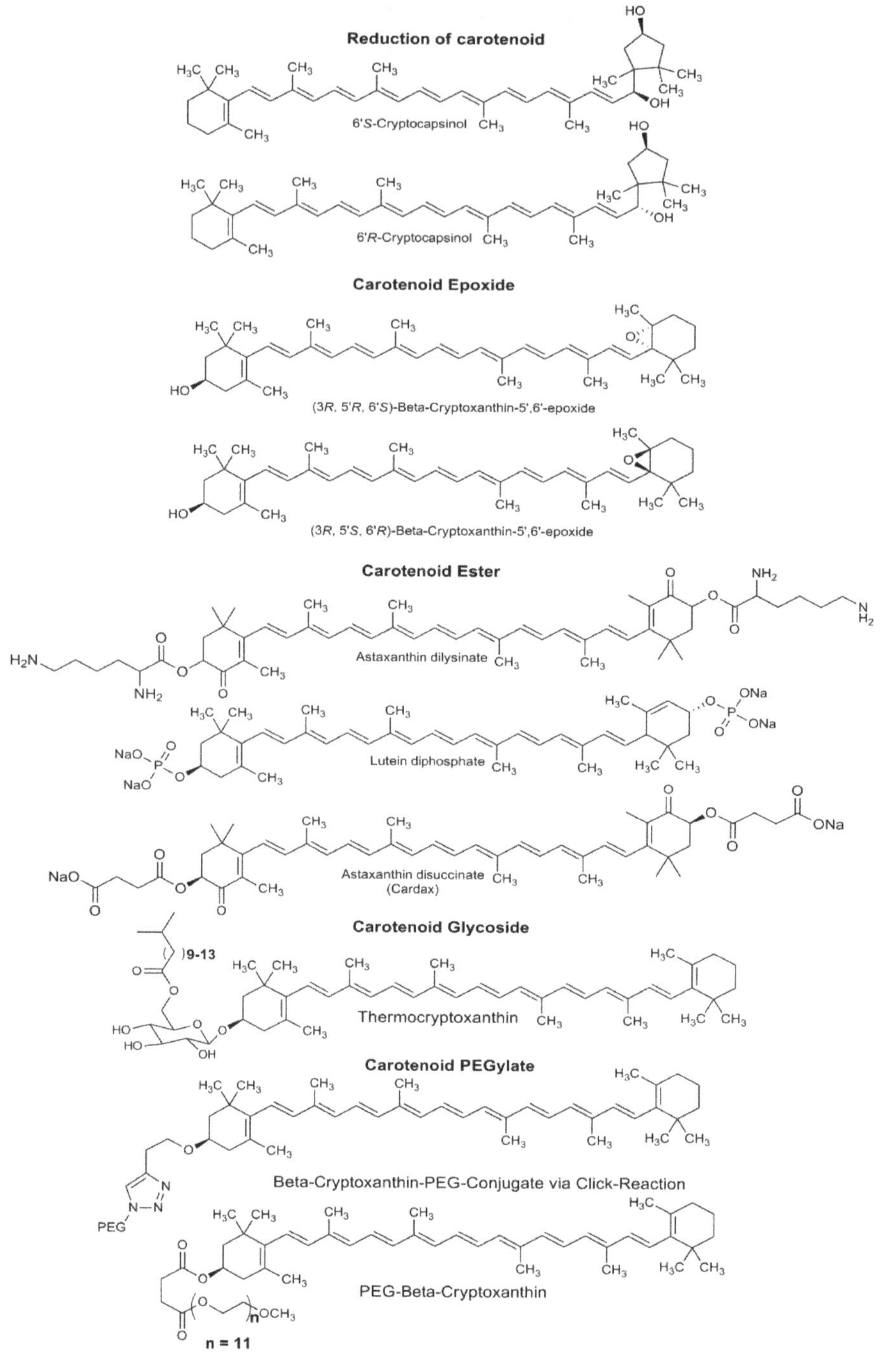

Figure 6. Types of carotenoid derivatives.

Reduced carotenoids: Similar to cryptocapsin and capsorubin, carotenoids are difficult to isolate or detect. However, the increased polarity of their reduced form can be utilized in their detection [76]. The reagent $NaBH_4$ in EtOH or EtOH/benzene is used to reduce the keto group of the carotenoid to generate two stereoisomeric alcohols (Figure 6) [76]. *Carotenoid epoxides:* Carotenoids are a source of vitamin A; however, when the β-ionone ring is epoxidized, the pro-vitamin A activity is lost [65,77]. This epoxidation is prepared using monoperoxyphthalic acid to produce two types of epoxides that can be separated through a chiral column (Figure 6) [77,78]. *Carotenoid esters*: Carotenoids, with the exception of bixin and crocin, are poor water-soluble molecules. The synthesis of carotenoid derivatives with water-soluble characteristics enables the therapeutic properties of this type of compound in aqueous solutions (e.g., Cardax) [75,79]. Esterification of carotenoids is most frequently performed using succinate, phosphates, and lysinates [74,75,80]. Succinate is prepared using succinic anhydride with

4-dimethylaminopyridine (DMAP) in dichloromethane (CH_2Cl_2) [39,80,81]. Meanwhile, phosphate is produced using lutein with dibenzyl phosphoroiodidate in CH_2Cl_2 [82]. Finally, preparation of the astaxanthin-amino acid conjugate can be achieved using $N^{\alpha\varepsilon}$-bis-(tert-butoxycarbonyl)-L-Lysine (BocLys(Boc)OH) with DMAP in CH_2Cl_2 and 1,3-diisopropylcarbodiimide (DIC), [83]. These types of carotenoid derivatives have been demonstrated to exhibit increased solubility in polar solvents when they are converted to sodium salt [82].

Carotenoid glycosides: This type of carotenoid derivative is found in nature in some microorganisms that are characterized by their resistance to heat, specifically the *Thermus* species. Thus, this type of compound is known as a thermoxanthin [75]. The presence of glycoside makes it more water soluble and amphiphilic. Yamano, et al. achieved synthesis of thermocryptoxanthin and thermozeaxanthin [84]. Glucosidation can be performed by combining glucosyl bromide with silver triflate (AgOTf) in some cases in the presence of N,N,N′,N′-tetramethylurea as a proton acceptor (Figure 6) [84]. *PEGylated carotenoids*: A polyethyleneglycol (PEG) conjugate is widely used for its pharmacokinetic properties and solubility in aqueous solution [39,74]. This type of carotenoid derivative is synthetized by coupling succinate with polyethylene glycols using dicyclohexylcarbodiimide (DCC) with DMAP in CH_2Cl_2 [81,85]. Another type of carotenoid derivative is produced by the azide-alkyne click reaction, which is well known for increasing water solubility (Figure 6) [75,86].

5. Neuroprotection by Carotenoids through Modulation of the App Pathway

Aβ peptide is formed by cleavage of amyloid precursor protein (APP), which is catabolized by secretases (α, β, and γ secretase), to form non-amyloidal and/or amyloidal products [87–89]. APP is a multidomain glycoprotein with signal peptide regions located at residues 1–17, two copper-binding sites at amino acids (aa) 124–189, and an E2 domain 376 where chromosome 21 produces eight isoforms of APP (695–770). The major isoform is APP 695. When the N-terminal region of APP is cleaved by β-secretase, secreted APP fragment beta (sAPPβ) is formed and γ-secretase transforms C-terminal fragment beta (CTFβ) in Aβ at the copper-binding site [90]. The non-amyloidogenic α-secretase belongs to the family of zinc metalloproteinases that cleaves APP at Lys687. Amyloidogenic aspartyl protease β-secretase cleaves at Met671, while γ-secretase cleaves at Val711 and Ala713 to form $A\beta_{40}$ and $A\beta_{42}$, respectively [90–93].

Several studies have demonstrated that carotenoids can inhibit Aβ aggregation [45,56,94–96]. Carotenoids such as lutein, lycopene, astaxanthin, fucoxanthin, cryptocapsin, and the apocarotenoid crocin have been demonstrated to inhibit $A\beta_{42}$ aggregation (Figure 7). Lutein, a hydroxylated carotenoid present in apricot extract, exhibits a strong inhibition of $A\beta_{42}$ fibril formation [56]. Katayama, et al. compared lutein with zeaxanthin, β-cryptoxanthin, β-carotene, and α-carotene, and found that lutein has the highest activity. The authors hypothesized that the number of hydroxyl groups plays an important role in the inhibition of Aβ aggregation [56]. Lycopene, an acyclic carotene found in tomatoes with a highly conjugated structure, has been shown to exhibit multiple benefits including inhibition of $A\beta_{42}$ formation [94–96]. Wang, et al. found that lycopene can reduce Aβ aggregation and inhibit the inflammatory response by suppressing microglia activation and increasing antioxidant enzyme activities [94]. Crocin, an unusual polar apocarotenoid found in *Crocus sativa* stigma, possesses an inhibitory activity similar to Aβ [43,97]. Papandreou, et al. found that trans-crocin-4 is the main apocarotenoid present in the perennial herb of the Iridaceous family [43]. Astaxanthin, a ketocarotenoid found in crustacean shells, is also considered to be a highly antioxidant molecule [62,98]. Lee, et al. found that astaxanthin can inhibit nitric oxide production in vitro and in vivo [98]. Fucoxanthin, an allene carotenoid found in marine microorganisms, have multiple therapeutic properties such as reduction of oxidative stress, decreased inflammation, decreased obesity effect, and inhibition of Aβ assembly [99,100]. Xiang, et al. demonstrated that fucoxanthin could inhibit Aβ assembly and that this inhibition is reinforced by hydrophobic interaction between this carotenoid and the Aβ peptide [100]. A recent study showed that fucoxanthin could inhibit β-secretase by hydrogen bonding with this enzyme [101]. Inhibition of this enzyme is another neuroprotective activity of carotenoids, and occurs by blocking the amyloidogenic pathway via inhibition of the initiation of APP cleavage to produce Aβ peptide [101]. Cryptocapsin is a ketocarotenoid with a non-conventional keto-kappa group found in *Pouteria sapota* [102,103]. We found that this carotenoid could potently inhibit $A\beta_{42}$ aggregation whereas cryptocapsin-5,6-epoxide, which is found in the same fruit, exhibited only a minor activity. Both carotenoids were compared with zeaxanthin, and the data demonstrated that cryptocapsin and zeaxanthin showed potent inhibition of $A\beta_{42}$ aggregation [25]. These results led us to conclude that hydroxyl and keto groups increase their activity while an epoxide group reduces it [25].

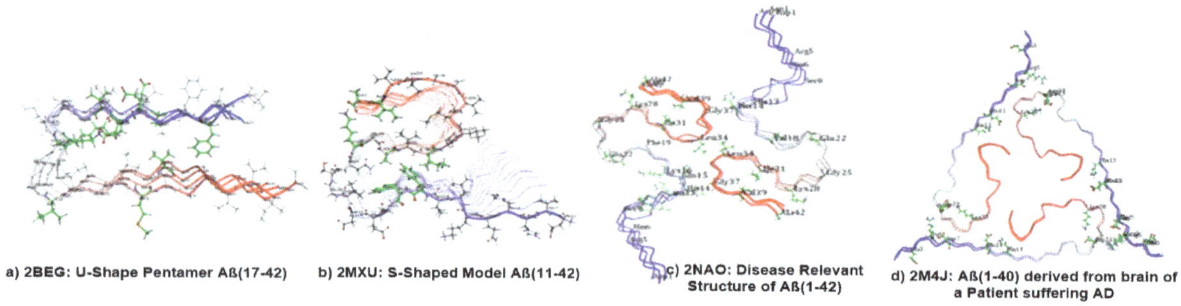

Figure 7. The Protein Data Bank (PDB) structures of four selected forms of Aβ fibrils are: (**a**) 2BEG including the $A\beta_{17–42}$ region; (**b**) 2MXU is characterized by the $A\beta_{11–42}$ region; (**c**) 2NAO is conformed by the $A\beta_{1–42}$ region; (**d**) 2M4J contains the $A\beta_{1–40}$ region.

Carotenoids are fascinating molecules that exhibit high antioxidant potential [104–106]. Lycopene, lutein, fucoxanthin, astaxanthin, cryptocapsin, and crocin are the most effective carotenoids in inhibiting Aβ aggregation. They have different structural characteristics, such as cyclic and acyclic structures, where the presence or absence of hydroxyl, epoxide, allenic, and keto groups is observed.

Our question is, when the process of aggregation begins, how does the carotenoid inhibit Aβ aggregation? We observed that a long chain of conjugated double bonds is present in these carotenoids (Figure 7), and that this polyene chain is responsible for their antioxidant activity by stabilization of radical species [52,107]. Nevertheless, how does the carotenoid inhibit Aβ aggregation? We observed that these carotenoids are oriented perpendicular to the Aβ peptide. This leads us to infer that the long polyene chain may block stacking of the peptide. Most likely the carotenoid conformation can be reinforced by the hydrogen bonding interactions or π-π stacking interactions that occur between the polar residues of the Aβ peptide, such as Glu22, Asp23, and Gly25, and the functional groups of the carotenoid (e.g., mainly the hydroxyl groups) [25]. Based on this observation, we conducted molecular docking analysis using five carotenoids with different structures and evaluated them against Aβ peptide aggregation.

6. Molecular Docking Analysis of Carotenoid and Apocarotenoid against Aβ Aggregation

Cryptocapsin, lutein, fucoxanthin, astaxanthin, and bixin were the carotenoids selected for molecular docking analysis. Because cryptocapsin was the most active in our experimental results, this compound was selected as our standard. Our objective was to perform structural analysis of carotenoids to evaluate how they prevent Aβ aggregation. Despite the fact that a vast number of carotenoids exist in nature, these five were selected based on their structural differences to examine whether these variations play a crucial role in Aβ aggregation.

We used a computational structure-based drug design and evaluated the possible interaction modes between different forms of Aβ fibrillar species, including $A\beta_{42}$ and $A\beta_{40}$, with carotenoid ligands like astaxanthin, bixin, cryptocapsin, fucoxanthin, and lutein retrieved from the PubChem database [108]. The molecular docking experiments were performed using CDOCKER, a docking protocol developed by Discovery Studio 3.5 (Accelrys, San Diego, CA, USA). The three-dimensional (3D) solution and solid state NMR structures of U-shaped pentamer $A\beta_{17–42}$ Protein Data Bank (PDB) identification (ID) were: 2BEG S-shaped Model $A\beta_{11–42}$; PDB ID: 2MXU Disease-Relevant structure of

$A\beta_{42}$; PDB ID: 2NAO and $A\beta_{40}$ derived from the brain of a patient suffering from AD; and PDB ID: 2M4J obtained from the RCSB PDB [109] (Figure 7).

The ligands and retrieved target PDB Aβ fibril NMR structures were minimized by using the conjugate gradient protocol and employing the CHARMm force field with Max Steps-2000 implemented in Discovery Studio 3.5 software (Accelrys, San Diego, USA).

The initial step was carried out by preparing different forms of Aβ fibrils and identifying the binding sites by using the Define and Edit binding site tool. The binding sites found are shown in Figure 8 as a set of points. Docking studies were carried out using the CDOCKER protocol under the Receptor-Ligand Interaction tools in Discovery Studio 3.5. CDOCKER is a powerful CHARMm-based docking method that has been shown to generate highly accurate docked poses [110].

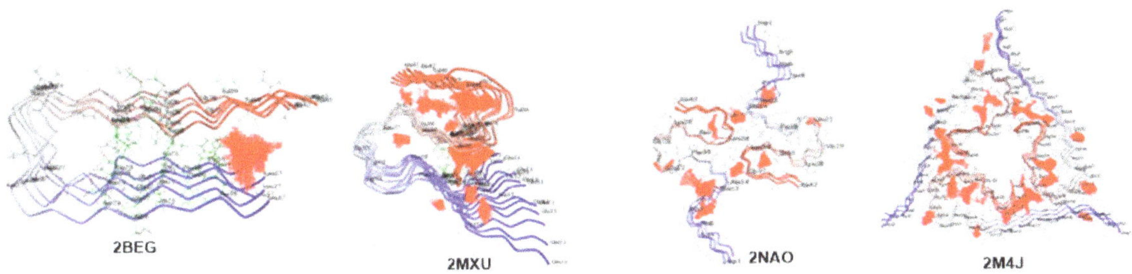

Figure 8. Probable receptor binding sites and alternative binding regions across different Aβ fibrils where ligand binding interactions can occur. Red dots correspond to the amino acid in the binding site.

The carotenoid ligands astaxanthin, bixin, cryptocapsin, fucoxanthin, and lutein (Figure 9) were docked onto the different forms of $A\beta_{42}$ and $A\beta_{40}$ fibrils. First, the Aβ fibril was held in a rigid conformation and the carotenoid ligands were allowed to flex during the refinement. Docking runs were adjusted to the 10–100 best outputs for evaluation of binding pose accuracy. Consequently, diverse poses are generated which adopted the random rigid body rotation and simulated annealing. Ligands displayed efficient docking with the generation of 10 conformers each. For each carotenoid ligand, the top 10 ligand binding poses were ranked according to their CDOCKER energies, which were calculated based upon the internal ligand strain energy and receptor-ligand interaction energy. The CDOCKER interaction signifies the energy of the non-bonded interaction that exists between the protein and ligand. It must be noted that, in both cases, greater CDOCKER energy and CDOCKER interaction energy values imply more favorable binding between the Aβ fibril and the ligand and therefore the best shape complementarity. The simulated docked complexes were studied based on the lowest binding affinity values (kcal/mol) and bonding interaction patterns (hydrogen, hydrophobic, and electrostatic). All ligand-protein interactions that exhibited stronger binding affinity and energies relative to individual targets are computed.

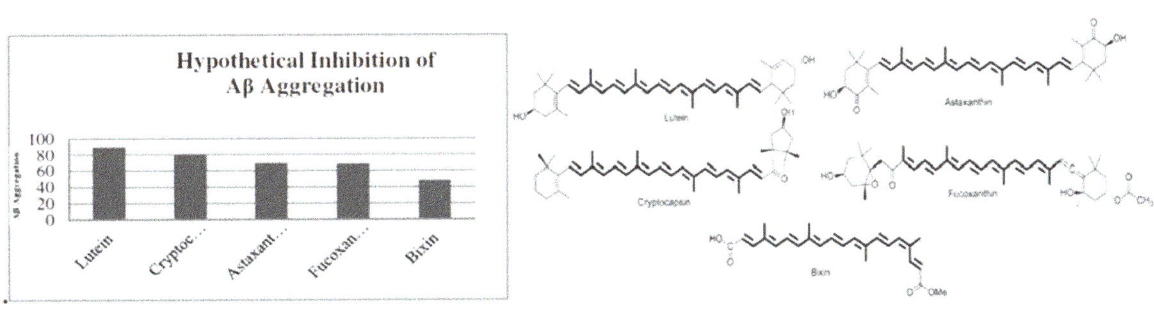

Figure 9. Hypothetical model of inhibition of Aβ aggregation by carotenoids and apocarotenoids. In this hypothetical inhibition of Aβ aggregation, lutein, a carotenoid with non-pro-vitamin A, showed the higher inhibition follow by cryptocapsin, a carotenoid with pro-vitamin A. After, astaxanthin and fucoxanthin, both of them are carotenoids with non-pro-vitamin A, and finally, Bixin, apocatenoid without pro-vitamin A.

It is interesting to understand that different types of structural polymorphism in the Aβ fibrils occur from the same polypeptide sequence in AD. These differences lead to variations in protofilament number, arrangement, and polypeptide conformations to numerous dissimilar patterns of inter- or intra-residue interactions. However, the most prevalent forms of Aβ peptides are $A\beta_{40}$ and $A\beta_{42}$ aa residues, with $A\beta_{42}$ being the more toxic form over $A\beta_{40}$. The higher toxicity of $A\beta_{42}$ chains may be explained by their ability to adopt three-stranded S-shaped antiparallel β-strands as a cylindrical barrel/pore-like structure when assembling as fibrils. In contrast, U-shaped configurations can only be observed for $A\beta_{40}$ peptides. Consistent with this, the patient-derived fibril structure of $A\beta_{40}$ chains possesses a three-fold symmetry which cannot take an S-shaped form but rather a U-shaped configuration that differs from other fibril polymorphs, which are more significant than other polymorphs for the pathology of AD. Hence, the present computational study is also intended to understand and appreciate the binding modes of carotenoids and their effect on fiber stability and fiber toxicity with four different forms of Aβ. The initial outcomes of the binding site analysis revealed that all four Aβ models exhibited interesting known binding sites and different small and large binding regions with uninformed size and depth across the Aβ fibril surface, where small molecule/large ligand binding interactions can occur. Docking studies of astaxanthin, bixin, cryptocapsin, fucoxanthin, and lutein binding with the selected model showed promising interactions of the ligands with each docked fibril. The ligand-protein complex was evaluated for hydrogen bond interactions and CDOCKER interaction (kcal/mol−1) energies.

Evaluating the interactions revealed that all the ligands exhibited strong interactions with residues such as Glu22, Val24, Gly25, Asp23, Ser26, Lys28, and Leu34, which participate in hydrogen bond formation (Table 1). Moreover, Ala21, Ile32, Gly33, Gly38, and Val39 participated through van der Waals interactions. Lutein showed the lowest CDOCKER energy (97.6659 kcal·mol−1), signifying greater interaction across 2BEG $A\beta_{42}$ fibrils. Irrespective of the binding energies projected for the ligands, all exhibited a similar binding mode pattern. Based on the data presented in Table 1, carotenoid-mediated inhibition of Aβ aggregation can be ranked as lutein > bixin > cryptocapsin > astaxanthin > fucoxanthin.

Table 1. Interactions of ligands with the U-shaped pentamer $A\beta_{17–42}$ using PDB ID: 2BEG.

Ligands	Highest -CDOCKER Energy (kcal/mol)	Highest -CDOCKER Interaction Energy (kcal/mol)	Amino Acid Residues Interacting with Aβ Chains	Common Residues Interacting Across all Ligands
Astaxanthin	−83.0351	−17.3682	Gly38, Val39	Ala21, Glu22 *, Val24 *, Gly25 *, Asp23 #, Ser26 #, Lys28 #, Ile32, Gly33; Leu34 *, Gly38, Val39
Bixin	−85.044	−127.336	Glu22 *	
Cryptocapsin	−83.6518	−14.4395	Leu34 *, Ile32, Gly33, Gly33	
Fucoxanthin	−69.4873	−39.3977	Asp23 #, Glu22, Ala21	
Lutein	−97.6659	−20.8785	Asp23 *, Val24 *,#, Gly25 *,#, Lys28 #, Ser26 #	

* Denotes main chain interactions and # specifies side chain interactions.

Similarly, this analysis revealed important interactions between carotenoids and 2MXU $A\beta_{11–42}$ (Table 2). All of these residues have been shown to interact with ligands via hydrogen bond formation while the remaining amino acids in the pocket display van der Waals interactions. Lutein (−60.6453 kcal/mol) exhibited the lowest CDOCKER energy. Regardless of their binding energies, all of the ligands exhibited a similar binding mode pattern with shared interacting residues such as Val12, His14, Ile32, Gly33, and Leu34. Based on the data in Table 2, carotenoid-mediated inhibition of Aβ aggregation can be ranked as lutein > cryptocapsin > fucoxanthin > astaxanthin > bixin.

Table 2. Interactions of ligands with the S-shaped model structure of $A\beta_{11-42}$ using PDB ID: 2MXU.

Ligands	Highest -CDOCKER Energy (kcal/mol)	Highest -CDOCKER Interaction Energy (kcal/mol)	Amino Acid Residues Interacting with Aβ Chains	Common Residues Interacting Across all Ligands
Astaxanthin	−36.1994	−60.0733	Val2, His14	
Bixin	10.2499	−45.5219	Leu34, Gly33	Val2, His14
Cryptocapsin	−44.9219	−60.0403	Gly33, Ile32, Gly33	Ile32, Gly33,
Fucoxanthin	−40.2796	−60.6453	Leu34, His14	Leu34
Lutein	−60.6453	−50.7407	His14	

Furthermore, the docking outcomes of the 2NAO-Disease-Relevant structure of $A\beta_{42}$ with carotenoids are shown in Table 3. These data reveal that all of the ligands form stable hydrogen bonds and van der Waals interactions. The other amino acid residues across the ligands participated via van der Waals interaction. However, cryptocapsin (−84.343 kcal/mol) and lutein (−88.1515 kcal/mol) exhibited the lowest CDOCKER energy. While all ligands share common interacting residues like Ser8, Glu11, Lys16 across the binding site of 2NAO. Based on the data in Table 3, carotenoid-mediated inhibition of Aβ aggregation can be ranked as lutein > cryptocapsin > astaxanthin > fucoxanthin > bixin.

Table 3. Interactions of ligands with the structures of Aβ (1–42) using PDB ID: 2NAO-Disease-Relevant.

Ligands	Highest -CDOCKER Energy (kcal/mol)	Highest -CDOCKER Interaction Energy (kcal/mol)	Amino Acid Residues Interacting with Aβ Chains	Common Residues Interacting Across all Ligands
Astaxanthin	−76.0481	−29.5232	Ser8, Glu11, Gly9 Tyr10	
Bixin	−74.169	−104.431	Glu22, Glu11	Ser8,
Cryptocapsin	−84.3430	−33.051	Lys16, Glu18	Glu11,
Fucoxanthin	−75.0944	−37.7015	Lys16, His13	Lys16
Lutein	−88.1515	−30.5548	Ser8	

Carotenoids also interact with 2M4J-$A\beta_{40}$ derived from the brain of a patient suffering from AD. As shown in Table 4, all of the ligands exhibited strong interactions with residues such as Glu28 and Gly37 through hydrogen bonding. The other amino acids participated by van der Waals interactions. Cryptocapsin (−101.782 kcal/mol) and lutein (−110.897 kcal/mol) exhibited the lowest CDOCKER energy. Based on the data in Table 4, carotenoid-mediated inhibition of Aβ aggregation can be ranked lutein > cryptocapsin > fucoxanthin > astaxanthin > bixin.

Table 4. Interactions of ligands with the structures of Aβ (1–40) derived from brain of a patient with AD using PDB ID: 2M4J.

Ligands	Highest -CDOCKER Energy (kcal/mol)	Highest -CDOCKER Interaction Energy (kcal/mol)	Amino Acid Residues Interacting with amyloid-β chains
Astaxanthin	−82.9702	−18.1365	-
Bixin	−22.6447	−16.4999	Lys28
Cryptocapsin	−101.782	−14.0123	Gly37
Fucoxanthin	−89.3804	−18.9031	Gly37
Lutein	−110.897	−16.1726	Gly37

A comparison of the different highest CDOCKER energy values allowed us to propose a hypothetical percentage of inhibition of Aβ aggregation by these five carotenoids (Figure 9). We observed that lutein was the most powerful carotenoid against Aβ aggregation followed by cryptocapsin. Astaxanthin and fucoxanthin showed moderate inhibition of Aβ aggregation. However, bixin, an apocarotenoid, displayed the lowest inhibition of Aβ aggregation. Therefore, we propose that carotenoids have greater potential to inhibit Aβ aggregation than apocarotenoids.

According to published literature, ligands which bind to the $A\beta_{16-20}$ region of $A\beta_{42}$ are capable of disrupting Aβ fibril formation. Likewise, studies have revealed that amino acid residues 16 to 20 in $A\beta_{16-20}$ are required for the self-association of Aβ peptides into Aβ fibrils. $A\beta_{16-20}$ forms an antiparallel β-sheet structure through binding to the homologous regions of amino acids 17–21 or 18–22 [111,112]. Similarly, it has been shown that $A\beta_{16-20}$ deletion, as the most important nucleation site, inhibits formation of the Aβ fibril [113]. Therefore, our docking analysis clearly indicates that ligands strongly interact in close contact with the 20–28 regions and hydrogen bonding at the Asp23-Lys28 salt bridge, resulting in disruption of the stability of the salt bridge and the oligomer structure as well as sheet breaking activity. Moreover, C-terminal residues such as Gly33, Met35, Val36, and Gly37 indicate that these ligands may disaggregate Aβ fibrils through their binding [111,113]. The data in Table 5 suggest that carotenoids and apocarotenoids can disrupt Aβ aggregation and the disaggregation pathway. Lutein can potentially inhibit oligomer formation due to interactions with residues 20–28 of the Aβ peptide, which are essential for oligomerization. Cryptocapsin has the potential to inhibit Aβ fibril formation due to interaction with residues 16–20. This carotenoid can also disaggregate Aβ fibrils through interaction with residues 33–37. Fucoxanthin is different from these carotenoids due to its potential to inhibit Aβ fibril formation, Aβ disaggregation, and oligomerization through interaction with residues 16–20, 24–28, and 33–37. Astaxanthin interacts with the Aβ peptide at amino acids 8–14, which are crucial for aggregation through interactions with metals such as Zn (II) and Cu (II) or Fe (II) and Al (III). This is a crucial metal-binding region [114]. However, we can hypothesize that its inhibition is based on disruption of hydrogen bond formation with residues 8–14 where this carotenoid has strong interactions with the polar residues of the Aβ peptide. Bixin, an apocarotenoid, has less contact with the Aβ peptide than carotenoids because it consists of half the number of carbons and possesses a cis conformation that reduces contact with the Aβ peptide. However, this apocarotenoid can interact with polar amino acids such as Glu11 and Glu22, Lys28, Gly33, and Leu34, indicating a potential for disrupting hydrogen bond formation with the Aβ peptide.

Table 5. Summary of interactions of the five compounds with the Aβ (1–42) sequence. Color code: astaxanthin (red), bixin (blue), cryptocapsin (purple), fucoxanthin (green), and lutein (yellow).

Ligands	8 S	9 G	10 Y	11 E	12 V	13 H	14 H	16 K	18 V	21 A	22 E	23 D	24 V	25 G	26 S	28 K	32 I	33 G	34 L	37 G	38 G	39 V
Astaxanthin	■	■	■	■	■		■														■	■
Bixin				■							■					■		■	■			
Cryptocapsin								■	■								■	■	■	■		
Fucoxanthin						■	■	■		■	■	■							■	■		
Lutein	■						■					■	■	■	■	■				■		

These results have allowed us to evaluate the inhibitory potential that carotenoids and apocarotenoids may possess. These data provide hints of their aggregation and disaggregation potential against Aβ formation. Some carotenoids can inhibit Aβ aggregation by interacting with residues in the regions of 8–14 and 16–20, which are essential for this procedure. On the other hand, there are carotenoids that can disaggregate Aβ fibrils by interacting with the 33–37 regions that are required for the fibrillation process. Nevertheless, there are carotenoids that can inhibit amino acids 23–28, which are essential for oligomerization. We also observed that there are carotenoids that may inhibit Aβ fibril aggregation and disaggregation.

Thus, we propose a plausible mechanism by which carotenoids inhibit Aβ aggregation and disaggregation. Our mechanism starts a proposal that the long chain of conjugated double bonds, characteristic of carotenoids, has a dual function. First, this polyene chain confers an antioxidant property to carotenoids by stabilizing radical species. Second, based on the planar structure of the polyene chain due to trans-configuration that is longer than the Aβ peptide, a perpendicular orientation may block self-aggregation of the peptide. The conformation of the carotenoid is reinforced by chemical interactions between the functional group of the carotenoid with polar residues of the Aβ peptide. For instance, all four carotenoids examined in this study share a similar polyene chain structure with trans-configuration. However, the apocarotenoid (bixin) has a short polyene chain with a *cis*-configuration. The carotenoid with a trans-configuration may have more potential to inhibit Aβ aggregation than a molecule with a *cis*-configuration. Another important difference that was observed is related to the quantity and positioning of hydroxyl groups within the molecule. For example, lutein, the most powerful carotenoid against Aβ aggregation, has two hydroxyl groups in the two β–ionone ring, specifically in the C_3 position. Cryptocapsin possesses one hydroxyl group in the 6-oxo-kappa end-group, specifically in the C_3 position. Astaxanthin has two hydroxyl groups in the C_3 position; however, this carotenoid is predicted to have lower potential for inhibiting Aβ aggregation than lutein. Therefore, it is possible that the keto-kappa groups and configuration of hydroxyl groups play a role in the inhibition of Aβ activity. Fucoxanthin has two hydroxyl groups but in different positions, as well as an epoxide group and an allene group that could influence the activity. The apocarotenoid bixin demonstrated the importance of the double-bond chain length in Aβ inhibition. These preliminary results allow us to propose a structure-activity relationship (SAR) where the double-bond chain is crucial for contact with the Aβ peptide. However, the hydroxyl group in the hydrogen bond interaction, along with their position and configuration in the molecule, is also important. Finally, the presence of epoxide, allene, and keto groups in the molecule may also affect Aβ inhibition.

In the published literature, little data exists showing the neuroprotective activity of carotenoids. While studies of these compounds have demonstrated their role in inhibiting the aggregation or disaggregation of Aβ fibrils, the underlying mechanism remains unknown. Thus, our proposed mechanism is based on two requirements: 1) blocking self-aggregation of the Aβ peptide by the length and configuration of the compound avoids self-assembly; and 2) the quantity and position of the hydroxyl groups are essential for interacting with the Aβ peptide/fibril through hydrogen bonding. Figure 10 is a schematic detailing the mechanism by which carotenoids can inhibit Aβ aggregation and disaggregation.

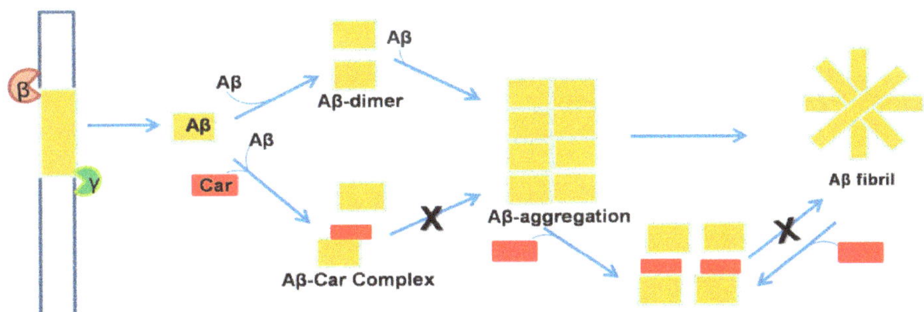

Figure 10. The hypothetical model to understand the role of carotenoids in the inhibition of $A\beta_{42}$ formation. β- and γ-secretases are the two enzymes that cleavage the amyloid precursor protein (APP) to form Aβ peptide. The aggregation of this peptide pass to dimer follows to oligomer until Aβ fibril. Carotenoids may potentially inhibit the APP pathway where carotenoids have been demonstrated to inhibit Aβ dimer, also oligomer, and also the disaggregation of Aβ fibril. Color code: Aβ (yellow), carotenoid (red), β-secretase (brown) and γ-secretase (green).

7. Aβ Aggregation and DNA Damage

While we focused on the neuroprotective activity of carotenoids especially for their role of inhibition of Aβ aggregation, this property is also important due to its potential effect on Aβ mediated genome instability. Previous studies have demonstrated a relationship between Aβ aggregation and DNA damage [11]. This raised the question whether the carotenoid compounds that inhibit Aβ aggregation also inhibit or prevent the DNA damage [11]. Indeed, studies have found that carotenoids can prevent the DNA damage [115–117]. This activity can be related to the type of carotenoid: the pro-vitamin A and non-vitamin A groups of carotenoids. The pro-vitamin A can be found in β-carotene and β-cryptoxanthin and lycopene, lutein, and astaxanthin possess the non-vitamin A property. Lutein can prevent the DNA damage when they exposed lutein to ultraviolet radiation using human neuroblastoma and rat trachea epithelial cells [118,119]. Future studies should investigate the protective effect of carotenoids on genome integrity, which could be important for both neurodegeneration and cancer prevention.

8. Conclusions and New Directions in Research

Carotenoids are natural products with a high therapeutic potential against neurodegenerative diseases, especially AD. For this reason, it is important to further explore comprehensively, mechanistic basis of carotenoids as a new source of therapeutic compounds in the fight against this devastating neurodegenerative disease. In this paper, we discussed the diversity of carotenoids found in nature and their high potential as therapeutic molecules involved in preventing multi-faceted toxic pathways of Aβ. Carotenoids are widely distributed in nature and exist in a variety of different types. However, only a few carotenoids have been characterized for their neuroprotective activity. We consider carotenoids as powerful natural compounds with nutraceutical and antioxidant properties that are critical in the fight against AD. Furthermore, most carotenoids can cross the blood-brain barrier. Future studies are in progress to evaluate the neuroprotective activity of carotenoids and their derivatives.

Author Contributions: Conceptualization, J.L.-B. and K.S.R.; Methodology, J.L.-B. and J.K.D.; Software, J.K.D.; Validation J.K.D., J.L.-B. and M.L.H.; Formal Analysis, J.K.D., J.L.-B. and M.L.H.; Data Curation, M.L.H.; Writing-Original Draft Preparation, J.L.-B. and J.K.D.; Writing-Review & Editing, J.L.-B., J.K.D., M.L.H, and K.S.R.; Visualization, J.L.-B., J.K.D., M.L.H, and K.S.R.; Supervision, K.S.R.; Project Administration, K.S.R.; Funding Acquisition, K.S.R.

Acknowledgments: J.L.-B. and K.S.R. are grateful to Melo Brain's Grant and MEF Nutritional Grant for support. J.L.-B. and K.S.R. also thank National Science System (SNI) of National Secretariat for Science, Technology, and Innovation of Panama (SENACYT) for support.

References

1. Hashimoto, M.; Rockenstein, E.; Crews, L.; Masliah, E. Role of protein aggregation in mitochondrial dysfunction and neurodegeneration in Alzheimer's and Parkinson's diseases. *Neuromol. Med.* **2003**, *4*, 21–36. [CrossRef]
2. Prado-Prado, F.; García, I. Review of theoretical studies for prediction of neurodegenerative inhibitors. *Mini Rev. Med. Chem.* **2012**, *12*, 452–466. [CrossRef] [PubMed]
3. Cho, J.K.; Ryu, Y.B.; Curtis-Long, M.J.; Ryu, H.W.; Yuk, H.J.; Kim, D.W.; Kim, H.J.; Lee, W.S.; Park, K.H. Cholinestrase inhibitory effects of geranylated flavonoids from Paulownia tomentosa fruits. *Bioorg. Med. Chem.* **2012**, *20*, 2595–2602. [CrossRef] [PubMed]
4. Majd, S.; Power, J.H.; Grantham, H.J.M. Neuronal response in Alzheimer's and Parkinson's disease: The effect of toxic proteins on intracellular pathways. *BMC Neurosci.* **2015**, *16*, 69. [CrossRef]
5. Wang, S.S.; Hung, Y.T.; Wen, W.S.; Lin, K.C.; Chen, G.Y. Exploring the inhibitory activity of short-chain phospholipids against amyloid fibrillogenesis of hen egg-white lysozyme. *Biochim. Biophys. Acta* **2011**, *1811*, 301–313. [CrossRef]
6. Lakey-Beitia, J.; Berrocal, R.; Rao, K.S.; Durant, A.A. Polyphenols as therapeutic molecules in Alzheimer's disease through modulating amyloid pathways. *Mol. Neurobiol.* **2015**, *51*, 466–479. [CrossRef]
7. Gadad, B.S.; Britton, G.B.; Rao, K.S. Targeting oligomers in neurodegenerative disorders: Lessons from α-synuclein, tau, and amyloid-β peptide. *J. Alzheimer's Dis.* **2011**, *24*, 223–232. [CrossRef]

8. Hegde, M.L.; Hegde, P.M.; Rao, K.S.; Mitra, S. Oxidative genome damage and its repair in neurodegenerative diseases: Function of transition metals as a double-edged sword. *J. Alzheimer's Dis.* **2011**, *24*, 183–198. [CrossRef]
9. Guerrero, E.; Padmaraju, V.; Hegde, M.L.; Britton, G.B.; Rao, K.S. Recent advances in α-synuclein functions, advanced glycation, and toxicity: Implications for Parkinson's disease. *Mol. Neurobiol.* **2013**, *47*, 525–536. [CrossRef]
10. Prakasam, A.; Muthuswamy, A.; Blonczy, Z.; Greig, N.H.; Fauq, A.; Rao, J.; Pappolla, M.A.; Sambamurti, K. Differential Accumulation of Secreted APP Metabolites in Ocular Fluids. *J. Alzheimer's Dis.* **2010**, *20*, 1243–1253. [CrossRef]
11. Suram, A.; Hegde, M.; Rao, K.S. A new evidence for DNA nicking property of amyloid b-peptide (1–42): Relevance to Alzheimer's disease. *Arch. Biochem. Biophys.* **2007**, *463*, 245–252. [CrossRef] [PubMed]
12. Rambaran, R.N.; Serpell, L.C. Amyloid fibrils Abnormal protein assembly. *Prion* **2008**, *2*, 112–117. [CrossRef] [PubMed]
13. Ramesh, B.N.; Raichurkar, K.P.; Shamasundar, N.M.; Rao, T.S.S.; Rao, K.S. Aβ(42) induced MRI changes in aged rabbit brain resembles AD brain. *Neurochem. Int.* **2011**, *59*, 637–642. [CrossRef] [PubMed]
14. Hardy, J.; Selkoe, D.J. The amyloid hypothesis of Alzheimer's disease: Progress and problems on the road to therapeutics. *Science* **2002**, *297*, 353–356. [CrossRef]
15. Chiang, K.; Koo, E. Emerging therapeutics for Alzheimer's disease. *Annu. Rev. Pharmacol. Toxicol.* **2014**, *54*, 381–405. [CrossRef]
16. Pillai, J.A.; Cummings, J.L. Clinical trials in predementia stages of Alzheimer disease. *Med. Clin. N. Am.* **2013**, *97*, 439–457. [CrossRef]
17. Schenk, D.; Basi, G.S.; Pangalos, M.N. Treatment strategies targeting amyloid β-protein. *Cold Spring Harb. Perspect. Med.* **2012**, *2*, a006387. [CrossRef]
18. Shi, M.; Caudle, W.M.; Zhang, J. Biomarker discovery in neurodegenerative diseases: A proteomic approach. *Neurobiol. Dis.* **2009**, *35*, 157–164. [CrossRef]
19. Kumar, G.P.; Khanum, F. Neuroprotective potential of phytochemicals. *Pharmacogn. Rev.* **2012**, *6*, 81–90. [CrossRef]
20. Fujiwara, H.; Tabuchi, M.; Yamaguchi, T.; Iwasaki, K.; Furukawa, K.; Sekiguchi, K.; Ikarashi, Y.; Kudo, Y.; Higuchi, M.; Saido, T.; et al. A traditional medicinal herb Paeonia suffruticosa and its active constituent 1,2,3,4,6-penta-O-galloyl-beta-D-glucopyranose have potent anti-aggregation effects on Alzheimer's amyloid beta proteins in vitro and in vivo. *J. Neurochem.* **2009**, *169*, 1648–1657. [CrossRef]
21. Ramesh, B.N.; Indi, S.S.; Rao, K.S. Anti-amyloidogenic property of leaf aqueous extract of Caesalpinia crista. *Neurosci. Lett.* **2010**, *475*, 110–114. [CrossRef] [PubMed]
22. Murillo, E.; Britton, G.B.; Durant, A.A. Antioxidant activity and polyphenol content in cultivated and wild edible fruits grown in Panama. *J. Pharm. Bioallied Sci.* **2012**, *4*, 313–317. [PubMed]
23. Obulesu, M.; Dowlathabad, M.R.; Bramhachari, P.V. Carotenoids and Alzheimer's disease: An insight into therapeutic role of retinoids in animal models. *Neurochem. Int.* **2011**, *59*, 535–541. [CrossRef] [PubMed]
24. Lakey-Beitia, J.; Gonzalez, Y.; Doens, D.; Stephens, D.E.; Santamaria, R.; Murillo, E.; Gutierrez, M.; Fernandez, P.L.; Rao, K.S.; Larionov, O.V.; et al. Assessment of Novel Curcumin Derivatives as Potent Inhibitors of Inflammation and Amyloid-Beta Aggregation in Alzheimer Disease. *J. Alzheimers Dis.* **2017**, *60*, S59–S68. [CrossRef] [PubMed]
25. Lakey-Beitia, J.; Doens, D.; Kumar, D.J.; Murillo, E.; Fernandez, P.L.; Rao, K.S.; Durant-Archibold, A.A. Anti-amyloid aggregation activity of novel carotenoids: Implications for Alzheimer's drug discovery. *Clin. Aging Interv.* **2017**, *12*, 815–822. [CrossRef]
26. Parker, R.S.; Swanson, J.E.; You, C.-S.; Edwards, A.J.; Huang, T. Bioavailability of carotenoids in human subjects. *Proc. Nutr. Soc.* **1999**, *58*, 155–162. [CrossRef]
27. Zern, T.L.; Fernandez, M.L. Cardioprotective Effects of Dietary Polyphenols. *J. Nutr.* **2005**, *135*, 2291–2294. [CrossRef]
28. Rivera Vélez, S.M. Guide for Carotenoid Identification in Biological Samples. *J. Nat. Prod.* **2016**, *79*, 1473–1484. [CrossRef]
29. Choi, S.K.; Osawa, A.; Maoka, T.; Hattan, J.I.; Ito, K.; Uchiyama, A.; Suzuki, M.; Shindo, K.; Misawa, N. 3-β-Glucosyl-3′-β-quinovosyl zeaxanthin, a novel carotenoid glycoside synthesized by Escherichia coli cells expressing the Pantoea ananatis carotenoid biosynthesis gene cluster. *Appl. Microbiol. Biotechnol.* **2013**, *97*, 8479–8486. [CrossRef]

30. Rao, A.V.; Rao, L.G. Carotenoids and human health. *Pharmacol. Res.* **2007**, *55*, 207–216. [CrossRef]
31. Polotow, T.G.; Poppe, S.C.; Vardaris, C.V.; Ganini, D.; Guariroba, M.; Mattei, R.; Hatanaka, E.; Martins, M.F.; Bondan, E.F.; Barros, M.P. Redox Status and Neuro Inflammation Indexes in Cerebellum and Motor Cortex of Wistar Rats Supplemented with Natural Sources of Omega-3 Fatty Acids and Astaxanthin: Fish Oil, Krill Oil, and Algal Biomass. *Mar. Drugs* **2015**, *13*, 6117–6137. [CrossRef] [PubMed]
32. Takaichi, S. Carotenoids in Algae: Distributions, Biosyntheses and Functions. *Mar. Drugs* **2011**, *9*, 1101–1118. [CrossRef] [PubMed]
33. Amorim-Carrilho, K.T.; Cepeda, A.; Fente, C.; Regal, P. Review of methods for analysis of carotenoids. *Trends Anal. Chem.* **2014**, *56*, 49–73. [CrossRef]
34. Cong, L.; Wang, C.; Chen, L.; Liu, H.; Yang, G.; He, G. Expression of phytoene synthase1 and Carotene Desaturase crtI Genes Result in an Increase in the Total Carotenoids Content in Transgenic Elite Wheat (Triticum aestivum L.). *J. Agric. Food Chem.* **2009**, *57*, 8652–8660. [CrossRef] [PubMed]
35. Bolhassani, A.; Khavari, A.; Bathaie, S.Z. Saffron and natural carotenoids: Biochemical activities and anti-tumor effects. *Biochim. Biophys. Acta* **2014**, *1845*, 20–30. [CrossRef] [PubMed]
36. Rodriguez-Concepcion, M.; Avalos, J.; Bonet, M.; Boronat, A.; Gomez-Gomez, L.; Hornero-Mendez, D.; Limon, M.; Meléndez-Martínez, A.; Olmedilla-Alonso, B.; Palou, A.; et al. A global perspective on carotenoids: Metabolism, biotechnology, and benefits for nutrition and health. *Prog. Lipid Res.* **2018**, *70*, 62–93. [CrossRef] [PubMed]
37. Failla, M.L.; Huo, T.; Thakkar, S.K. In vitro screening of relative bioaccessibility of carotenoids from foods. *Asia Pac. J. Clin. Nutr.* **2008**, *17*, 200–203. [PubMed]
38. Marin, E.; Nussaume, L.; Quesada, A.; Gonneau, M.; Sotta, B.; Hugueney, P.; Frey, A.; Marion-Poll, A. Molecular identification of zeaxanthin epoxidase of Nicotiana plumbaginifolia, a gene involved in abscisic acid biosynthesis and corresponding to the ABA locus of Arabidopsis thaliana. *EMBO J.* **1996**, *15*, 2331–2342. [CrossRef]
39. Háda, M.; Nagy, V.; Gulyás-Fekete, G.; Deli, J.; Agócs, A. Towards Carotenoid Dendrimers: Carotenoid Diesters and Triesters with Aromatic Cores. *Helv. Acta* **2010**, *93*, 1149–1155. [CrossRef]
40. Shaish, A.; Harari, A.; Kamari, Y.; Soudant, E.; Harats, D.; Ben-Amotz, A. A carotenoid algal preparation containing phytoene and phytofluene inhibited LDL oxidation in vitro. *Plant Foods Hum. Nutr.* **2008**, *63*, 83–86. [CrossRef]
41. Chisté, R.C.; Freitas, M.; Mercadante, A.Z.; Fernandes, E. Carotenoids inhibit lipid peroxidation and hemoglobin oxidation, but not the depletion of glutathione induced by ROS in human erythrocytes. *Life Sci.* **2014**, *99*, 52–60. [CrossRef] [PubMed]
42. Pérez-Gálvez, A.; Mínguez-Mosquera, M.I. Esterification of xanthophylls and its effect on chemical behavior and bioavailability of carotenoids in the human. *Nutr. Res.* **2005**, *25*, 631–640. [CrossRef]
43. Papandreou, M.A.; Kanakis, C.D.; Polissiou, M.G.; Efthimiopoulos, S.; Cordopatis, P.; Margarity, M.; Lamari, F.N. Inhibitory Activity on Amyloid-Beta Aggregation and Antioxidant Properties of Crocus sativus Stigmas Extract and Its Crocin Constituents. *J. Agric. Food Chem.* **2006**, *54*, 8762–8768. [CrossRef]
44. Firdous, A.P.; Preethi, K.C.; Kuttan, R. Antioxidant potential of meso-zeaxanthin a semi synthetic carotenoid. *Food Chem.* **2010**, *119*, 1096–1101. [CrossRef]
45. Sachdeva, A.K.; Chopra, K. Lycopene abrogates Aβ(1-42)-mediated neuroinflammatory cascade in an experimental model of Alzheimer's disease. *J. Nutr. Biochem.* **2015**, *26*, 736–744. [CrossRef]
46. Britton, G. Functions of Intact Carotenoids. In *Carotenoids*; Birkhäuser: Basel, Switzerland, 2008; Volume 4, pp. 189–212.
47. Kopsell, D.A.; Kopsell, D.E. Accumulation and bioavailability of dietary carotenoids in vegetable crops. *Trends Plant Sci.* **2006**, *11*, 499–507. [CrossRef]
48. Hirschberg, J. Carotenoid biosynthesis in flowering plants. *Curr. Opin. Plant Biol.* **2001**, *4*, 210–218. [CrossRef]
49. Chemler, J.A.; Yan, Y.; Koffas, M.A.G. Biosynthesis of isoprenoids, polyunsaturated fatty acids and flavonoids in Saccharomyces cerevisiae. *Microb. Cell Fact.* **2006**, *5*, 20. [CrossRef]
50. Werner, S.; Böhm, V. Bioaccessibility of carotenoids and vitamin e from pasta: Evaluation of an in vitro digestion model. *J. Agric. Food Chem.* **2011**, *59*, 1163–1170. [CrossRef]
51. Wolak, T.; Hamias, R.; Volvich, L.; Paran, E. Carotenoids and flavonoids synergistically attenuate inflammation in endothelial cells induced by TNF-α. *J. Am. Soc. Hypertens.* **2014**, *8*, e77. [CrossRef]
52. Britton, G. Structure and properties of carotenoids in relation to function. *FASEB J.* **1995**, *15*, 1551–1558. [CrossRef]

53. Britton, G.; Khachik, F. Carotenoids in Food. In *Carotenoids*; Birkhäuser: Basel, Switzerland, 2009; Volume 5, pp. 45–66.
54. Britton, G.; Liaaen-Jensen, S.; Pfander, H. Natural Functions. In *Carotenoids*; Birkhäuser: Basel, Switzerland, 2008; pp. 1–370.
55. Rodriguez-Amaya, D.B. *A Guide to carotenoid Analysis in Foods*; ILSI Press: Washington, DC, USA, 2001; pp. 1–64.
56. Katayama, S.; Ogawa, H.; Nakamura, S. Apricot carotenoids possess potent anti-amyloidogenic activity in vitro. *J. Agric. Food Chem.* **2011**, *59*, 12691–12696. [CrossRef] [PubMed]
57. Faulks, R.M.; Southon, S. Challenges to understanding and measuring carotenoid bioavailability. *Biochim. Biophys. Acta* **2005**, *1740*, 95–100. [CrossRef] [PubMed]
58. Vershinin, A. Biological functions of carotenoids-diversity and evolution. *Biofactors* **1999**, *10*, 99–104. [CrossRef] [PubMed]
59. Hornero-Méndez, D.; Gómez-Ladrón De Guevara, R.; Mínguez-Mosquera, M.I. Carotenoid biosynthesis changes in five red pepper (Capsicum annuum L.) cultivars during ripening. Cultivar selection for breeding. *J. Agric. Food Chem.* **2000**, *48*, 3857–3864. [CrossRef] [PubMed]
60. Maiani, G.; Castón, M.J.P.; Catasta, G.; Toti, E.; Cambrodón, I.G.; Bysted, A.; Granado-Lorencio, F.; Olmedilla-Alonso, B.; Knuthsen, P.; Valoti, M.; et al. Carotenoids: Actual knowledge on food sources, intakes, stability and bioavailability and their protective role in humans. *Mol. Nutr. Food Res.* **2009**, *53*, S194–218. [CrossRef]
61. Murillo, E.; Giuffrida, D.; Menchaca, D.; Dugo, P.; Torre, G.; Meléndez-Martinez, A.J.; Mondello, L. Native carotenoids composition of some tropical fruits. *Food Chem.* **2013**, *140*, 825–836. [CrossRef]
62. Che, H.; Li, Q.; Zhang, T.; Wang, D.; Yang, L.; Xu, J.; Yanagita, T.; Xue, C.; Chang, Y.; Wang, Y. The effects of astaxanthin and docosahexaenoic acid-acylated astaxanthin on Alzheimer's disease in APP/PS1 double transgenic mice. *J. Agric. Food Chem.* **2018**, *66*, 4948–4957. [CrossRef]
63. Moise, A.R.; Al-Babili, S.; Wurtzel, E.T. Mechanistic aspects of carotenoid biosynthesis. *Chem. Rev.* **2014**, *114*, 164–193. [CrossRef]
64. Kita, M.; Kato, M.; Ban, Y.; Honda, C.; Yaegaki, H.; Ikoma, Y.; Moriguchi, T. Carotenoid accumulation in Japanese apricot (Prunus mume Siebold & Zucc.): Molecular analysis of carotenogenic gene expression and ethylene regulation. *J. Agric. Food Chem.* **2007**, *55*, 3414–3420.
65. Gulyás-Fekete, G.; Murillo, E.; Kurtán, T.; Papp, T.; Illyés, T.-Z.; Drahos, L.; Visy, J.; Agócs, A.; Turcsi, E.; Deli, J. Cryptocapsinepoxide-type carotenoids from red mamey, Pouteria sapota. *J. Nat. Prod.* **2013**, *76*, 607–614. [CrossRef] [PubMed]
66. Scotter, M.J.; Wilson, L.A.; Appleton, G.P.; Castle, L. Analysis of Annatto (Bixa orellana) Food Coloring Formulations. Determination of Aromatic Hydrocarbon Thermal Degradation Products by Gas Chromatography. *J. Agric. Food Chem.* **2000**, *48*, 484–488. [CrossRef] [PubMed]
67. Murillo, E.; Nagy, V.; Agócs, A.; Deli, J. Carotenoids with κ -End Group. In *Carotenoids*; Nova Science Publishers: New York, NY, USA, 2013; pp. 1–78.
68. Gaweska, H.; Fitzpatrick, P.F. Structures and Mechanism of the Monoamine Oxidase Family. *Biomol. Concepts* **2011**, *2*, 365–377. [CrossRef]
69. Deli, J.; Molnár, P.; Matus, Z.; Tóth, G. Carotenoid composition in the fruits of red paprika (Capsicum annuum var. lycopersiciforme rubrum) during ripening; biosynthesis of carotenoids in Red Paprika. *J. Agric. Food Chem.* **2001**, *49*, 1517–1523. [CrossRef]
70. Wallar, B.J.; Lipscomb, J.D. Dioxygen Activation by Enzymes Containing Binuclear Non-Heme Iron Clusters. *Chem. Rev.* **1996**, *96*, 612–625. [CrossRef]
71. Baik, M.; Newcomb, M.; Friesner, R.A.; Lippard, S.J. Mechanistic Studies on the Hydroxylation of Methane by Methane Monooxygenase. *Chem. Rev.* **2003**, *103*, 2385–2419. [CrossRef]
72. Yun, D.; Garcia-Serres, R.; Chicalese, B.M.; An, Y.H.; Huynh, B.H.; Bollinger, J.M. (μ-1,2-Peroxo)diiron(III/III) Complex as a Precursor to the Diiron (III/IV) Intermediate X in the Assembly of the Iron-radical Cofactor of Ribonucleotide Reductase from Mouse. *Biochemistry* **2007**, *46*, 1925–1932. [CrossRef]
73. Demming-Adams, B.; Adams, W.W., III. The role of xanthophyll cycle carotenoids in the protection of photosynthesis. *Trends Plant Sci.* **1996** *1*, 21–26. [CrossRef]
74. Háda, M.; Petrovics, D.; Nagy, V.; Böddi, K.; Deli, J.; Agócs, A. The first synthesis of PEG–carotenoid conjugates. *Tetrahedron Lett.* **2011**, *52*, 3195–3197. [CrossRef]

75. Háda, M.; Nagy, V.; Deli, J.; Agócs, A. Hydrophilic carotenoids: Recent progress. *Molecules* **2012**, *17*, 5003–5012. [CrossRef]
76. Deli, J.; Ősz, E.; Molnár, P.; Zsila, F.; Simonyi, M.; Tóth, G. Reduction of Capsorubin and Cryptocapsin. *Helv. Chim. Acta* **2001**, *84*, 3810–3817. [CrossRef]
77. Turcsi, E.; Murillo, E.; Kurtán, T.; Szappanos, Á.; Illyés, T.-Z.; Gulyás-Fekete, G.; Agócs, A.; Avar, P.; Deli, J. Isolation of β-Cryptoxanthin-epoxides, Precursors of Cryptocapsin and 3′-Deoxycapsanthin, from Red Mamey (Pouteria sapota). *J. Agric. Food Chem.* **2015**, *63*, 6059–6065. [CrossRef] [PubMed]
78. Molnar, P.; Deli, J.; Matma, Z.; Totha, G.; Steckb, A.; Pfanderb, H. Partial Synthesis and Characterization of the Mono-and Diepoxides of p-Cryptoxanthin. *Helv. Chim. Acta* **1997**, *80*, 221–229. [CrossRef]
79. Cardounel, A.J.; Dumitrescu, C.; Zweier, J.L.; Lockwood, S.F. Direct superoxide anion scavenging by a disodium disuccinate astaxanthin derivative: Relative efficacy of individual stereoisomers versus the statistical mixture of stereoisomers by electron paramagnetic resonance imaging. *Biochem. Biophys. Res. Commun.* **2003**, *307*, 704–712. [CrossRef]
80. Frey, D.A.; Kataisto, E.W.; Ekmanis, J.L.; O'Malley, S.; Lockwood, S.F. The Efficient Synthesis of Disodium Disuccinate Astaxanthin (Cardax). *Org. Process Res. Dev.* **2004**, *8*, 796–801. [CrossRef]
81. Háda, M.; Nagy, V.; Takátsy, A.; Deli, J.; Agócs, A. Dicarotenoid esters of bivalent acids. *Tetrahedron Lett.* **2008**, *49*, 3524–3526. [CrossRef]
82. Nadolski, G.; Cardounel, A.J.; Zweier, L.; Lockwood, S.F. The synthesis and aqueous superoxide anion scavenging of water-dispersible lutein esters. *Bioorg. Med. Chem. Lett.* **2006**, *16*, 775–781. [CrossRef]
83. Jackson, H.L.; Cardounel, A.J.; Zweier, L.; Lockwood, S.F. Synthesis, characterization, and direct aqueous superoxide anion scavenging of a highly water-dispersible astaxanthin-amino acid conjugate. *Bioorg. Med. Chem. Lett.* **2004**, *14*, 3985–3991. [CrossRef]
84. Yamano, Y.; Sakai, Y.; Hara, M.; Ito, M. Carotenoids and related polyenes. Part 9. 1 Total synthesis of thermozeaxanthin and thermocryptoxanthin and the stabilizing effect of thermozeaxanthin on liposomes. *J. Chem. Soc. Perkin Trans. 1* **2013**, *2*, 2006–2013.
85. Neises, V.B.; Steglich, W. Einfaches Verfahren zur Veresterung von Carbonsäuren. *Angew. Chem.* **1978**, *90*, 556–557. [CrossRef]
86. Shi, W.; Dolai, S.; Rizk, S.; Hussain, A.; Tariq, H.; Averick, S.; L'Amoreaux, W.; El Ldrissi, A.; Banerjee, P.; Raja, K. Synthesis of monofunctional curcumin derivatives, clicked curcumin dimer, and a PAMAM dendrimer curcumin conjugate for therapeutic applications. *Org. Lett.* **2007**, *9*, 5461–5464. [CrossRef] [PubMed]
87. Convertino, M.; Pellarin, R.; Catto, M.; Carotti, A.; Caflisch, A. 9,10-Anthraquinone hinders beta β-aggregation: How does a small molecule interfere with Aβ-peptide amyloid fibrillation? *Protein Sci.* **2009**, *18*, 792–800. [PubMed]
88. Shih, P.H.; Wu, C.H.; Yeh, C.T.; Yen, G.C. Protective effects of anthocyanins against amyloid β-peptide-induced damage in neuro-2A cells. *J. Agric. Food Chem.* **2011**, *59*, 1683–1689. [CrossRef] [PubMed]
89. Esler, W.P.; Wolfe, M.S. A portrait of Alzheimer secretases-new features and familiar faces. *Science* **2001**, *293*, 1449–1454. [CrossRef]
90. Zhou, Y.; Suram, A.; Venugopal, C.; Prakasam, A.; Lin, S.; Su, Y.; Li, B.; Paul, S.M.; Sambamurti, K. Geranylgeranyl pyrophosphate stimulates gamma-secretase to increase the generation of Abeta and APP-CTFgamma. *FASEB J.* **2008**, *22*, 47–54. [CrossRef]
91. Hamley, I.W. The amyloid beta peptide: A chemist's perspective. Role in Alzheimer's and fibrillization. *Chem. Rev.* **2012**, *112*, 5147–5192. [CrossRef]
92. Venugopal, C.; Demos, C.M.; Rao, K.S.; Pappolla, M.A. Beta-secretase: Structure, function, and evolution. *CNS Neurol. Disord. Drug Targets* **2008**, *7*, 278–294. [CrossRef]
93. Rajendran, L.; Schneider, A.; Schlechtingen, G.; Weidlich, S.; Ries, J.; Braxmeier, T.; Schwille, P.; Schulz, J.B.; Schroeder, C.; Simons, M.; et al. Efficient inhibition of the Alzheimer's disease β-secretase by membrane targeting. *Science* **2008**, *320*, 520–523. [CrossRef]
94. Wang, J.; Li, L.; Wang, Z.; Cui, Y.; Tan, X.; Yuan, T.; Liu, Q.; Liu, Z.; Liu, X. Supplementation of lycopene attenuates lipopolysaccharide-induced amyloidogenesis and cognitive impairments via mediating neuroinflammation and oxidative stress. *J. Nutr. Biochem.* **2018**, *56*, 16–25. [CrossRef]
95. Reboul, E.; Borel, P.; Abou, L.; Charbonnier, M.; Caris-Veyrat, C.; Goupy, P.; Lairon, D. Human Nutrition and Metabolism Enrichment of Tomato Paste with 6% Tomato Peel Increases Lycopene and Beta-Carotene Bioavailability in Men. *J. Nutr.* **2005** *135*, 790–794. [CrossRef]

96. Cho, K.S.; Shin, M.; Kim, S.; Lee, S.B. Recent Advances in Studies on the Therapeutic Potential of Dietary Carotenoids in Neurodegenerative Diseases. *Oxid. Med. Cell. Longev.* **2018**, *2018*, 4120458. [CrossRef] [PubMed]
97. Ghahghaei, A.; Bathaie, S.Z.; Kheirkhah, H.; Bahraminejad, E. The protective effect of crocin on the amyloid fibril formation of Aβ42 peptide in vitro. *Cell. Mol. Biol. Lett.* **2013**, *18*, 328–339. [CrossRef] [PubMed]
98. Lee, D.-H.; Lee, Y.J.; Kwon, K.H. Neuroprotective Effects of Astaxanthin in Oxygen-Glucose Deprivation in SH-SY5Y Cells and Global Cerebral Ischemia in Rat. *J. Clin. Biochem. Nutr.* **2010**, *47*, 121–129. [CrossRef] [PubMed]
99. Zhang, Y.; Wu, H.; Wen, H.; Fang, H.; Hong, Z.; Yi, R.; Liu, R. Simultaneous Determination of Fucoxanthin and Its Deacetylated Metabolite Fucoxanthinol in Rat Plasma by Liquid Chromatography-Tandem Mass Spectrometry. *Mar. Drugs* **2015**, *13*, 6521–6536. [CrossRef] [PubMed]
100. Xiang, S.; Liu, F.; Lin, J.; Chen, H.; Huang, C.; Chen, L.; Zhou, Y.; Ye, L.; Zhang, K.; Jin, J.; et al. Fucoxanthin Inhibits β-Amyloid Assembly and Attenuates β-Amyloid Oligomer-Induced Cognitive Impairments. *J. Agric. Food Chem.* **2017**, *65*, 4092–4102. [CrossRef]
101. Jung, H.; Ali, M.; Choi, R.; Jeong, H.; Chung, H.; Choi, J. Kinetics and molecular docking studies of fucosterol and fucoxanthin, BACE1 inhibitors from brown algae Undaria pinnatifida and Ecklonia stolonifera. *Food Chem. Toxicol.* **2016**, *89*, 104–111. [CrossRef]
102. Murillo, E.; Mclean, R.; Britton, G.; Agócs, A.; Nagy, V.; Deli, J. Sapotexanthin, an A-Provitamin Carotenoid from Red Mamey (Pouteria sapota). *J. Nat. Prod.* **2011**, *74*, 283–285. [CrossRef]
103. Chacón-Ordóñez, T.; Esquivel, P.; Jiménez, V.M.; Carle, R.; Schweiggert, R.M. Deposition Form and Bioaccessibility of Keto-carotenoids from Mamey Sapote (Pouteria sapota), Red Bell Pepper (Capsicum annuum), and Sockeye Salmon (Oncorhynchus nerka) Filet. *J. Agric. Food Chem.* **2016**, *64*, 1989–1998. [CrossRef]
104. Miyake, S.; Kobayashi, S.; Tsubota, K.; Ozawa, Y. Phase II enzyme induction by a carotenoid, lutein, in a PC12D neuronal cell line. *Biochem. Biophys. Res. Commun.* **2014**, *446*, 535–540. [CrossRef]
105. Nishino, A.; Yasui, H.; Maoka, T. Reaction of Paprika Carotenoids, Capsanthin and Capsorubin, with Reactive Oxygen Species. *J. Agric. Food Chem.* **2016**, *64*, 4786–4792. [CrossRef]
106. Nakagawa, K.; Kiko, T.; Miyazawa, T.; Sookwong, P.; Tsuduki, T.; Satoh, A.; Miyazawa, T. Amyloid β-induced erythrocytic damage and its attenuation by carotenoids. *FEBS Lett.* **2011**, *585*, 1249–1254. [CrossRef] [PubMed]
107. Maksimov, G.V.; Volkov, V.V.; Parshina, E.Y.; Akhalaia, M.I.; Kozlova, O.V.; Derinskaya, E.V.; Revin, V.V.; Rubin, A.B. Investigation of carotenoid conformations in myelin nerve upon changes in oxygen content. *Biochem. Biophys. Mol. Biol.* **2007**, *417*, 324–326. [CrossRef] [PubMed]
108. Kim, S.; Thiessen, P.; Bolton, E.; Chen, J.; Fu, G.; Gindulyte, A.; Han, L.; He, J.; He, S.; Shoemaker, B.; et al. PubChem Substance and Compound databases. *Nucleic Acids Res.* **2016**, *44*, D1202–D1213. [CrossRef]
109. Berman, H.; Westbrook, J.; Feng, Z.; Gilliland, G.; Bhat, T.; Weissig, H.; Shindyalov, I.; Bourne, P. The Protein Data Bank. *Nucleic Acids Res.* **2000**, *28*, 235–242. [CrossRef]
110. Momany, F.A.; Rone, R. Validation of the general purpose QUANTA® 3.2/CHARMm® force field. *J. Comput. Chem.* **1992**, *13*, 888–900. [CrossRef]
111. Tjernberg, L.O.; Na, J.; Lindqvist, F.; Johansson, J.; Karlstro, A.R.; Thyberg, J. Arrest of Beta-Amyloid Fibril Formation by a Pentapeptide Ligand. *J. Biol. Chem.* **1996**, *271*, 8545–8548. [CrossRef]
112. Kumar, J.; Namsechi, R.; Sim, V.L. Structure-Based Peptide Design to Modulate Amyloid Beta Aggregation and Reduce Cytotoxicity. *PLoS ONE* **2015**, *12*, e0129087. [CrossRef]
113. Hetényi, C.; Körtvélyesi, T.; Penke, B. Mapping of Possible Binding Sequences of Two Beta-Sheet Breaker Peptides on Beta Amyloid Peptide of Alzheimer's Disease. *Bioorg. Med. Chem.* **2002**, *10*, 1587–1593. [CrossRef]
114. Kepp, K.P. Alzheimer's disease: How metal ions define β-amyloid function. *Coord. Chem. Rev.* **2017**, *351*, 127–159. [CrossRef]
115. Azqueta, A.; Collins, A.R. Carotenoids and DNA damage. *Mutat. Res. Mol. Mech. Mutagen.* **2012**, *733*, 4–13. [CrossRef]
116. Torbergsen, A.C.; Collins, A.R. Recovery of human lymphocytes from oxidative DNA damage; the apparent enhancement of DNA repair by carotenoids is probably simply an antioxidant effect. *Eur. J. Nutr.* **2000**, *39*, 80–85. [CrossRef] [PubMed]

117. Zhao, X.; Aldini, G.; Johnson, E.J.; Rasmussen, H.; Kraemer, K.; Woolf, H.; Musaeus, N.; Krinsky, N.I.; Russell, R.M.; Yeum, K. Modification of lymphocyte DNA damage by carotenoid supplementation in postmenopausal women 1-4. *Am. J. Clin. Nutr.* **2018**, *83*, 163–169. [CrossRef] [PubMed]
118. Serpeloni, J.M.; Mazzaron, G.; Friedmann, J.; Zerlotti, A.; Lourdes, M.; Bianchi, P.; Pires, M.; Greggi, L. Dietary carotenoid lutein protects against DNA damage and alterations of the redox status induced by cisplatin in human derived HepG2 cells. *Toxicol. In Vitro* **2012**, *26*, 288–294. [CrossRef] [PubMed]
119. Santocono, M.; Zurria, M.; Berrettini, M.; Fedeli, D.; Falcioni, G. Influence of astaxanthin, zeaxanthin and lutein on DNA damage and repair in UVA-irradiated cells. *J. Photochem. Photobiol. B Biol.* **2006**, *85*, 205–215. [CrossRef]

3

Chlorella sorokiniana Extract Improves Short-Term Memory in Rats

Maria Grazia Morgese [1], Emanuela Mhillaj [2], Matteo Francavilla [3,4], Maria Bove [2], Lucia Morgano [1], Paolo Tucci [1], Luigia Trabace [1,*,†] and Stefania Schiavone [1,†]

Department of Clinical and Experimental Medicine, University of Foggia, Foggia 71121, Italy;
mariagrazia.morgese@unifg.it (M.G.M.); luciamorgano@alice.it (L.M.); paolo.tucci@unifg.it (P.T.);
2 stefania.schiavone@unifg.it (S.S.)
Department of Physiology and Pharmacology, "Sapienza" University of Rome, Rome 00185, Italy;
3 emanuela.mhillaj@uniroma1.it (E.M.); maria.bove@uniroma1.it (M.B.)
STAR Agroenergy Research Group, University of Foggia, Via Gramsci, 89-91, Foggia 71121, Italy;
4 matteo.francavilla@unifg.it
* Institute of Marine Science, National Research Council, via Pola 4, Lesina 71010, Italy
Correspondence: luigia.trabace@unifg.it
† These authors contributed equally to this work.

Academic Editor: Derek J. McPhee

Abstract: Increasing evidence shows that eukaryotic microalgae and, in particular, the green microalga *Chlorella*, can be used as natural sources to obtain a whole variety of compounds, such as omega (ω)-3 and ω-6 polyunsatured fatty acids (PUFAs). Although either beneficial or toxic effects of *Chlorella sorokiniana* have been mainly attributed to its specific ω-3 and ω-6 PUFAs content, the underlying molecular pathways remain to be elucidated yet. Here, we investigate the effects of an acute oral administration of a lipid extract of *Chlorella sorokiniana*, containing mainly ω-3 and ω-6 PUFAs, on cognitive, emotional and social behaviour in rats, analysing possible underlying neurochemical alterations. Our results showed improved short-term memory in *Chlorella sorokiniana*-treated rats compared to controls, without any differences in exploratory performance, locomotor activity, anxiety profile and depressive-like behaviour. On the other hand, while the social behaviour of *Chlorella sorokiniana*-treated animals was significantly decreased, no effects on aggressivity were observed. Neurochemical investigations showed region-specific effects, consisting in an elevation of noradrenaline (NA) and serotonin (5-HT) content in hippocampus, but not in the prefrontal cortex and striatum. In conclusion, our results point towards a beneficial effect of *Chlorella sorokiniana* extract on short-term memory, but also highlight the need of caution in the use of this natural supplement due to its possible masked toxic effects.

Keywords: *Chlorella sorokiniana*; short-term memory; emotional behaviour; serotonin; noradrenaline; hippocampus

1. Introduction

Increasing evidence shows that algae, and in particular eukaryotic microalgae, can be used as natural sources to obtain a number of food and non-food products [1,2]. Moreover, because of the high cost of microalgae production technology, academia and industry are looking for new applications of algae extracts/products that could contribute to increase the economic value of biomass with a "biorefinery" approach [3]. Within the food science and nutrition field, the identification and characterization of new bioactive compounds, which are able to confer additional health benefits beyond the basic nutritional and energetic requirements in order to maintain and promote consumers' health and prevent chronic diseases is, at present, a hot-topic [2]. Considering the tremendous market value of the functional food industry, valued in 168 billion dollars just in the US in 2010 [4], it is easy to understand the enormous interest in the identification of new compounds, extracts and products that, once their efficacy has been proved with scientific evidence, can be produced at a larger scale. Among them, there is a whole variety of compounds, such as polyunsatured fatty acids (PUFAs), which are widely known to exert pharmacological or nutraceutical effects [5]. In particular, the PUFA composition in many species of the green microalga *Chlorella*, belonging to the phylum *Chlorophyta*, has been well characterized and the correlations between cultivation, conditions and percentages of fatty acids have been the focus of many studies [6]. Among all the *Chlorella* strains, the *Chlorella sorokiniana* has been shown to be the most suitable one to extract omega (ω)-3 and ω-6 PUFAs, mainly by biorefinery-based production methods [7–9]. Together with their beneficial effects against cardiovascular system disorders and their protective actions on uncontrolled cellular proliferation, ω-3 PUFAs have been demonstrated to be important physiological components of total brain lipid amount and to play a crucial role in several neurological functions, such as neurogenesis, neurotransmission and protection against oxidative stress-induced cerebral damage [10,11]. Further on, they are precursors of molecules involved in the modulation of cerebral immune and inflammatory processes [12,13]. Reduced dietary ω-3 PUFAs content has been shown to be associated with impaired cognitive and behavioural performance [14] and correlated to the development of depressive and anxiety-like symptoms [15]. In this context, we have recently demonstrated that lifelong nutritional ω-3 PUFAs deficiency evokes depressive-like state through soluble β amyloid (βA) involvement in rats [16]. Accordingly, ω-3 PUFAs have been also demonstrated to have important neuroprotective effects in both rodent models of neurodegenerative diseases [17,18] and human clinical investigations [19,20]. On the other hand, the role of ω-6 PUFA in brain maturation and development is much less studied. It is known that the main ω-6 derivative, arachidonic acid (AA), crucially contributes to several physiological functions, acting both as an important precursor of bioactive mediators and as an activator of protein kinases and ion channels involved in the processes of synaptic transmission [21]. Recently, the involvement of a ω-6 PUFA-enriched diet in enhancing plasma levels of βA has been reported in rodents [16]. In addition, a high ω-6/ω-3 ratio appears to be particularly unfavorable for proper central nervous system functioning [22]. Importantly, *Chlorella sorokiniana* is marketed in the US as a dietary supplement for weight control and protection against cancer, oxidative-stress and age-dependent cognitive impairment, as well as metabolic and cardiovascular diseases [23]. On the other hand, some recent reports have shown side toxic effects following dietary supplementation with *Chlorella sorokiniana*, such as gastrointestinal disorders, allergic reactions and increased skin sensitivity to the sun, elevation in plasma levels of uric acid and, more rarely, tubulointerstitial nephritis and psychotic symptoms development [24–26]. Although both the beneficial or toxic effects of *Chlorella sorokiniana* have been attributed to its specific ω-3 and ω-6 PUFAs content [23], the underlying molecular pathways remain to be elucidated yet. The aim of the present study was to investigate the effects of an acute oral administration of a lipid extract, containing mainly ω-3 and ω-6 PUFAs, obtained from monoxenic strain of *Chlorella sorokiniana* on the cognitive, emotional and social behaviour in rats and to identify the possible underlying neurochemical alterations. By using a double experimental approach (extraction and chemical characterization of the total lipid component on one hand and analysis of its activity on behaviour and neurochemistry on the other hand), we demonstrated specific behavioural effects of *Chlorella sorokiniana* lipid extract in rats, together with a specific brain region neuromodulatory activity.

2. Results

2.1. Chemical Characterization of Chlorella Sorokiniana Extract

The algal biomass showed a total lipids (TL) content of 21% dry weight (d.w.), which was composed mainly by fatty acids (42% d.w.) and unsaponified fraction (UF) (19% d.w.). The remaining 39% d.w. was composed by water-soluble compounds including short polypeptides, glycerol, monomeric sugars and salts. The bioactivity of the TL fraction was characterized in terms of chemical composition of its two main components: unsaturated fatty acids (UFs, Table 1) and fatty acid methyl esters (FAMEs, Table 2).

The most abundant UF compounds were 3,7,11,15-tetramethyl-2-hexadecen-1-ol and ergosterol. As shown in Table 2, FAMEs belonging to the C_{16} and C_{18} carbon chain groups were the most abundant, and accounted for 92% of the total FAMEs detected, according to previously reported results [27,28]. Among them, PUFAs showed a concentration of 286.7 mg·g^{-1} TL, while monounsaturated (MUFA) and saturated (SFA) fatty acids were found in lower concentrations. PUFAs were composed by ω-3 (169.5 mg·g^{-1} TL) and ω-6 (114.6 mg·g^{-1} TL) fatty acids in a ratio of 1 to 1.5 (ω-3 to ω-6). α-Linolenic acid and (Z,Z,Z)-7,10,13-hexadecatrienoic acid were the predominant ω-3 fatty acids, while linoleic acid and (Z,Z)-7,10-hexadecadienoic acid were the most abundant ω-6 fatty acids.

Table 1. UFs of the TL fraction extracted from *Chlorella sorokiniana*.

Compound	UF (mg·g^{-1} TL)
10-Heneicosene (c,t)	
2-Dexyl-1-decanol	3.24
3,7,11,15-Tetramethyl-2-hexadecen-1-ol acetate (isomer)	0.43
3,7,11,15-Tetramethyl-2-hexadecen-1-ol acetate (isomer)	0.22
3,7,11,15-Tetramethyl-2-hexadecen-1-ol acetate (isomer)	0.32
3,7,11,15-Tetramethyl-2-hexadecen-1-ol	64.26
Squalene	1.23
Not Identified	8.55
α-Tocopherol	2.72
(22*E*)-Ergosta-5,7,9(11),22-tetraen-3-ol	6.23
(3β,22*E*)-Ergosta-5,8,22-trien-3-ol	9.16
Ergosterol	43.36
(3β)-Ergosta-5,8-dien-3-ol	7.12
(3β,5α)-Ergost-7-en-3-ol	21.56

Table 2. FAMEs of the TL fraction extracted from *Chlorella sorokiniana*.

Compound	FAMEs (mg·g^{-1} TL)
Omega 3	169.53
(Z,Z,Z)-7,10,13-Hexadecatrienoic acid methyl ester	69.24
α-Linolenic acid methyl ester	100.29
Omega 6	116.66
(Z,Z)-7,10-Hexadecadienoic acid methyl ester	35.56
(Z,Z)-9,12-Heptadecadienoic acid methyl ester	2.06
Linoleic acid methyl ester	79.04
Saturated	58.60
Dodecanoic acid methyl ester	0.02
Tridecanoic acid methyl ester	0.02
Tetradecanoic acid methyl ester	1.27
Methyl 13-methyltetradecanoate	0.35
Pentadecanoic acid methyl ester	0.60
Hexadecanoic acid methyl ester	43.88
15-Methylhexadecanoic acid methyl ester	1.68
Heptadecanoic acid methyl ester	1.84
Methyl stearate	6.17
Eicosanoic acid methyl ester	1.53
Heneicosanoic acid methyl ester	0.16
Docosanoic acid methyl ester	0.36
Tricosanoic acid methyl ester	0.07
Tetracosanoic acid methyl ester	0.15
Pentacosanoic acid methyl ester	0.12
Hexacosanoic acid methyl ester	0.38
Monounsaturated	54.29

Table 2. *Cont.*

Compound	FAMEs ($mg \cdot g^{-1}$ TL)
Methyl myristoleate	0.25
cis-7-Tetradecenoic acid methyl ester	0.72
(Z-13-Methyltetradec-9-enoic acid methyl ester	0.37
Methyl palmitoleate	20.50
(Z)-7-Hexadecenoic acid methyl ester	2.03
(*E*)-9-Hexadecenoic acid methyl ester	2.88
(Z)-9-Heptadecenoic acid methyl ester	2.95
Oleic acid methyl ester	24.47
Methyl 9-eicosenoate	0.13

2.2. Effects of Acute Oral Administration of Chlorella Extract on Cognition and Short-Term Memory

The effects of an acute *Chlorella sorokiniana* administration on cognition and short-term memory were assessed by performing the Novel Object Recognition (NOR) test. Results showed that the discrimination index was significantly increased in *Chlorella sorokiniana*-treated rats compared to controls (Figure 1a, unpaired t-test; $p < 0.05$). Moreover, both *Chlorella sorokiniana*- and vehicle-treated rats exhibited the same exploratory performances in the NOR test, with a significant difference in total time spent exploring the new object rather than the familiar one (Figure 1b, Two-way ANOVA; $F_{(1,28)} = 37.33$, $p < 0.0001$, followed by Bonferroni's multiple comparisons test; familiar vs. novel object; $p < 0.001$ and $p < 0.01$ for *Chlorella sorokiniana* extract and vehicle, respectively).

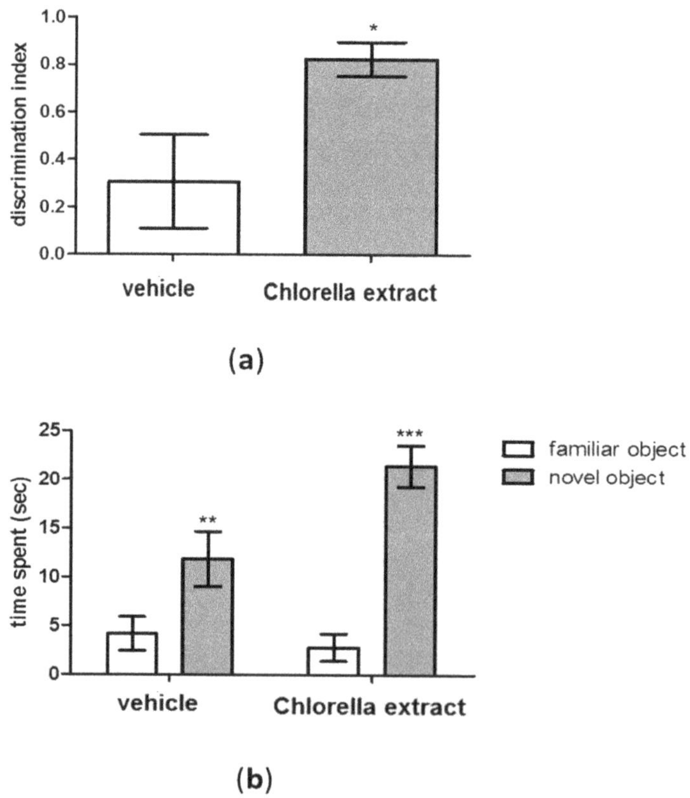

Figure 1. The NOR test in male Wistar rats after *Chlorella sorokiniana* extract or vehicle administration. (**a**) discrimination index and (**b**) time spent in the NOR test of male Wistar rats after *Chlorella sorokiniana* extract (Chlorella extract, 30 mg/kg/mL dark bar) or vehicle (sunflower oil 1 mL/kg, empty bar) administration. Data are expressed as mean ± SEM (n = 8 per group); (**a**) t-test * $p < 0.05$ vs. vehicle-treated rats; (**b**) Two-way ANOVA followed by Bonferroni's multiple comparisons test. ** $p < 0.01$ vs. familiar object and *** $p < 0.001$ vs. familiar object for vehicle- and for *Chlorella sorokiniana*-treated rats, respectively.

2.3. Effects of Acute Oral Administration of Chlorella Sorokiniana Extract on Locomotion

As shown in Figure 2a,b, there were no significant differences in the number of entries into closed and open arms between *Chlorella sorokiniana*- and vehicle-treated rats in the Elevated Plus Maze (EPM) test (unpaired *t*-test; n.s.). Moreover, as reported in Figure 2c, no statistical differences were found in total exploration time in the NOR test between *Chlorella sorokiniana*- and vehicle-treated rats (unpaired *t*-test; n.s.). Since this lack of effect on locomotion could have been induced by a muscle damage, and since the appearance of creatine-kinase M-type (CKM) in blood has been generally considered to be a marker of skeletal muscle damage, we measured plasma CKM concentrations in *Chlorella sorokiniana*- and vehicle-treated rats. Results showed no difference between experimental groups (unpaired *t*-test; n.s.; Figure 2d), thus confirming that *Chlorella sorokiniana* administration did not affect locomotor activity, at least under our experimental conditions.

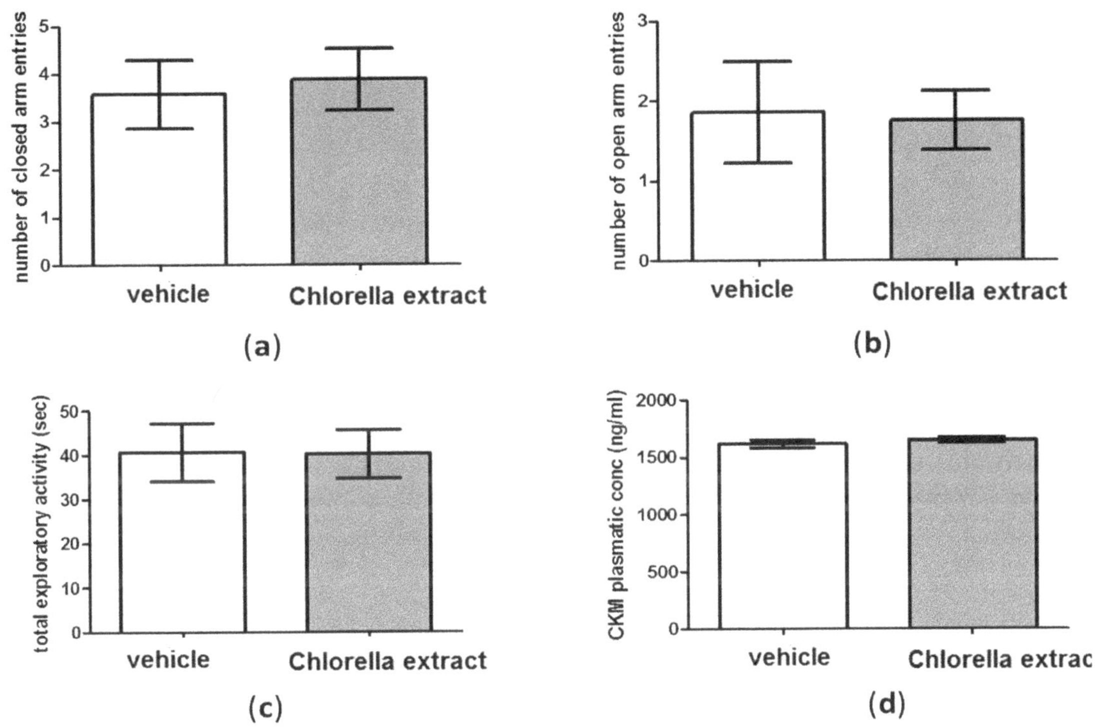

Figure 2. Evaluation of locomotion parameters in male Wistar rats after *Chlorella sorokiniana* extract or vehicle administration. (**a**) Number of closed arms entries and (**b**) number of open arms entries in the elevated plus-maze test; (**c**) total exploratory activity in the novel object recognition test; (**d**) plasma CKM concentrations Wistar rats after *Chlorella sorokiniana* extract (Chlorella extract, 30 mg/kg/mL dark bar) or vehicle (sunflower oil 1 mL/kg, empty bar) administration. Data are expressed as mean ± SEM (n = 8 per group).

2.4. Effects of Acute Oral Administration of Chlorella sorokiniana Extract on Emotional Profile

We did not detect changes in anxiety- and depressive-like behaviour between *Chlorella sorokiniana*- and vehicle-treated groups in EPM and Forced Swimming Test (FST). Indeed, as shown in Figure 3a–d, no significant differences were found in the time spent into open and closed arms and in the entries frequency into open and closed arms (unpaired *t*-test; n.s.) between experimental groups in the EPM test. Likewise, no differences in the immobility, swimming and struggling frequency in *Chlorella sorokiniana*-treated rats, compared to controls, were reported in the FST (Figure 3e,g unpaired *t*-test; n.s.).

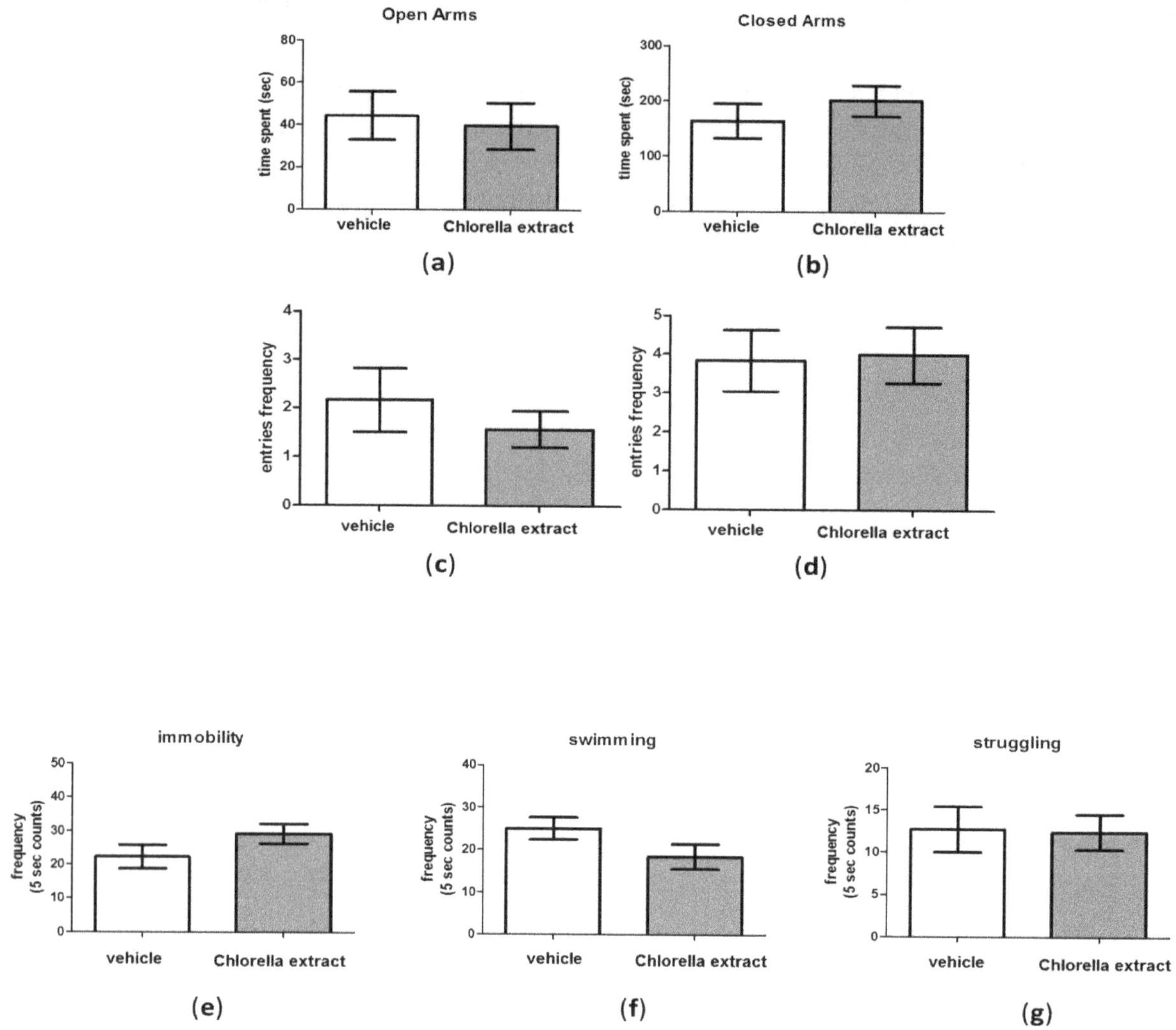

Figure 3. The forced swimming test and elevated plus maze test in male Wistar rats after *Chlorella sorokiniana* extract or vehicle administration. (**a**) Amount of time spent in open and (**b**) closed arms, (**c**) the entries frequency into open and (**d**) closed arms in the EPM test; (**e**) Immobility; (**f**) swimming and (**g**) struggling frequency in the FST. Male Wistar rats were treated with *Chlorella sorokiniana* extract (Chlorella extract, 30 mg/kg/mL dark bar) or vehicle (sunflower oil 1 mL/kg, empty bar) administration. Data are expressed as mean ± SEM ($n = 8$ per group).

2.5. Effects of Acute Oral Administration of Chlorella sorokiniana Extract on Central Monoamine Content

In order to corroborate behavioural results with neurochemical data, we measured serotonin (5-HT) and noradrenaline (NA) content in hippocampus (HIPP), prefrontal cortex (PFC) and striatum (STR) of *Chlorella sorokiniana*- and vehicle-treated animals. Hippocampal 5-HT content was significantly increased in *Chlorella sorokiniana*-treated rats compared to controls animals (Figure 4b, unpaired *t*-test; $p < 0.05$). Similarly, we found that hippocampal NA concentrations were significantly higher in animals that received *Chlorella sorokiniana* administration compared to controls (Figure 4a, unpaired *t*-test; $p < 0.05$). On the other hand, no differences between *Chlorella sorokiniana*- and vehicle-treated animals were found in PFC and STR with respect to NA and 5-HT contents (Figure 4c–e, unpaired *t*-test; n.s.).

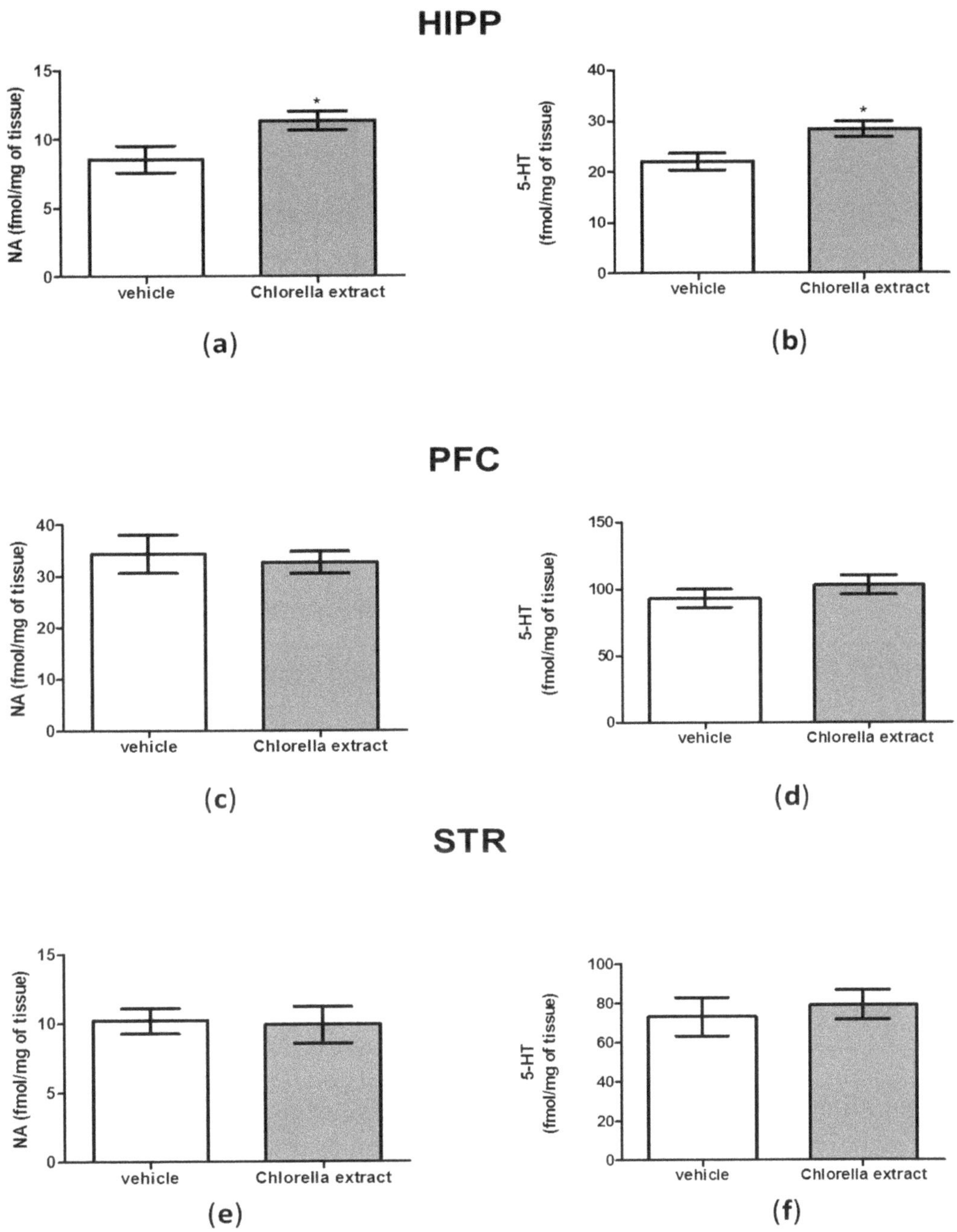

Figure 4. Monoamine quantification in male Wistar rats after *Chlorella sorokiniana* extract or vehicle administration. NA and 5-HT levels in HIPP (**a** and **b**); PFC (**c** and **d**); STR (**e** and **f**) of male Wistar rats after *Chlorella sorokiniana* extract (Chlorella extract, 30 mg/kg/mL dark bar) or vehicle (sunflower oil 1 mL/kg, empty bar) administration. Data are expressed as mean ± SEM ($n = 8$ per group); (**a**) *t*-test * $p < 0.05$ vs. vehicle-treated rats and (**b**) *t*-test * $p < 0.05$ vs. vehicle-treated rats.

2.6. Effects of Acute Oral Administration of Chlorella sorokiniana Exctract on Social Behaviour

Results showed that social behaviour was significantly decreased in *Chlorella sorokiniana*-treated animals with respect to controls (Figure 5a, unpaired *t*-test; $p < 0,05$), while no differences were found in aggressive behaviour between *Chlorella sorokiniana*- and vehicle-treated rats (Figure 5b, unpaired *t*-test; n.s.).

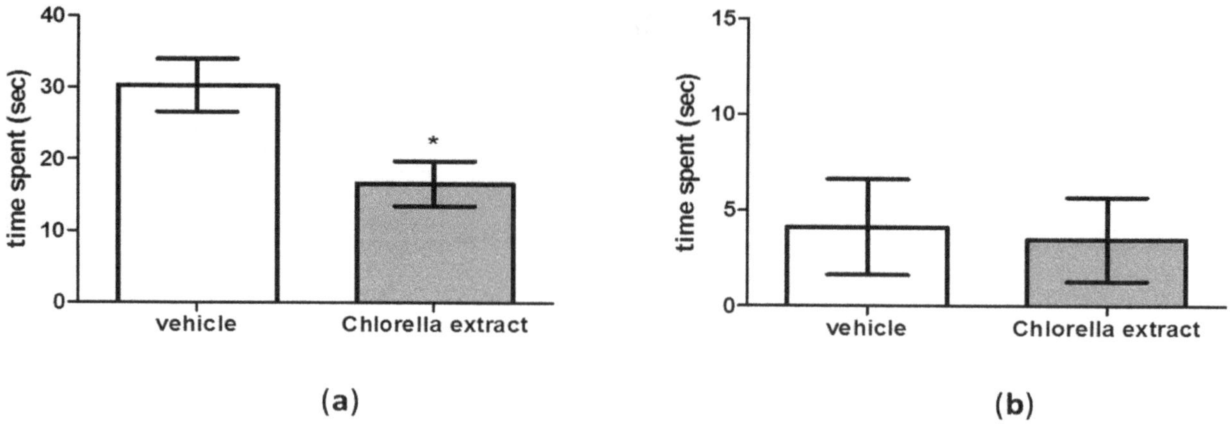

Figure 5. The social interaction test in male Wistar rats after *Chlorella sorokiniana* extract or vehicle administration. (**a**) Time spent performing social and (**b**) time spent performing aggressive behaviour. Male Wistar rats were treated with *Chlorella sorokiniana* extract (Chlorella extract, 30 mg/kg/mL dark bar) or vehicle (sunflower oil 1 mL/kg, empty bar) administration. Data are expressed as mean ± SEM ($n = 8$ per group); (**a**) *t*-test * $p < 0.05$ vs. vehicle-treated rats.

3. Discussion

In the present study we found that an acute oral administration of *Chlorella sorokiniana* lipid extract was able to significantly improve memory performance in rats. This behavioural outcome was corroborated by neurochemical data indicating a significant increase in NA and 5-HT at the hippocampal level.

In previous studies, *Chlorella sorokiniana* was reported to be an attractive source of bioactive compounds, foods, feeds and fuels [27,29,30]. Those findings make *Chlorella sorokiniana* an interesting and challenging biomass that could be used to find new and more valuable bioactive molecules.

Interestingly, we found that the lipidic fraction extracted from *Chlorella sorokiniana*, rich in PUFA of either ω-3 and ω-6 families, induced in rats an increased interest in exploring a novel object in respect to a previously encountered familiar one. This test represents a simple and reproducible behavioural assay primarily based on innate and spontaneous exploratory behaviour in rodent without the use of any reinforcement paradigm or stressful stimuli. It has been demonstrated that the NOR test allows one to study either short or long term memory, depending on the behavioural paradigm chosen [31]. In our experimental conditions, by using an intertrial interval of 1 minute, we tested the effect of treatment on short-term memory. We found for the first time that the lipidic fraction of *Chlorella sorokiniana*, particularly rich in linoleic and α linolenic acids (ALA), can improve memory function after a single oral administration. In searching of putative targets, peroxisome proliferator-activated receptors (PPAR) can be suitable candidates. Indeed, linoleic acid and linolenic acids have been reported to directly bind PPARα and γ receptors [23]. Activation of these intracellular receptors has been shown to improve memory and cognition in several animal models, either after global cerebral ischemia [32], or in diabetes-induced cognitive dysfunction [33], or in transgenic mice model of mental retardation [34].

In particular, activation of PPARγ receptors at a hippocampal level was shown to improve brain derived neurotrophic factor (BDNF) expression [33], and to rescue the long-term potentiation (LTP) induction by restoring α-amino-3-hydroxy-5-methyl-4-isoxazolepropionic acid (AMPA) receptor expression and extracellular signal–regulated kinases-cAMP response element-binding protein (ERK-CREB) activities [34]. In further agreement, transient transfection of constitutively active PPARγ plasmid in hippocampal neuronal cells was reported to be able to increase BDNF, AMPA, and *N*-methyl-D-aspartate (NMDA) receptors expression and spine formation [34]. On the other hand, ALA, the most concentrated fatty acids in *Chlorella sorokiniana* extract, was hypothesized to modulate NMDA functioning and BDNF release by influencing membrane fluidity [35]. Indeed, ALA can markedly increase membrane fluidity that correspond to a better efficiency in formation of lipid rafts in neuronal membranes [36]. Lipid raft composition, and thus lipid micro-environments on the cell surface, by favouring specific protein-protein interactions can influence the activation of signaling cascades [37]. Such an enhanced efficiency of transmembrane signaling would result in increased activated NMDA receptors, which are part of lipid raft [38]. This event would lead to higher calcium influx and initiation of signal transduction pathways ending up to activation of nuclear factor kappa B (NF-κB) via the canonical pathway which then translocates to the nucleus, ultimately leading to increased BDNF mRNA and protein levels [39–41]. Enhanced intracellular BDNF would result in its higher secretion, thereby binding to its receptors Tropomyosin receptor kinase B (TrkB), and thus controlling synaptic function [42]. Our results are in line with the findings of other studies reporting that short term supplementation with ω-3 PUFA can improve brain cognitive function by altering α-synuclein, calmodulin and transthyretin genes expression in the HIPP [43]. It has been shown that α-synuclein can regulate the homeostasis of monoamines in synapses, through modulatory interactions of the protein with monoaminergic transporters, particularly for NA [44,45]. The NA transporter (NET) is the primary mechanism of NA reuptake and termination of noradrenergic transmission [46,47]. Thus, it can be speculated that PUFA present in our *Chlorella sorokiniana* fraction, by altering α-synuclein, may modulate NET efficiency leading to increased NA levels. Indeed, in our experimental conditions, we found a significant increase in NA content only at hippocampal level. Otherwise, modulation of plasmalemma fluidity and lipid raft composition could explain such neurochemical alteration. Indeed, as previously hypothesized, increased NMDA receptor signaling may explain the increased NA release, considering that in rat hippocampal synaptosome preparations, NMDA agonists were shown to enhance NA release [48]. On the other hand, it should be taken into account that increased neurotransmitter contents can also reflect a reduction in their release or an increase in their storage. In this regard, very few data are available concerning the effects of PUFA rich extract on 5-HT and NA increased storage. Reduction in dopamine vesicle density in the rat frontal cortex has been reported after ω-3 PUFA deficiency [49], although a mechanism involving an alteration in vesicle density would appear hardly applicable in our experimental conditions considering the short overlap between drug exposure and time of measurement. In any case, we cannot completely rule out such hypothesis and further studies are necessary to elucidate this possible mechanism.

Our neurochemical result endorses the behavioural outcome on short-term memory. Indeed, we found increased NA and 5-HT content only in the HIPP, a brain area important for both spatial memory and non-spatial objects or items experienced, as a form of event memory [50–52]. It was reported that NA controls multiple brain functions, such as attention, perception, arousal, sleep, learning, and memory. The HIPP is innervated by noradrenergic projections and hippocampal neurons express β-adrenergic receptors (β-AR). These receptors modulate long-lasting forms of synaptic potentiation, such as LTP, a neuronal process crucially involved in long-term storage of spatial and contextual memories [53]. Furthermore NA, by acting on hippocampal β-AR, was shown to regulate spatial memories and in particular the content and persistence of synaptic information storage in the hippocampal subfields. In addition, activation of these receptors is graded according to the novelty or saliency of the experience [54]. Likewise, it has been shown that stimulation of adenylate cyclase following β-AR activation is the putative mechanism through which NA produces LTP in the dentate gyrus of the HIPP [55].

On the other hand, 5-HT was also increased after *Chlorella sorokiniana* administration. Serotonergic neurotransmission is responsible for regulating hippocampal plasticity and electrical activity, as well as hippocampal-dependent behaviours and cognitive performance [56]. In particular, it has been shown that by acting at 5-HT_{1A} receptors at hippocampal level, increased 5-HT levels can improve memory performance [57]. Thus, we can hypothesize that the increase in 5-HT content in the HIPP of treated rats could neurochemically underline the improvement of short-term memory induced by *Chlorella sorokiniana* lipidic fraction.

On the other hand, considering the short duration of the exposure to algal fraction we cannot exclude that any central neurochemical alterations found actually reflect peripheral activation. In this regard, PPAR are highly expressed in epithelial cells of colon and, to a lesser degree, in macrophages and lymphocytes [58]. Furthermore, peripheral release of hormones after food intake has been associated to beneficial effect on memory formation [59].

Ultimately, it has been demonstrated that gut microbiota is actually able to metabolize PUFA and derived metabolites can accumulate in plasma of treated mice [60]. In this light, alteration in cognitive function have been found after gut microbial perturbation while memory enhancement was described after probiotic treatment (see [61] for a review). Therefore, further studies aimed at elucidating possible peripheral effects at the gut level are warranted.

On the other hand, we evaluated the emotional profile in rats after *Chlorella sorokiniana* administration and no alterations in depressive-like or anxiety-like behaviours were retrieved, as revealed by FST and EPM, respectively, although a different strain of *Chlorella*, *Chlorella vulgaris*, has been proposed as adjuvant therapy in depressed and anxious medicated patients [62]. However, discrepancies can be justified on the basis of the different algal strains, algal harvesting and culture biorefinery processes and thus different fatty acid compositions. It is well known that impaired serotonergic neurotransmission in the PFC area is central to depressive disorders [63] and increases in cortical 5-HT and NA have been related to higher swimming and struggling frequencies, respectively, in the FST [64,65]. Thus, the absence of neurochemical alterations in PFC are in line with the absence of alterations found in the FST outcomes. In addition, our behavioural outcomes were validated by the fact that no locomotion alterations were found after *Chlorella sorokiniana* extract administration, as revealed by total exploration time in NOR test, CKM plasma levels and full entries in EPM.

Finally, we found that *Chlorella sorokiniana* administration, while it did not affect aggressive behaviour as indicated by a lack of alteration in noradrenergic content in PFC [66], it reduced the social behaviour. This behavioural paradigm can be used to study sociability [67]. Previous studies have negatively correlated fronto-cortical 5-HT metabolism with this behavioural trait [67], although conflicting results have been reported [68,69]. On the other hand, increase in 5-HT release at a hippocampal level has been linked to decreased social behaviour in rats, but according to the authors, such neurochemical modifications cannot be considered the only explanation [70]. Accordingly, in our conditions, while no alterations in PFC were noted, a significant increase was found in serotonergic hippocampal content, possibly explaining the behavioural outcome. However, it should be noted that differences in methodological procedures, such as sample collection and processing, timing after last behavioural testing, and rat strains could account for some of the variance observed across the literature, thus future studies in this direction are surely warranted in order to evaluate the safety profile of our algal extract.

In conclusion, we have described for the first time the beneficial effect of lipidic fraction of *Chlorella sorokiniana* on short-term memory after acute administration. *Chlorella sorokiniana* is marketed in the US as a dietary supplement for age-dependent cognitive impairment [23] and is generally considered safe. Although our study supports this evidence, our data also indicate that attention should be paid to the use of this natural supplement for its possible masked toxic effects.

4. Experimental Section

4.1. Microalgae Cultivation

Monoxenic strain of *Chlorella sorokiniana* (UTEX 2805) was phototrophically cultivated in an outdoor closed vertical tubular photobioreactor (PBR) (400 L volume) at the STAR*Facility Centre of the University of Foggia (Foggia, Italy), and grown in Bold Basal medium during the period from April 2015 and June 2015, under a solar radiation (PAR) that ranged between 700 and 930 $W \cdot m^{-2}$. Flow rate of air was 10 $L \cdot W \cdot min^{-1}$, while CO_2 was injected on pH demand ($pH_{set\ point}$ = 8.00). The temperature in the PBR ranged between 18 and 25 °C. All the parameters were monitored online by SCADA Software (Version 2.0.1, Aqualgae SL, Vigo, Spain). The algal growth rate was monitored each day by measuring the optical absorbance at 550 nm. The PBR operated in a semi-continuous way with a dilution rate of 0.25 day^{-1} and a mean productivity of 25.12 g $m^{-2} \cdot day^{-1}$. The harvested culture was daily centrifuged using a semi-continuous centrifuge (Westfalia, GEA Westfalia Separator Group GmbH, Oelde, Germany). The dewatered algal biomass was then freeze-dried and stored at −20 °C.

4.2. Extract and PUFA Characterization

Lipids from freeze-dried algal biomass were extracted as previously reported by Francavilla et al. [71]. TL were saponified and the saponified mixture was then transferred into a separatory funnel, and the Teflon tube was washed with 40 mL of Milli-Q (Millipore, Milan, Italy) water. The unsaponified matter in the combined solution was then extracted four times with 20 mL of n-hexane. The hexane phases were combined, dried overnight with sodium sulphate, filtered and evaporated. The UF was analysed by means of gas chromatography-mass spectrometry (GC-MS, IT-240, Agilent Technologies, Santa Clara, CA, USA), as previously described by Francavilla et al. [72]. Hydroalcoholic residue of extraction process of UF was acidified until pH 1 by adding HCl 2 M and extracted three times with 25 mL of *n*-hexane. The hexane phases were combined, dried with sodium sulphate anhydrous, filtered and evaporated. The yellowish viscous liquid obtained (fatty acids) was treated with 10 mL of freshly prepared 5% methanolic HCl in a Teflon tube for microwave. This mixture was carefully mixed and the tube was closed under nitrogen and then heated for 20 min in a microwave oven (MARS 6, CEM Corporation, Buckingham, UK) at 80 °C. After cooling to room temperature, 5 mL of 6% aqueous K_2CO_3 were added and the mixture was extracted four times with 20 mL of *n*-hexane. The hexane phases were then combined, dried with sodium sulphate anhydrous, filtered and evaporated. The process yielded a yellowish viscous liquid (FAMEs) that was weighed and stored at −20 °C until GC-MS analysis. FAMEs were analysed by GC-MS/MS equipment at 110 °C for 5 min, followed by a 2 $°C \cdot min^{-1}$ ramp up to 260 °C, followed by 5 min at 260 °C. The injector temperature was 250 °C and the injected volume was 1 μL. FAME peaks were identified by comparison of their retention times and mass spectra with those of a standard mixture (PUFA C4-C24, Supelco, Bellafonte, PA, USA), whereas they were quantified by using calibration curves made with PUFA C4-C24 standard (Supelco) and using C15:0 FAME (Supelco) as internal standard.

4.3. Animals and Treatment

Adult male Wistar rats (Harlan, S. Pietro al Natisone, Udine, Italy) weighing 250–300 g were used in this study. They were housed at constant room temperature (22 ± 1 °C) and relative humidity (55% ± 5%) under a 12 h light/dark cycle with ad libitum access to food and water. Procedures involving animals and their care were conducted in conformity with the institutional guidelines of the Italian Ministry of Health (D.L. 26/2014), the Guide for the Care and Use of Mammals in Neuroscience and Behavioural Research (National Research Council 2004), the Directive 2010/63/EU of the European Parliament and of the Council of 22 September 2010 on the protection of animals used for scientific purposes and to ARRIVE guidelines. "3Rs" were pursuit in every experimental procedure. Animal welfare was daily monitored through the entire period of experimental procedures. No signs of distress were evidenced and all efforts were made to minimize the number of animals used and their suffering.

Two experimental groups were considered: control animals treated with sunflower oil as vehicle and rats administered the *Chlorella sorokiniana* extract by gavage at the dose of 30 mg/kg diluted in 1 mL of sunflower oil. Behavioral and neurochemical experiments were performed 40 min after oral administration of *Chlorella sorokiniana* extract. Behavioral and neurochemical protocols were carried out in separate subset of animals in order to avoid confounding factors derived by carry over effects.

4.4. NOR Test

The NOR test was performed according to Giustino at al. [73]. Briefly, rats were submitted to two habituation sessions where they were allowed for 5 min to explore the apparatus (circular arena, 75 cm diameter). 24 h after the last habituation, a session of two 3-min trials, separated by a 1-min intertrial interval (retention interval), was carried out. The discrimination index was calculated using the following formula: (N − F) / (N + F) (N = times spent in exploration of the novel object during the choice trial; F = times spent in exploration of the familiar object in the choice trial) [74].

4.5. FST

The FST was performed according to Porsolt et al. [75]. On the first test day, animals were placed individually in inescapable Perspex cylinders (diameter 23 cm; height 70 cm), filled with a constant maintained 25 ± 1 °C temperature water at a height of 30 cm [65]. During the pre-conditioning period, animals were observed for 15 min. Then, rats were removed and dried before to be returned to their home cages. Twenty-four hours later, each rat was positioned on the water-filled cylinder for 5 min. This session was video-recorded and subsequently scored by an observer blind to the treatment groups. During the test sessions, the time spent in performing the following behaviours was measured: struggling (time spent in tentative of escaping), swimming (time spent moving around the cylinder) and immobility (time spent remaining afloat making only the necessary movements to keep its head above the water).

4.6. Social Interaction Test

The social interaction procedure was adapted from File et al. [76], as previously described [77]. The test was performed in a circular open arena (made of dark plastic; diameter 60 cm; height 31 cm), unfamiliar to the animals and placed in a deemed lit room. On the day of testing, all rats were weighed, and pairs were assigned on the basis of weight and treatment. More specifically, *Chlorella sorokiniana*-treated rats were tested with vehicle-treated partners on the basis of weight, ensuring that they did not differ by more than 10 g. The animals were marked on their back and placed head to head simultaneously in the arena, and their behaviour was recorded for 10 min by a camera mounted vertically above the test arena. During quantification, the observer, who was blinded to the experimental conditions, scored the total time that each rat spent performing the following behaviours: sniffing (sniffing several body parts of the other rat, including the anogenital region), following (moving towards and following behind the other rat around the arena), climbing (climbing over and under the conspecific's back), kicking and boxing. The defined social interactions included the following: sniffing, following and climbing the partner as social behaviour and boxing and kicking as aggressive behaviour parameters.

4.7. EPM Test

The EPM test was performed according to Pellow et al. [77]. The apparatus consisted of two opposite Plexiglas open arms (50 cm × 10 cm) without side walls and two closed arms (50 cm × 10 cm × 40 cm) extending horizontally at right angles from a central area (10 cm × 10 cm). The maze was situated in a separate brightly lit room illuminated with four, 32-W fluorescent overhead lights that produced consistent illumination within the room. The apparatus had similar levels of illumination on both the open and closed arms. The maze was elevated to a height of 50 cm in the lit room. At the beginning of the experiment, the rat was placed in the central platform facing an open arm and allowed to explore the maze for 5 min. The following parameters were analyzed: number and frequency of entries into open and closed arms and the time spent in open and closed arms. An arm entry was counted when the hind paws were placed on the open arm.

4.8. Post-Mortem Tissue Analysis

Rats were euthanized and brains were immediately removed and cooled on ice for dissection of HIPP, PFC and STR regions, according to the atlas of Paxinos and Watson [78]. Tissues were frozen and stored at −80 °C until analysis was performed.

4.8.1. Monoamine Quantification

5-HT and NA concentrations were determined by high performance liquid chromatography (HPLC) coupled with an electrochemical detector (Ultimate ECD, Dionex Scientific, Milan, Italy), as previously described [16]. Separation was performed by using a LC18 reverse phase column (Kinetex, 150 mm × 3 mm, ODS 5 μm; Phenomenex, Castel Maggiore, Bologna, Italy). The detection was accomplished by a thin-layer amperometric cell (Dionex, Thermo Scientific, Milan, Italy) with a 5 mm diameter glassy carbon electrode at a working potential of 0.400 V vs. Pd. The mobile phase used was 75 mM NaH_2PO_4, 1.7 mM octane sulfonic acid, 0.3 mM EDTA, acetonitrile 10%, in distilled water, buffered at pH 3.0. The flow rate was maintained by an isocratic pump (LC-10 AD, Shimadzu, Kyoto, Japan) at 0.6 mL/min. Data were acquired and integrated using Chromeleon software (version 6.80, Dionex, San Donato Milanese, Italy).

4.8.2. Measurement of Plasma Levels of Creatine-Kinase M-Type

Measurement of plasma levels of CKM was performed by using an enzyme-linked immunosorbent assay (ELISA) kit provided by Abcam (Cambridge, UK). Assays were performed according to the manufacturer's instructions. Each sample analysis was performed in duplicate to avoid inter-assay variations.

4.9. Blindness of the Study

All analyses were performed blind with respect to the treatment delivery. The blinding of the data was maintained until the analysis and the collection of data was terminated.

4.10. Statistical Analysis

All statistical analysis were performed using Graph Pad 5.0 for Windows (GraphPad Software, La Jolla, CA, USA). All data were tested for normality by performing the Bartlett Test. Data were analyzed by unpaired Student's *t*-test or two-way analysis of variance (ANOVA), followed by Bonferroni's *post-hoc* test. Data were expressed as mean ± standard error of mean (SEM). Differences were considered significant only when *p*-values were less than 0.05.

Acknowledgments: This study was supported by Ali. Fun to L.T. and F.I.R. form Apulia Region to M.G.M., M.F. and S.S.

Author Contributions: Study design: L.T., M.G.M. and S.S. Study conduct: E.M., M.F., M.B. and P.T. Data collection: M.G.M., M.F., E.M., M.B. and P.T. Data analysis: S.S., M.G.M., E.M., M.B. and P.T. Data interpretation: S.S., M.G.M., E.M., P.T., L.T. Drafting manuscript: S.S., M.G.M., E.M. and L.T. Revising manuscript content: S.S., M.G.M., E.M., M.B., P.T., L.M., M.F. and L.T. All Authors approve the final version of the manuscript. L.T. takes responsibility for the integrity of the data analysis.

References

1. Draaisma, R.B.; Wijffels, R.H.; Slegers, P.M.; Brentner, L.B.; Roy, A.; Barbosa, M.J. Food commodities from microalgae. *Curr. Opin. Biotechnol.* **2013**, *24*, 169–177. [CrossRef] [PubMed]
2. Sanchez-Camargo Adel, P.; Montero, L.; Stiger-Pouvreau, V.; Tanniou, A.; Cifuentes, A.; Herrero, M.; Ibanez, E. Considerations on the use of enzyme-assisted extraction in combination with pressurized liquids to recover bioactive compounds from algae. *Food Chem.* **2016**, *192*, 67–74. [CrossRef] [PubMed]
3. Francavilla, M.; Manara, P.; Kamaterou, P.; Monteleone, M.; Zabaniotou, A. Cascade approach of red macroalgae gracilaria gracilis sustainable valorization by extraction of phycobiliproteins and pyrolysis of residue. *Bioresour. Technol.* **2015**, *184*, 305–313. [CrossRef] [PubMed]
4. Khan, M.I.; Anjum, F.M.; Sohaib, M.; Sameen, A. Tackling metabolic syndrome by functional foods. *Rev. Endocr. Metab. Disord.* **2013**, *14*, 287–297. [CrossRef] [PubMed]
5. Zhao, Y.; Wang, M.; Lindstrom, M.E.; Li, J. Fatty acid and lipid profiles with emphasis on *n*-3 fatty acids and phospholipids from ciona intestinalis. *Lipids* **2015**, *50*, 1009–1027. [CrossRef] [PubMed]

6. Zou, S.; Fei, C.; Song, J.; Bao, Y.; He, M.; Wang, C. Combining and comparing coalescent, distance and character-based approaches for barcoding microalgaes: A test with *Chlorella*-like species (chlorophyta). *PLoS ONE* **2016**, *11*. [CrossRef] [PubMed]
7. Dong, T.; Wang, J.; Miao, C.; Zheng, Y.; Chen, S. Two-step in situ biodiesel production from microalgae with high free fatty acid content. *Bioresour. Technol.* **2013**, *136*, 8–15. [CrossRef] [PubMed]
8. Doughman, S.D.; Krupanidhi, S.; Sanjeevi, C.B. ω-3 Fatty acids for nutrition and medicine: Considering microalgae oil as a vegetarian source of epa and dha. *Curr. Diabetes Rev.* **2007**, *3*, 198–203. [CrossRef] [PubMed]
9. Gouveia, L.; Oliveira, A.C. Microalgae as a raw material for biofuels production. *J. Ind. Microbiol. Biotechnol.* **2009**, *36*, 269–274. [CrossRef] [PubMed]
10. Tapiero, H.; Ba, G.N.; Couvreur, P.; Tew, K.D. Polyunsaturated fatty acids (PUFA) and eicosanoids in human health and pathologies. *Biomed. Pharmacother.* **2002**, *56*, 215–222. [CrossRef]
11. Innis, S.M.; Jacobson, K. Dietary lipids in early development and intestinal inflammatory disease. *Nutr. Rev.* **2007**, *65*, S188–S193. [CrossRef] [PubMed]
12. Orr, S.K.; Bazinet, R.P. The emerging role of docosahexaenoic acid in neuroinflammation. *Curr. Opin. Investig. Drugs* **2008**, *9*, 735–743. [PubMed]
13. Labrousse, V.F.; Nadjar, A.; Joffre, C.; Costes, L.; Aubert, A.; Gregoire, S.; Bretillon, L.; Laye, S. Short-term long chain omega3 diet protects from neuroinflammatory processes and memory impairment in aged mice. *PLoS ONE* **2012**, *7*, e36861. [CrossRef] [PubMed]
14. Singh, M. Essential fatty acids, dha and human brain. *Indian J. Pediatr.* **2005**, *72*, 239–242. [CrossRef] [PubMed]
15. Lang, U.E.; Beglinger, C.; Schweinfurth, N.; Walter, M.; Borgwardt, S. Nutritional aspects of depression. *Cell. Physiol. Biochem.* **2015**, *37*, 1029–1043. [CrossRef] [PubMed]
16. Morgese, M.G.; Tucci, P.; Mhillaj, E.; Bove, M.; Schiavone, S.; Trabace, L.; Cuomo, V. Lifelong nutritional ω-3 deficiency evokes depressive-like state through soluble β amyloid. *Mol. Neurobiol.* **2016**, 1–11. [CrossRef] [PubMed]
17. Stavrovskaya, I.G.; Bird, S.S.; Marur, V.R.; Baranov, S.V.; Greenberg, H.K.; Porter, C.L.; Kristal, B.S. Dietary ω-3 fatty acids do not change resistance of rat brain or liver mitochondria to Ca^{2+} and/or prooxidants. *J. Lipids* **2012**, *2012*, 797105. [CrossRef] [PubMed]
18. Kawashima, A.; Harada, T.; Kami, H.; Yano, T.; Imada, K.; Mizuguchi, K. Effects of eicosapentaenoic acid on synaptic plasticity, fatty acid profile and phosphoinositide 3-kinase signaling in rat hippocampus and differentiated PC12 cells. *J. Nutr. Biochem.* **2010**, *21*, 268–277. [CrossRef] [PubMed]
19. Eriksdotter, M.; Vedin, I.; Falahati, F.; Freund-Levi, Y.; Hjorth, E.; Faxen-Irving, G.; Wahlund, L.O.; Schultzberg, M.; Basun, H.; Cederholm, T.; et al. Plasma fatty acid profiles in relation to cognition and gender in Alzheimer's disease patients during oral ω-3 fatty acid supplementation: The omegad study. *J. Alzheimers Dis.* **2015**, *48*, 805–812. [CrossRef] [PubMed]
20. Freund-Levi, Y.; Vedin, I.; Hjorth, E.; Basun, H.; Faxen Irving, G.; Schultzberg, M.; Eriksdotter, M.; Palmblad, J.; Vessby, B.; Wahlund, L.O.; et al. Effects of supplementation with ω-3 fatty acids on oxidative stress and inflammation in patients with alzheimer's disease: The omegad study. *J. Alzheimers Dis.* **2014**, *42*, 823–831. [PubMed]
21. Sullivan, E.L.; Riper, K.M.; Lockard, R.; Valleau, J.C. Maternal high-fat diet programming of the neuroendocrine system and behavior. *Horm Behav.* **2015**, *76*, 153–161. [CrossRef] [PubMed]
22. Farahani, S.; Motasaddi Zarandy, M.; Hassanzadeh, G.; Shidfar, F.; Jalaie, S.; Rahimi, V. The effect of low ω-3/ω-6 ratio on auditory nerve conduction in rat pups. *Acta Med. Iran.* **2015**, *53*, 346–350. [PubMed]
23. Chou, Y.C.; Prakash, E.; Huang, C.F.; Lien, T.W.; Chen, X.; Su, I.J.; Chao, Y.S.; Hsieh, H.P.; Hsu, J.T. Bioassay-guided purification and identification of PPARα/γ agonists from *Chlorella sorokiniana*. *Phytother. Res.* **2008**, *22*, 605–613. [CrossRef] [PubMed]
24. Yim, H.E.; Yoo, K.H.; Seo, W.H.; Won, N.H.; Hong, Y.S.; Lee, J.W. Acute tubulointerstitial nephritis following ingestion of chlorella tablets. *Pediatr. Nephrol.* **2007**, *22*, 887–888. [CrossRef] [PubMed]
25. Mizoguchi, T.; Takehara, I.; Masuzawa, T.; Saito, T.; Naoki, Y. Nutrigenomic studies of effects of chlorella on subjects with high-risk factors for lifestyle-related disease. *J. Med. Food* **2008**, *11*, 395–404. [CrossRef] [PubMed]

26. Selvaraj, V.; Singh, H.; Ramaswamy, S. Chlorella-induced psychosis. *Psychosomatics* **2013**, *54*, 303–304. [CrossRef] [PubMed]
27. Parsaeimehr, A.; Sun, Z.; Dou, X.; Chen, Y.F. Simultaneous improvement in production of microalgal biodiesel and high-value α-linolenic acid by a single regulator acetylcholine. *Biotechnol. Biofuels* **2015**, *8*, 11. [CrossRef] [PubMed]
28. Ngangkham, M.; Ratha, S.K.; Prasanna, R.; Saxena, A.K.; Dhar, D.W.; Sarika, C.; Prasad, R.B. Biochemical modulation of growth, lipid quality and productivity in mixotrophic cultures of *Chlorella sorokiniana*. *Springerplus* **2012**, *1*, 33. [CrossRef] [PubMed]
29. Cordero, B.F.; Obraztsova, I.; Couso, I.; Leon, R.; Vargas, M.A.; Rodriguez, H. Enhancement of lutein production in *Chlorella sorokiniana* (Chorophyta) by improvement of culture conditions and random mutagenesis. *Mar. Drugs* **2011**, *9*, 1607–1624. [CrossRef] [PubMed]
30. Chen, C.Y.; Chang, H.Y. Lipid production of microalga *Chlorella sorokiniana* cy1 is improved by light source arrangement, bioreactor operation mode and deep-sea water supplements. *Biotechnol. J.* **2016**, *11*, 356–362. [CrossRef] [PubMed]
31. Tucci, P.; Mhillaj, E.; Morgese, M.G.; Colaianna, M.; Zotti, M.; Schiavone, S.; Cicerale, M.; Trezza, V.; Campolongo, P.; Cuomo, V.; et al. Memantine prevents memory consolidation failure induced by soluble α amyloid in rats. *Front. Behav. Neurosci.* **2014**, *8*, 332. [CrossRef] [PubMed]
32. Xuan, A.G.; Chen, Y.; Long, D.H.; Zhang, M.; Ji, W.D.; Zhang, W.J.; Liu, J.H.; Hong, L.P.; He, X.S.; Chen, W.L. PPARα agonist fenofibrate ameliorates learning and memory deficits in rats following global cerebral ischemia. *Mol. Neurobiol.* **2015**, *52*, 601–609. [CrossRef] [PubMed]
33. Kariharan, T.; Nanayakkara, G.; Parameshwaran, K.; Bagasrawala, I.; Ahuja, M.; Abdel-Rahman, E.; Amin, A.T.; Dhanasekaran, M.; Suppiramaniam, V.; Amin, R.H. Central activation of PPAR-γ ameliorates diabetes induced cognitive dysfunction and improves bdnf expression. *Neurobiol. Aging* **2015**, *36*, 1451–1461. [CrossRef] [PubMed]
34. Zhou, L.; Chen, T.; Li, G.; Wu, C.; Wang, C.; Li, L.; Sha, S.; Chen, L.; Liu, G.; Chen, L. Activation of PPARγ ameliorates spatial cognitive deficits through restoring expression of ampa receptors in seipin knock-out mice. *J. Neurosci.* **2016**, *36*, 1242–1253. [CrossRef] [PubMed]
35. Blondeau, N.; Lipsky, R.H.; Bourourou, M.; Duncan, M.W.; Gorelick, P.B.; Marini, A.M. α-Linolenic acid: An ω-3 fatty acid with neuroprotective properties-ready for use in the stroke clinic? *Biomed. Res. Int.* **2015**, *2015*, 519830. [CrossRef] [PubMed]
36. Basiouni, S.; Stockel, K.; Fuhrmann, H.; Schumann, J. Polyunsaturated fatty acid supplements modulate mast cell membrane microdomain composition. *Cell. Immunol.* **2012**, *275*, 42–46. [CrossRef] [PubMed]
37. Simons, K.; Toomre, D. Lipid rafts and signal transduction. *Nat. Rev. Mol. Cell. Biol.* **2000**, *1*, 31–39. [CrossRef] [PubMed]
38. Besshoh, S.; Chen, S.; Brown, I.R.; Gurd, J.W. Developmental changes in the association of nmda receptors with lipid rafts. *J. Neurosci. Res.* **2007**, *85*, 1876–1883. [CrossRef] [PubMed]
39. Marini, A.M.; Rabin, S.J.; Lipsky, R.H.; Mocchetti, I. Activity-dependent release of brain-derived neurotrophic factor underlies the neuroprotective effect of *N*-methyl-D-aspartate. *J. Biol. Chem.* **1998**, *273*, 29394–29399. [CrossRef] [PubMed]
40. Blondeau, N.; Widmann, C.; Lazdunski, M.; Heurteaux, C. Activation of the nuclear factor-kappab is a key event in brain tolerance. *J. Neurosci.* **2001**, *21*, 4668–4677. [PubMed]
41. Lipsky, R.H.; Xu, K.; Zhu, D.; Kelly, C.; Terhakopian, A.; Novelli, A.; Marini, A.M. Nuclear factor kappab is a critical determinant in *N*-methyl-D-aspartate receptor-mediated neuroprotection. *J. Neurochem.* **2001**, *78*, 254–264. [CrossRef] [PubMed]
42. Jiang, X.; Tian, F.; Mearow, K.; Okagaki, P.; Lipsky, R.H.; Marini, A.M. The excitoprotective effect of *N*-methyl-D-aspartate receptors is mediated by a brain-derived neurotrophic factor autocrine loop in cultured hippocampal neurons. *J. Neurochem.* **2005**, *94*, 713–722. [CrossRef] [PubMed]
43. Sopian, N.F.; Ajat, M.; Shafie, N.I.; Noor, M.H.; Ebrahimi, M.; Rajion, M.A.; Meng, G.Y.; Ahmad, H. Does short-term dietary ω-3 fatty acid supplementation influence brain hippocampus gene expression of zinc transporter-3? *Int. J. Mol. Sci.* **2015**, *16*, 15800–15810. [CrossRef] [PubMed]
44. Wersinger, C.; Jeannotte, A.; Sidhu, A. Attenuation of the norepinephrine transporter activity and trafficking via interactions with α-synuclein. *Eur. J. Neurosci.* **2006**, *24*, 3141–3152. [CrossRef] [PubMed]

45. Jeannotte, A.M.; Sidhu, A. Regulation of the norepinephrine transporter by α-synuclein-mediated interactions with microtubules. *Eur. J. Neurosci.* **2007**, *26*, 1509–1520. [CrossRef] [PubMed]
46. Nelson, J.C. Synergistic benefits of serotonin and noradrenaline reuptake inhibition. *Depress. Anxiety* **1998**, *7* (Suppl. 1), 5–6. [CrossRef]
47. Smythies, J. Section III. The norepinephrine system. *Int. Rev. Neurobiol.* **2005**, *64*, 173–211. [PubMed]
48. Pittaluga, A.; Raiteri, M. *N*-methyl-D-aspartic acid (NMDA) and non-NMDA receptors regulating hippocampal norepinephrine release. I. Location on axon terminals and pharmacological characterization. *J. Pharmacol. Exp. Ther.* **1992**, *260*, 232–237. [PubMed]
49. Zimmer, L.; Delpal, S.; Guilloteau, D.; Aioun, J.; Durand, G.; Chalon, S. Chronic *n*-3 polyunsaturated fatty acid deficiency alters dopamine vesicle density in the rat frontal cortex. *Neurosci. Lett.* **2000**, *284*, 25–28. [CrossRef]
50. Broadbent, N.J.; Squire, L.R.; Clark, R.E. Spatial memory, recognition memory, and the hippocampus. *Proc. Natl. Acad. Sci. USA* **2004**, *101*, 14515–14520. [CrossRef] [PubMed]
51. Cohen, S.J.; Munchow, A.H.; Rios, L.M.; Zhang, G.; Asgeirsdottir, H.N.; Stackman, R.W., Jr. The rodent hippocampus is essential for nonspatial object memory. *Curr. Biol.* **2013**, *23*, 1685–1690. [CrossRef] [PubMed]
52. Takano, M. Vasculitis of the retina. It's treatment and light-coagulation for the hemorrhage of retinal vein obstruction. *Nihon Ganka Kiyo* **1971**, *22*, 889–897. [PubMed]
53. O'Dell, T.J.; Connor, S.A.; Guglietta, R.; Nguyen, P.V. β-adrenergic receptor signaling and modulation of long-term potentiation in the mammalian hippocampus. *Learn. Mem.* **2015**, *22*, 461–471. [CrossRef] [PubMed]
54. Hagena, H.; Hansen, N.; Manahan-Vaughan, D. β-adrenergic control of hippocampal function: Subserving the choreography of synaptic information storage and memory. *Cereb. Cortex* **2016**, *26*, 1349–1364. [CrossRef] [PubMed]
55. Stanton, P.K.; Sarvey, J.M. Depletion of norepinephrine, but not serotonin, reduces long-term potentiation in the dentate gyrus of rat hippocampal slices. *J. Neurosci.* **1985**, *5*, 2169–2176. [PubMed]
56. Nichols, D.E.; Nichols, C.D. Serotonin receptors. *Chem. Rev.* **2008**, *108*, 1614–1641. [CrossRef] [PubMed]
57. Glikmann-Johnston, Y.; Saling, M.M.; Reutens, D.C.; Stout, J.C. Hippocampal 5-HT_{1A} receptor and spatial learning and memory. *Front. Pharmacol.* **2015**, *6*, 289. [CrossRef] [PubMed]
58. Dubuquoy, L.; Rousseaux, C.; Thuru, X.; Peyrin-Biroulet, L.; Romano, O.; Chavatte, P.; Chamaillard, M.; Desreumaux, P. PPARγ as a new therapeutic target in inflammatory bowel diseases. *Gut* **2006**, *55*, 1341–1349. [CrossRef] [PubMed]
59. Gomez-Pinilla, F. Brain foods: The effects of nutrients on brain function. *Nat. Rev. Neurosci.* **2008**, *9*, 568–578. [CrossRef] [PubMed]
60. Druart, C.; Neyrinck, A.M.; Vlaeminck, B.; Fievez, V.; Cani, P.D.; Delzenne, N.M. Role of the lower and upper intestine in the production and absorption of gut microbiota-derived PUFA metabolites. *PLoS ONE* **2014**, *9*, e87560. [CrossRef] [PubMed]
61. Cryan, J.F.; O'Mahony, S.M. The microbiome-gut-brain axis: From bowel to behavior. *Neurogastroenterol. Motil.* **2011**, *23*, 187–192. [CrossRef] [PubMed]
62. Panahi, Y.; Badeli, R.; Karami, G.R.; Badeli, Z.; Sahebkar, A. A randomized controlled trial of 6-week chlorella vulgaris supplementation in patients with major depressive disorder. *Complement. Ther. Med.* **2015**, *23*, 598–602. [CrossRef] [PubMed]
63. Krishnan, V.; Nestler, E.J. The molecular neurobiology of depression. *Nature* **2008**, *455*, 894–902. [CrossRef] [PubMed]
64. Detke, M.J.; Rickels, M.; Lucki, I. Active behaviors in the rat forced swimming test differentially produced by serotonergic and noradrenergic antidepressants. *Psychopharmacology (Berl.)* **1995**, *121*, 66–72. [CrossRef] [PubMed]
65. Cryan, J.F.; Holmes, A. The ascent of mouse: Advances in modelling human depression and anxiety. *Nat. Rev. Drug Discov.* **2005**, *4*, 775–790. [CrossRef] [PubMed]
66. Cambon, K.; Dos-Santos Coura, R.; Groc, L.; Carbon, A.; Weissmann, D.; Changeux, J.P.; Pujol, J.F.; Granon, S. Aggressive behavior during social interaction in mice is controlled by the modulation of tyrosine hydroxylase expression in the prefrontal cortex. *Neuroscience* **2010**, *171*, 840–851. [CrossRef] [PubMed]
67. Tonissaar, M.; Philips, M.A.; Eller, M.; Harro, J. Sociability trait and serotonin metabolism in the rat social interaction test. *Neurosci. Lett.* **2004**, *367*, 309–312. [CrossRef] [PubMed]

68. Duxon, M.S.; Starr, K.R.; Upton, N. Latency to paroxetine-induced anxiolysis in the rat is reduced by co-administration of the 5-HT_{1A} receptor antagonist way100635. *Br. J. Pharmacol.* **2000**, *130*, 1713–1719. [CrossRef] [PubMed]
69. Kenny, P.J.; Cheeta, S.; File, S.E. Anxiogenic effects of nicotine in the dorsal hippocampus are mediated by 5-HT_{1A} and not by muscarinic m1 receptors. *Neuropharmacology* **2000**, *39*, 300–307. [CrossRef]
70. File, S.E.; Zangrossi, H., Jr.; Andrews, N. Social interaction and elevated plus-maze tests: Changes in release and uptake of 5-HT and GABA. *Neuropharmacology* **1993**, *32*, 217–221. [CrossRef]
71. Francavilla, M.; Trotta, P.; Luque, R. Phytosterols from dunaliella tertiolecta and dunaliella salina: A potentially novel industrial application. *Bioresour. Technol.* **2010**, *101*, 4144–4150. [CrossRef] [PubMed]
72. Francavilla, M.; Colaianna, M.; Zotti, M.; Morgese, M.G.; Trotta, P.; Tucci, P.; Schiavone, S.; Cuomo, V.; Trabace, L. Extraction, characterization and in vivo neuromodulatory activity of phytosterols from microalga dunaliella tertiolecta. *Curr. Med. Chem.* **2012**, *19*, 3058–3067. [CrossRef] [PubMed]
73. Giustino, A.; Beckett, S.; Ballard, T.; Cuomo, V.; Marsden, C.A. Perinatal cocaine reduces responsiveness to cocaine and causes alterations in exploratory behavior and visual discrimination in young-adult rats. *Brain Res.* **1996**, *728*, 149–156. [CrossRef]
74. Giovannini, M.G.; Bartolini, L.; Kopf, S.R.; Pepeu, G. Acetylcholine release from the frontal cortex during exploratory activity. *Brain Res.* **1998**, *784*, 218–227. [CrossRef]
75. Porsolt, R.D.; Bertin, A.; Jalfre, M. Behavioral despair in mice: A primary screening test for antidepressants. *Arch. Int. Pharmacodyn. Ther.* **1977**, *229*, 327–336. [PubMed]
76. File, S.E. The use of social interaction as a method for detecting anxiolytic activity of chlordiazepoxide-like drugs. *J. Neurosci. Methods* **1980**, *2*, 219–238. [CrossRef]
77. Tucci, P.; Morgese, M.G.; Colaianna, M.; Zotti, M.; Schiavone, S.; Cuomo, V.; Trabace, L. Neurochemical consequence of steroid abuse: Stanozolol-induced monoaminergic changes. *Steroids* **2012**, *77*, 269–275. [CrossRef] [PubMed]
78. Paxinos, G.; Watson, C. *The Rat Brain in Stereotaxic Coordinates*, 4th ed.; Academic Press: San Diego, CA, USA, 1998.

4

Extracts from Traditional Chinese Medicinal Plants Inhibit Acetylcholinesterase, a Known Alzheimer's Disease Target

Dorothea Kaufmann [1,*], Anudeep Kaur Dogra [2], Ahmad Tahrani [1], Florian Herrmann [1] and Michael Wink [1]

1 Institute of Pharmacy and Molecular Biotechnology, Department of Biology, Ruprecht Karls University Heidelberg, Heidelberg 69120, Germany; mad.rani@gmail.com (A.T.); Florian.Herrmann@t-online.de (F.H.); wink@uni-hd.de (M.W.)

2 Centre for Pharmacognosy and Phytotherapy, The School of Pharmacy, University of London, 29-39 Brunswick Square, London WC1N 1AX, UK; anudeep.k.dogra@gmail.com

* Correspondence: d.kaufmann@uni-heidelberg.de

Academic Editor: Luigia Trabace

Abstract: Inhibition of acetylcholinesterase (AChE) is a common treatment for early stages of the most general form of dementia, Alzheimer's Disease (AD). In this study, methanol, dichloromethane and aqueous crude extracts from 80 Traditional Chinese Medical (TCM) plants were tested for their in vitro anti-acetylcholinesterase activity based on Ellman's colorimetric assay. All three extracts of *Berberis bealei* (formerly *Mahonia bealei*), *Coptis chinensis* and *Phellodendron chinense*, which contain numerous isoquinoline alkaloids, substantially inhibited AChE. The methanol and aqueous extracts of *Coptis chinensis* showed IC_{50} values of 0.031 µg/mL and 2.5 µg/mL, therefore having an up to 100-fold stronger AChE inhibitory activity than the already known AChE inhibitor galantamine (IC_{50} = 4.33 µg/mL). Combinations of individual alkaloids berberine, coptisine and palmatine resulted in a synergistic enhancement of ACh inhibition. Therefore, the mode of AChE inhibition of crude extracts of *Coptis chinensis*, *Berberis bealei* and *Phellodendron chinense* is probably due to of this synergism of isoquinoline alkaloids. All extracts were also tested for their cytotoxicity in COS7 cells and none of the most active extracts was cytotoxic at the concentrations which inhibit AChE. Based on these results it can be stated that some TCM plants inhibit AChE via synergistic interaction of their secondary metabolites. The possibility to isolate pure lead compounds from the crude extracts or to administer these as nutraceuticals or as cheap alternative to drugs in third world countries make TCM plants a versatile source of natural inhibitors of AChE.

Keywords: acetylcholinesterase; acetylcholinesterase inhibitor; isoquinoline alkaloids; berberine; coptisine; palmatine; Alzheimer's; *Coptis*; natural products; Traditional Chinese Medicine

---

1. Introduction

With more than 46 million people suffering from Alzheimer's disease (AD) worldwide [1], this neuro-degenerative disorder is the most common form of dementia in elderly people [2]. The progressive degenerative brain syndromes connected to dementia affect memory, thinking, behaviour and emotion. Typical symptoms include loss of memory and difficulties to perform previously routine tasks. Patients also have problems with finding the right words or understand what people are saying and they often undergo personality and mood changes [3]. During the progression of AD, the death of nerve cells in the cerebral cortex leads to a shrinkage of the brain. In consequence, gaps develop in the temporal lobe and hippocampus, where new information is stored and retrieved. These lesions affect the ability to remember, think, speak and make decisions [3].

Brain processing speed and memory is determined by the neurotransmitter acetylcholine (ACh). A low level of ACh results in impaired learning and memory as well as general "slow thinking". Furthermore, a deficiency of ACh seems to be directly correlated to AD [4]. The level of ACh in the brain of patients suffering from AD is greatly reduced compared to the healthy patients. In late stages of AD, levels of ACh have declined by up to 85% [5]. This decrease results from the inability to synthesise enough ACh for sufficient transmission of information. Furthermore, ACh is broken down in the synaptic cleft by acetylcholinesterase (AChE). Therefore, one way to elevate ACh levels in the brain is to inhibit AChE. The breakdown of ACh is decreased and more ACh is available to bind to ACh receptors resulting in an improvement of cognitive function [6,7]. AChE inhibitors are still the first choice of drugs for the treatment of AD. The AChE inhibitors galantamine and rivastigmine are used in mild to moderate stages of the disease; donepezil is the drug of choice for all stages. This therapy is no longer considered to be only symptomatic, but also disease modifying [8,9]. Another option is memantine, which is an antagonist of the *N*-methyl-D-aspartate receptor and prescribed for moderate to severe cases of AD either as single compound or in combination with donepezil. Although all of these therapies improve the length and quality of life of the patients, they are only symptomatic and fail to cure the disease [10,11].

Various plant-derived compounds are already used for the treatment of AD. The most prominent examples are physostigmine, galantamine (Reminyl®) and huperzine A, but more than 150 different plant species in various preparations and mixtures have been used in the context of age related CNS disorders [12–15]. We have also already showed the anti-AChE activity of myrtenal, a monoterpene derived from *Taxus baccata* [16]. Therefore, it can be assumed that plants are still a promising source of new bioactive compounds with anti-AChE activity.

This study investigates the use of plants from Traditional Chinese Medicine (TCM), a complete medical system used to diagnose, treat and prevent illness for thousands of years, as inhibitors of AChE. Eighty of the most commonly used TCM plants were tested for their in vitro inhibitory activity of AChE. Contrary to the approach of isolating single compounds from plants our idea was to use complex extracts. These consist of a wide variety of different secondary metabolites, usually belonging to different chemical classes. These chemical compounds can interfere with their targets in a pleiotropic manner. The overall effect is sometimes not only additive, but even synergistic. This means that the overall effect of a mixture is greater than the sum of the individual effects [17,18].

We were able to show that three of the TCM plants, which contain isoquinoline alkaloids, substantially inhibited AChE. The most remarkable finding was that the alkaloid containing methanol extract of *Coptis chinensis* showed a 100-fold more powerful AChE inhibition than galantamine. The mode of action of the highly active extracts is probably due to synergistic interactions, which could be shown when individual alkaloids, such as berberine, coptisine and palmatine (which occur in the extracts) were combined.

2. Results

2.1. Inhibition of Acetylcholinesterase by Extracts from TCM Plants

In this study methanol, dichloromethane and aqueous crude extracts from 80 TCM plants were tested for their in vitro anti-acetylcholinesterase activity. Physostigmine and galantamine, both known acetylcholinesterase inhibitors [19], were used as the positive controls. The extracts of *Berberis bealei* Carrière, Berberidaceae (formerly *Mahonia bealei*; Shi Da Gong Lao), *Coptis chinensis* Franch, Ranunculaceae (Huang Lian) and *Phellodendron chinense* Scheid., Rutaceae (Huang Bai) showed the highest inhibition of AChE activity. None of these extracts was cytotoxic in COS7 cells at their respective AChE inhibitory concentrations (Table 1) suggesting their potential therapeutic application. A high ratio between the IC_{50} in COS7 cells and corresponding AChE inhibition denotes a beneficial therapeutic profile of the compound. IC_{50} values for all other plant extracts are listed in Table 2.

Table 1. AChE inhibitory (AChEi) activity and cytotoxicity in COS7 cells of the most active TCM plant extracts. All data are expressed as mean ± standard deviation; all experiments were carried out in triplicates and repeated independently. (AChE assay: $n = 3$; $n = 9$ for *Coptis chinensis* samples. Cytotoxicity: $n = 3$).

Sample	IC_{50} AChE Inhibition (mg/mL)	IC_{50} COS7 (µg/mL)	Ratio IC_{50} COS7/AChE
Berberis bealei MeOH	34.10 ± 4.89	35.37 ± 4.21	1.0
Berberis bealei CH_2Cl_2	9.99 ± 1.18	13.36 ± 1.76	1.3
Berberis bealei H_2O	87.77 ± 4.11	270.0 ± 13.5	3.1
Coptis chinensis MeOH	0.031 ± 0.002	3.72 ± 0.74	120
Coptis chinensis CH_2Cl_2	8.13 ± 0.90	39.57 ± 4.87	4.9
Coptis chinensis H_2O	2.5 ± 0.61	118.3 ± 7.4	47
Phellodendron chinense MeOH	8.03 ± 0.98	85.52 ± 11.90	10
Phellodendron chinense CH_2Cl_2	6.34 ± 1.37	71.33 ± 6.87	11
Phellodendron chinense H_2O	84.83 ± 1.84	282.9 ± 15.3	3.3
Berberine	1.48 ± 0.07	-	-
Coptisine	1.27 ± 0.06	-	-
Palmatine	5.21 ± 0.48	-	-
Physostigmine	2.24 ± 0.27	-	-
Galantamine	4.33 ± 0.21	-	-

2.2. Phytochemical Analysis of Most Active Extracts

Literature lists the alkaloids berberine, coptisine and palmatine as the main compounds of *Berberis bealei* [20–24], *Coptis chinensis* [25–27] and *Phellodendron chinense* [28]. Therefore HPLC and LC-MS was used to confirm the presence of these alkaloids. Figure 1 illustrates the HPLC profile of the methanol extract of *Coptis chinensis* and lists the alkaloids detected in the different crude extracts of the three most active species. Berberine and palmatine were found in all nine extracts; coptisine only in the crude extracts of *Coptis chinensis*. Total alkaloids were highest in the methanol extract of *Coptis chinensis* and lowest in the aqueous extract of *Berberis bealei*. Berberine is the main alkaloid of all extracts of *Coptis chinensis* and *Phellodendron chinense*. The main alkaloid of *Berberis bealei* is palmatine.

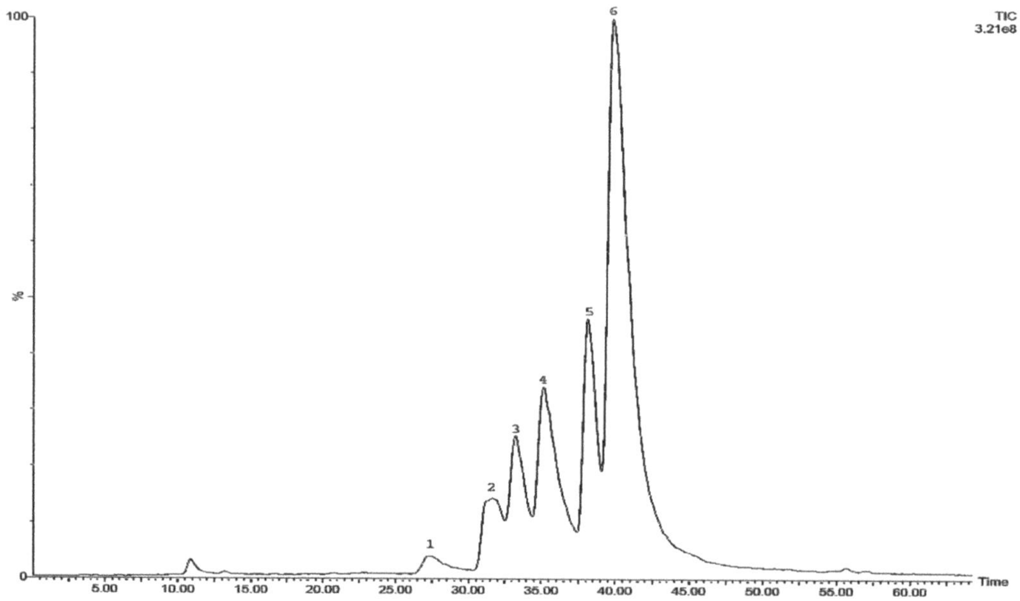

Figure 1. HPLC-MS total ion current chromatogram of a methanol extract of *Coptis chinensis*. Peaks: 1: Tetradehydroscoulerine / tetrahydrocheilanthifolinium ($m/z = 322$); 2: columbamine ($m/z = 338$); 3: epiberberine ($m/z = 336$); 4: coptisine ($m/z = 320$); 5: palmatine ($m/z = 352$); 6: berberine ($m/z = 336$).

Table 2. AChE inhibitory activity and cytoxicity in COS7 cells of TCM plant extracts.

Family/Plant	Chinese Name	DNA	AChE (IC_{50} (μg/mL))			COS7 (IC_{50} (μg/mL))		
			MeOH	CH_2Cl_2	H_2O	MeOH	CH_2Cl_2	H_2O
Acanthaceae	-	-	-	-	-	-	-	-
Andrographis paniculata	Chuan Xin Lian	Family	NA	NA	NA	344.7 ± 13.3	104.7 ± 5.2	255.6 ± 11.9
Amaranthaceae	-	-	-	-	-	-	-	-
Celiosa cristata	Ji Guan hua	Genus	NA	NA	NA	28.43 ± 2.87	136.00 ± 8.40	263.9 ± 12.3
Apiaceae	-	-	-	-	-	-	-	-
Bupleurum chinense	Chai Hu	Genus	NA	NA	NA	358.7 ± 19.8	87.12 ± 3.67	15.60 ± 11.76
Bupleurum marginatum	Nan Chai Hu	Genus	NA	NA	NA	576.0 ± 31.2	67.41 ± 5.23	350.7 ± 17.5
Centella asiatica	Lei Gong Gen	Species	NA	NA	NA	392.8 ± 78.2	64.97 ± 4.85	325.8 ± 12.1
Saposhnikovia divaricata	Fang Feng	Genus	NA	NA	NA	1575 ± 147	46.00 ± 2.64	153.0 ± 7.7
Selinum monnieri	She Chuang Zi	Family	NA	NA	NA	120.0 ± 11.7	37.02 ± 2.39	339.7 ± 11.1
Araliaceae	-	-	-	-	-	-	-	-
Eleutherococcus senticosus	Ci Wu Jia	Species	NA	NA	NA	190.1 ± 18.4	61.49 ± 5.98	130.5 ± 7.5
Panax ginseng	Ren Shen	Species	NA	NA	NA	510.8 ± 29.5	47.76 ± 5.82	151.7 ± 8.9
Panax notoginseng	San Qi	Species	NA	NA	NA	229.5 ± 19.5	6.47 ± 0.89	182.3 ± 9.1
Arecaceae	-	-	-	-	-	-	-	-
Areca catechu	Bing Lang	n/a	NA	NA	NA	31.02 ± 2.69	117.02 ± 7.33	16.60 ± 2.01
Apogynaceae	-	-	-	-	-	-	-	-
Cyanchum paniculatum	Liao Diao Zhu	Genus	NA	NA	NA	227.7 ± 16.9	114.25 ± 6.78	220.7 ± 7.6
Asparagaceae	-	-	-	-	-	-	-	-
Polygonatum humile	Huan Jjing	Species	NA	NA	NA	147.4 ±15.4	53.94 ± 4.67	298.4 ± 13.6
Asteraceae	-	-	-	-	-	-	-	-
Arcticum lappa	Niu Bang	Species	NA	NA	NA	1813 ± 225	344.25 ± 12.31	355.5 ± 12.6
Artemisia annua	Huang Hua Hao	n/a	NA	NA	NA	201.1 ± 8.7	34.57 ± 3.18	288.6 ± 11.4
Artemisia capillaris	Yin Chen Hao	Genus	NA	NA	NA	215.4 ± 9.3	29.49 ± 2.56	201.9 ± 9.5
Centipeda minima	Ebu Shi Cao	n/a	NA	NA	NA	54.21 ± 4.98	10.44 ± 1.70	55.64 ± 4.62
Chrysanthemum indicum	Ye Ju Hua	Genus	NA	NA	NA	287.2 ± 9.8	63.58 ± 5.78	320.9 ± 14.3
Chrysanthemum morifolium	Ju Hua	Genus	NA	NA	NA	166.7 ± 8.4	42.88 ± 3.96	760.4 ± 28.3
Eclipta prostata	Han Lian Cao	Species	NA	NA	NA	186.1 ± 12.8	112.06 ± 9.65	291.7 ± 13.9
Senecio scandens	Qian Li Guang	Genus	NA	NA	NA	126.2 ± 12.2	143.54 ± 9.64	114.2 ± 6.7
Siegesbeckia orientalis	Xi Xian Cao	Family	NA	NA	NA	84.4 ± 7.5	17.78 ± 1.94	159.2 ± 7.4
Taraxum officinale	Pu Gong Ying	Species	NA	NA	NA	485.3 ± 17	177.16 ± 8.45	156.9 ± 6.3
Berberidaceae	-	-	-	-	-	-	-	-
Berberis bealei	Shi Da Gong Lao	Species	34.10 ± 4.89	9.99 ± 1.18	87.77 ± 4.11	35.37 ± 4.21	13.36 ± 1.76	270.0 ± 13.5
Dysosma versipellis	Ba Jiao Lian	n/a	NA	NA	NA	54.90 ± 4.69	49.95 ± 5.29	1276 ± 39

Table 2. *Cont.*

Family/Plant	Chinese Name	DNA	AChE (IC_{50} (μg/mL))			COS7 (IC_{50} (μg/mL))		
			MeOH	CH_2Cl_2	H_2O	MeOH	CH_2Cl_2	H_2O
Epimedium koreanum	Yin Yang Huo	Species	NA	NA	NA	0.37 ± 0.03	3.60 ± 0.56	140.8 ± 6.2
Brassicaceae	-	-	-	-	-	-	-	-
Isatis indigotica rhizome	Ban Langen	Family	NA	NA	NA	324.4 ± 17.8	42.38 ± 4.54	557.2 ± 27.2
Isatis indigotica leaf	Daq Qing Ye	Family	NA	NA	NA	90.62 ± 11.37	0.64 ± 0.07	93.51 ± 4.73
Capsella bursa-pastoris	Ji Cai	Species	NA	NA	NA	29.82 ± 3.87	120.82 ± 7.89	234.2 ± 11.6
Caprifoliaceae	-	-	-	-	-	-	-	-
Lonicera confusa	Ren Dong Teng	Genus	NA	NA	NA	118.9 ± 12.8	58.99 ± 5.13	446.8 ± 21.2
Crassulacea	-	-	-	-	-	-	-	-
Sedum rosea	Hong Jing Tian	Species	NA	NA	NA	87.42 ± 7.43	74.67 ± 6.54	61.97 ± 4.12
Cupressaceae	-	-	-	-	-	-	-	-
Platycladus orientalis	Ce Bai Ye	Species	NA	NA	NA	158.7 ± 12.4	21.80 ± 2.91	97.78 ± 56.53
Dryopteridaceae	-	-	-	-	-	-	-	-
Cyrtomium fortunei	Guang Zhong	Species	NA	NA	NA	348.7 ± 26.5	132.13 ± 5.03	30.42 ± 2.45
Ephedraceae	-	-	-	-	-	-	-	-
Ephedra sinica	Ma Huang	Species	NA	NA	NA	36.76 ± 3.93	41.82 ± 4.85	69.15 ± 5.98
Equisetaceae	-	-	-	-	-	-	-	-
Equisetum hiemale	Mu Zei	Species	NA	NA	NA	243.5 ± 17.1	35.76 ± 3.50	265.9 ± 12.3
Euphorbiaceae	-	-	-	-	-	-	-	-
Croton tiglium	Ba Dou	n/a	NA	NA	NA	222.1 ± 18.4	225.98 ± 10.69	166.2 ± 5.7
Fabaceae	-	-	-	-	-	-	-	-
Abrus cantonensis	Ji Gu Cao	Genus	NA	NA	NA	733.1 ± 42.6	129.45 ± 7.65	575.2 ± 24.4
Acacia catechu	Er Cha	n/a	NA	NA	NA	34.86 ± 2.55	31.56 ± 3.78	35.71 ± 3.86
Cassia tora	Jue Ming Zi	Genus	NA	NA	NA	75.95 ± 6.50	189.15 ± 8.43	481.3 ± 19.4
Desmodium styracifolium	Guang Jin Qian Cao	Genus	NA	NA	NA	104.1 ± 9.35	139.86 ± 5.50	333.5 ± 13.9
Glycyrrhiza inflata	Gan Cao	Species	NA	333 ± 9	NA	126.8 ± 11.2	6.97 ± 1.43	583.9 ± 21.3
Spatholobus suberectus	Ji Xue Teng	Genus	NA	NA	NA	54.87 ± 4.89	154.66 ± 6.72	16.63 ± 1.32
Sutherlandia frutescens	n/a	n/a	NA	NA	NA	352.0 ± 29.5	259.37 ± 9.39	857.3 ± 26.8
Geraniaceae	-	-	-	-	-	-	-	-
Geranium wilfordii	Loa Guan Cao	Genus	NA	NA	NA	169.8 ± 16.4	17.02 ± 1.80	225.8 ± 9.6
Ginkgoaceae	-	-	-	-	-	-	-	-
Ginkgo biloba	Yin Xing	Species	NA	1003 ± 15	NA	260.1 ± 24.21	15.40 ± 1.34	450.8 ± 21.3
Hypericaceae	-	-	-	-	-	-	-	-
Hypericum japonicum	Tian Ji Huang	Genus	NA	NA	NA	100.9 ± 9.0	10.83 ± 0.53	151.8 ± 13.9

Table 2. *Cont.*

Family/Plant	Chinese Name	DNA	AChE (IC_{50} (μg/mL))			COS7 (IC_{50} (μg/mL))		
			MeOH	CH_2Cl_2	H_2O	MeOH	CH_2Cl_2	H_2O
Iridaceae	-	-	-	-	-	-	-	-
Belamcanda chinensis	She Gan	Species	NA	NA	NA	319.5 ± 28.4	89.25 ± 7.32	222.1 ± 12.7
Lamiaceae	-	-	-	-	-	-	-	-
Mentha haplocalyx	Bo He	Genus	NA	NA	NA	147.8 ± 12.3	34.16 ± 3.35	285.7 ± 14.6
Prunella vulgaris	Xia Ku Cao	Species	NA	NA	NA	494.5 ± 45.7	90.48 ± 6.47	21.57 ± 2.90
Scutellaria baicalensis	Huang Qin	Species	NA	NA	NA	28.88 ± 2.65	287.98 ± 8.93	46.41 ± 3.96
Lauraceae	-	-	-	-	-	-	-	-
Cinnamomum cassia	Gui Zhi	Genus	1027 ± 16	953 ± 12	NA	108.4 ± 9.8	23.20 ± 2.76	453.9 ± 21.5
Loranthaceae	-	-	-	-	-	-	-	-
Taxillus chinensis	Sang Ji Sheng	Family	NA	NA	NA	378.2 ± 32.4	68.65 ± 7.42	181.7 ± 9.2
Lythraceae	-	-	-	-	-	-	-	-
Punica granatum	Shi Liu	Species	NA	NA	NA	218.6 ± 16.3	126.64 ± 8.64	8.608 ± 1.432
Magnoliaceae	-	-	-	-	-	-	-	-
Magnolia officinalis	Hou Pu	Species	320 ± 9	183 ± 6	NA	13.12 ± 0.97	5.45 ± 1.37	73.01 ± 5.42
Melanthiaceae	-	-	-	-	-	-	-	-
Paris polyphylla	Qi Ye Yi Zhi Hua	Species	NA	NA	NA	5.52 ± 0.39	24.07 ± 2.82	38.49 ± 2.47
Myrisinaceae	-	-	-	-	-	-	-	-
Lysimachia christinae	Jin Qian Cao	Genus	NA	NA	NA	436.3 ± 36.6	137.39 ± 6.39	152.2 ± 8.4
Myrtaceae	-	-	-	-	-	-	-	-
Eucalyptus robusta	An Shu	n/a	NA	NA	NA	15.21 ± 0.62	n/a	94.19 ± 5.99
Oleaceae	-	-	-	-	-	-	-	-
Fraxinus chinensis	Qin Pi	n/a	NA	NA	NA	38.72 ± 6.59	39.23 ± 4.11	193.2 ± 11.6
Ophioglossacea	-	-	-	-	-	-	-	-
Ophioglossum vulgatum	Yi Zhi Jian	Species	NA	NA	NA	68.70 ± 11.42	62.87 ± 6.58	344.0 ± 13.4
Orchideaceae	-	-	-	-	-	-	-	-
Dendrobium loddigesii	Shi Hu	Species	NA	NA	NA	61.65 ± 15.36	25.74 ± 2.94	104.3 ± 6.3
Paeoniaceae	-	-	-	-	-	-	-	-
Paeonia lactiflora	Chi Shao	Genus	NA	NA	NA	309.8 ± 24.7	34.06 ± 4.60	148.2 ± 6.1
Pedaliaceae	-	-	-	-	-	-	-	-
Harpagophytum procumbens	n/a	n/a	NA	NA	NA	217.2 ± 18.53	15.89 ± 2.25	242.9 ± 12.6
Poaceae	-	-	-	-	-	-	-	-
Cymbopogon distans	Yun Xian Cao	Genus	NA	NA	NA	17.88 ± 1.16	114.57 ± 8.63	257.8 ± 13.2
Polygonaceae	-	-	-	-	-	-	-	-
Fallopia multiflora	He Shou Wu	Genus	NA	523 ± 11	NA	48.87 ± 4.62	107.74 ± 7.94	61.32 ± 5.61

Table 2. *Cont.*

Family/Plant	Chinese Name	DNA	AChE (IC_{50} (μg/mL))			COS7 (IC_{50} (μg/mL))		
			MeOH	CH_2Cl_2	H_2O	MeOH	CH_2Cl_2	H_2O
Polygonum cuspidatum	Hu Zhang	Species	NA	NA	NA	19.59 ± 2.23	2.85 ± 0.87	39.81 ± 3.84
Rheum officinale	Da Huang	Species	NA	NA	NA	3.53 ± 0.80	n/a	51.59 ± 5.48
Ranunculaceae	-	-	-	-	-	-	-	-
Coptis chinensis	Huang Lian	Species	0.031 ± 0.002	8.13 ± 0.90	2.5 ± 0.61	3.72 ± 0.74	39.57 ± 4.87	118.3 ± 7.4
Rosaceae	-	-	-	-	-	-	-	-
Rosa chinensis	Yu Ji Hua	n/a	NA	NA	NA	36.76 ± 3.45	141.55 ± 9.52	24.32 ± 2.86
Rosa laevigata	Jin Ying Zi	n/a	NA	NA	NA	13.30 ± 2.21	151.80 ± 9.79	93.61 ± 7.30
Sanguisorba officinalis	Di Yu	Species	NA	NA	NA	1100 ± 97	26.77 ± 3.58	20.55 ± 2.59
Rubiaceae	-	-	-	-	-	-	-	-
Hedyotis diffusa	Bai Hua She She Cao	Genus	NA	NA	NA	418.1 ± 34.8	45.35 ± 4.12	158.7 ± 9.2
Rutaceae	-	-	-	-	-	-	-	-
Evodia lepta	San Cha Ku	Family	NA	NA	NA	5.13 ± 0.75	42.06 ± 4.65	419.3 ± 19.4
Evodia rutaecarpa	Wu Zhu Yu	n/a	NA	NA	NA	427.7 ± 37.2	8.78 ± 1.78	1176 ± 34
Phellodendron chinense	Huang Bai	Genus	8.03 ± 0.98	6.34 ± 1.37	84.83 ± 1.84	85.52 ± 11.90	71.33 ± 6.87	282.9 ± 15.3
Saururaceae	-	-	-	-	-	-	-	-
Houttuynia cordata	Yu Xing Cao	Species	NA	NA	NA	63.95 ± 5.98	48.26 ± 5.19	633.3 ± 17.8
Schisandraceae	-	-	-	-	-	-	-	-
Kadsura longipedunculata	Zi Ging Pi	Species	NA	NA	NA	43.92 ± 2.59	1.88 ± 0.94	6.812 ± 1.678
Selaginellaceae	-	-	-	-	-	-	-	-
Selaginella tamariscina	Juan Bai	Species	NA	NA	NA	150.9 ± 13.34	98.83 ± 8.62	103.9 ± 6.
Valerianaceae	-	-	-	-	-	-	-	-
Patrinia scabiosaefolia	Bai Jiang	Genus	NA	NA	NA	15.96 ± 2.69	38.77 ± 2.87	38.49 ± 3.73
Verbenaceae	-	-	-	-	-	-	-	-
Verbena officinalis	Ma Bian Cao	Species	NA	NA	NA	37.76 ± 4.42	145.91 ± 9.06	93.94 ± 5.97
Violaceae	-	-	-	-	-	-	-	-
Viola yezoensis	Zi Hua Di Ding Cao	Genus	NA	NA	NA	19.19 ± 1.45	60.87 ± 5.49	135.6 ± 6.4
Zingiberaceae	-	-	-	-	-	-	-	-
Alpinia galanga	Hong Dou Kou	n/a	NA	NA	NA	53.48 ± 4.92	5.76 ± 1.53	952.2 ± 31.2
Alpinia oxaphylla	Yi Zhi Ren	Species	NA	NA	NA	110.2 ± 9.5	30.40 ± 2.81	105.8 ± 7.5

All data are expressed as mean ± standard deviation; all experiments were carried out in triplicates and repeated independently. (AChE assay: $n = 3$; $n = 9$ for *Coptis chinensis* samples. Cytotoxicity: $n = 3$). Samples were considered to be inactive (NA) in the AChE assay if they showed less than 80% inhibition of AChE activity at a concentration of 1250 μg/mL. For some plants not all extracts could be prepared, these samples are marked n/a (not analysed).

2.3. *Inhibition of Acetylcholinesterase by Pure Substances*

Plants produce a high diversity of secondary metabolites representing a complex mixture of compounds belonging to several chemical classes. The mode of action of most plants cannot be attributed to one single chemical compound, but to the pleiotropic effects of the secondary metabolites contained in the plant [29]. To understand the potential mode of action of the aforementioned TCM plants, the isolated alkaloids berberine, coptisine and palmatine were tested for their individual inhibition of AChE (Table 1). It is notable that none of the three alkaloids inhibits AChE as strong as the crude methanol extract of *Coptis chinensis*.

2.4. *Inhibition of ACh is Based on Synergism*

The finding that none of the tested alkaloids showed an equally strong AChE inhibitory effect as the crude methanol extract of *Coptis chinensis* led to the assumption that the mode of action of this crude extract could be based on synergism of individual alkaloids. Therefore, synergism studies were carried out: the AChE assay was conducted with a dilution series of one of the isolated alkaloids (1st alkaloid) in combination with a steady IC_{30} concentration of the other alkaloids (2nd alkaloid). Data is shown in Table 3. Comparing the FIC values obtained at constant concentrations of the 2nd alkaloid with varying concentrations of the 1st alkaloid showed decreasing FIC values by increasing the concentration of the 1st alkaloid. In some of the tested combinations an FIC value of ≤ 0.5 was observed, which signifies a synergistic effect.

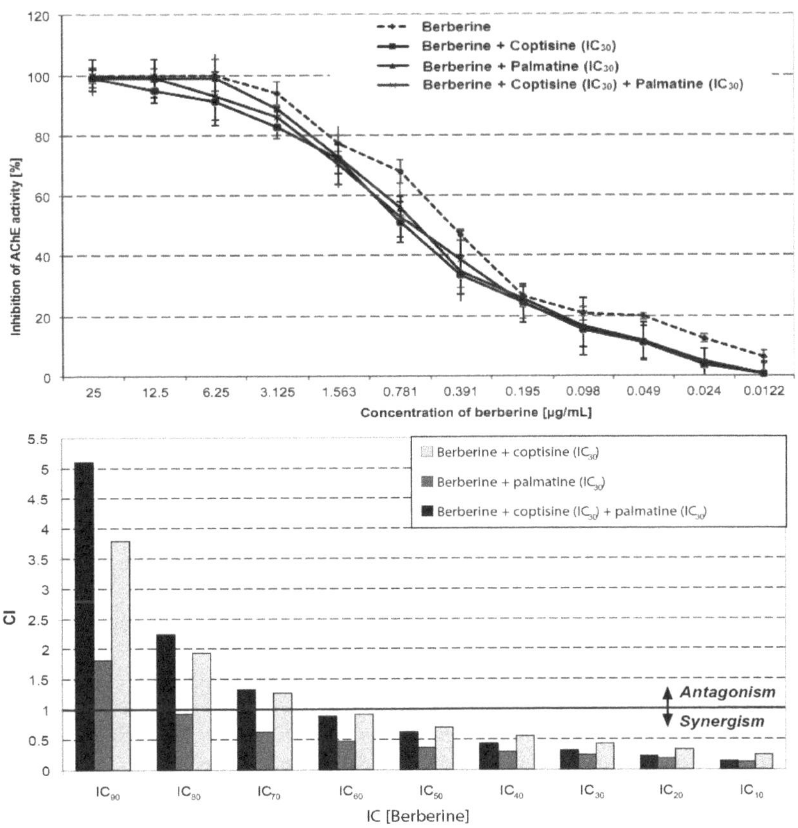

Figure 2. AChE inhibitory effect and synergistic effects of berberine in combination with coptisine and palmatine. The combination of berberine with other alkaloids inhibits ACh stronger than berberine alone (**top**); The combination index (CI) increases with higher concentrations of berberine (**bottom**). Data is shown as mean ± SD from three individual experiments, each carried out in triplicates.

Table 3. AChE inhibitory activity of combinations of berberine, coptisine and palmatine. The 1st alkaloid (italics) was diluted in 1:1 steps; the 2nd alkaloid was used in a steady IC_{30} concentration. All IC values are stated in (μg/mL). A combination index (CI) < 1.0 (bold) indicates synergism. All data is shown as mean ± SD from three independent experiments, each carried out as a triplicate.

Sample	IC_{10}	IC_{20}	IC_{30}	IC_{40}	IC_{50}	IC_{60}	IC_{70}	IC_{80}	IC_{90}
Berberine	0.27	0.51	0.76	1.08	1.48	2.02	2.85	4.32	8.09
Berberine + coptisine IC_{30}	0.051	0.11	0.18	0.28	0.4	0.59	0.9	1.5	3.22
CI	**0.24**	**0.33**	**0.43**	**0.55**	**0.7**	**0.91**	1.26	1.92	3.79
Berberine + palmatine IC_{30}	0.031	0.08	0.15	0.24	0.37	0.59	0.96	1.75	4.33
CI	**0.12**	**0.18**	**0.24**	**0.29**	**0.36**	**0.47**	**0.62**	**0.92**	1.81
Berberine + coptisine IC_{30} + palmatine IC_{30}	0.027	0.066	0.12	0.19	0.31	0.48	0.78	1.42	3.47
CI	**0.14**	**0.22**	**0.32**	**0.43**	**0.62**	**0.88**	1.32	2.24	5.1
Coptisine	0.6	0.79	0.95	1.11	1.27	1.46	1.69	2.04	2.68
Coptisine + berberine IC_{30}	0.12	0.26	0.44	0.67	1	1.49	2.3	3.91	8.67
CI	**0.36**	**0.67**	1.04	1.49	2.11	2.98	4.39	7.06	14.6
Coptisine + palmatine IC_{30}	0.13	0.3	0.52	0.82	1.23	1.86	2.9	5.01	11.4
CI	**0.25**	**0.47**	**0.7**	**0.98**	1.33	1.82	2.57	3.93	7.6
Coptisine + berberine IC_{30} + palmatine IC_{30}	0.13	0.29	0.47	0.73	1.08	1.6	2.44	4.11	8.97
CI	**0.43**	**0.83**	1.25	1.83	2.59	3.67	5.37	8.63	17.8
Palmatine (μg/mL)	1.73	2.6	3.4	4.25	5.21	6.39	7.97	10.4	15.7
Palmatine + berberine IC_{30}	0.25	0.67	1.28	2.18	3.54	5.77	9.81	18.7	49.6
CI	**0.47**	1.14	2.06	3.38	5.34	8.49	14.1	26.4	68.5
Palmatine + coptisine IC_{30}	0.37	0.96	1.82	3.08	5	8.11	13.7	26.1	68.8
CI	**0.44**	**0.76**	1.1	1.49	1.97	2.6	3.54	5.13	8.99
Palmatine + berberine IC_{30} + coptisine IC_{30}	0.43	1.06	1.95	3.2	5.05	7.97	13.1	24	59.8
CI	1.27	2.92	5.19	8.33	12.9	20.12	32.7	59.2	145

The most apparent synergistic effect was found in the experiments in which coptisine and palmatine were combined with berberine (Figure 2, Table 3). Here, synergy was detected up to IC_{60} concentration of berberine combined with the IC_{30} concentration of coptisine or palmatine. At higher concentrations of berberine, FIC values between 0.5 and 1.0 indicate an additive effect.

In the experiments where coptisine and palmatine were used as 1st alkaloids synergy was only observed at very low concentrations of the 1st alkaloid. Again, FIC values decreased with increasing concentrations of the 1st alkaloid. At high concentrations of the 1st alkaloid even antagonistic effects of the alkaloids analysed were noted.

3. Discussion

Nature offers a high diversity of chemical compounds that might be beneficial as potential treatments for human diseases. Therefore, this study aimed at elucidating the potential of 80 TCM plants as inhibitors of acetylcholinesterase, a known Alzheimer target. For that purpose, inhibition of acetylcholinesterase was observed in a high-throughput enzymatic assay. Furthermore, cytotoxicity in COS7 cells was assessed and potential synergistic effects of the chemical compounds contained in the TCM plant extracts were evaluated. In contrast to other research approaches where natural products are used as lead compounds and modified synthetically [30,31] we concentrated on the question if a crude extract comprised of various constituents has benefits over the isolated single components of it.

A range of secondary plant metabolites has shown anti-cholinesterase activity including alkaloids, flavonoids and lignans with alkaloids being the largest group of ACh inhibitors [32,33]. The strong inhibitory activity of alkaloids is associated with their similarity to ACh. Many alkaloids have a positively-charged nitrogen which can bind in the gorge of active site of actetylcholinesterase [34].

Several plant drugs are used to treat deficits in memory and symptoms of AD, including *Coptis chinensis* [25,35], *Magnolia officinalis* [36–38], *Cinnamomum cassia* [39] and most commonly, *Ginkgo biloba*. Ginkgo is the most popular plant for the treatment of memory-affiliated problems although no direct anti-acetylcholinesterase activity has been observed so far. In this study none of the crude plant extracts of *Ginkgo biloba* showed any substantial AChE inhibitory activity. The same accounts for *Magnolia officinalis* with only meagre AChE inhibitory activity.

The AChE inhibitory activity of the root of *Coptis chinensis* (Coptidis rhizoma) and its isolated alkaloids has been discussed earlier [25] but the mode of action has not been described so far. Here, a distinctive anti-AChE effect was observed in all three extracts. These effects might be credited to berberine, the main alkaloid of *Coptis chinensis*, as well as the other protoberberine alkaloid coptisine and the benzo[c]phenanthridine alkaloid palmatine (Figure 3). Both the methanol and the aqueous extracts show a stronger inhibition of AChE than galantamine. Remarkably, the methanol extract exhibits an AChE inhibition that is 100-fold stronger than the one observed for galantamine. Usually plants contain a complex profile of secondary metabolites therefore the effect of a plant extract usually cannot be accredited to one single compound. Also synergistic effects have to be taken into account [17,18]. When comparing the IC_{50} values of the crude plant extracts to the IC_{50} values of the pure alkaloids berberine, coptisine and palmatine it strikes out that the methanol extract is much more active than any of the pure alkaloids tested. This suggests that not berberine alone causes the AChE inhibitory activity but rather the combination of alkaloids and other chemical compounds that apparently act synergistically. This study provides evidence that the AChE inhibitory effect of the alkaloids berberine, coptisine and palmatine is clearly synergistic (Table 3, Figure 1). The strongest synergism was observed for the combination of berberine and coptisine. Also the combination of berberine with coptisine and palmatine together produced strong synergistic effects.

LC-MS analysis indicated that in *Coptis chinensis* berberine is the main alkaloid followed by coptisine and palmatine. Therefore, it can be assumed that the strong AChE inhibition of this drug is based on synergistic action of these alkaloids. Furthermore, the methanol extract of *Coptis chinensis* has the highest concentration of alkaloids of all extracts tested, which might explain its extremely strong inhibition of AChE.

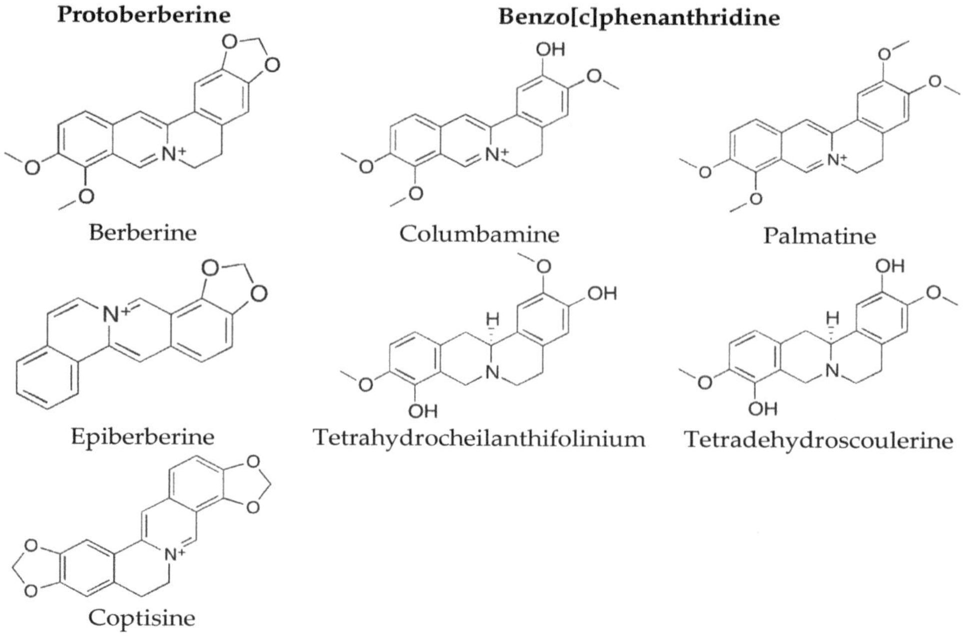

Figure 3. Alkaloids contained in *Coptis chinensis*.

Berberis bealei comprises of a variety of bioactive secondary metabolites such as protoberberine alkaloids like berberine, columbamine, jatrorrhizine and palmatine [20–24]. All three crude extracts showed an apparent inhibition of AChE. The dichloromethane extract contains the largest amount of alkaloids of the extracts of *Berberis bealei* and also shows the strongest AChE inhibitory activity. The very low IC_{50} of the dichloromethane extract points to the fact that the combination of palmatine and berberine enhances the AChE inhibition. Here, this synergistic effect of this combination is clearly proven but the presence of other compounds like flavonoids or saponins has to be taken into account as well.

The main constituents of *Phellodendron chinense* are isoquinoline alkaloids such as berberine, palmatine, jatrorrhizine and sesquiterpene lactones [28]. So far it can be stated that the active component is largely the alkaloid berberine [40]. All three extracts inhibited AChE substantially. Again, AChE inhibitory activity of these three extracts can be accredited to synergy. In all extracts berberine is the main alkaloid and the synergism experiments hint to the fact that the combination with palmatine increases the AChE inhibitory activity. Compared to *Coptis chinensis*, the AChE inhibitory activity of *Phellodendron chinense* is significantly lower which might be credited to the absence of coptisine in this extract.

Of the TCM plants analysed in this study, *Coptis chinensis, Berberis bealei* and *Phellodendron chinense* seem to be the most promising candidates for an apparent inhibition of AChE activity as all three crude plant extracts show a distinctive inhibitory effect. Most striking of all results is the finding that the methanol extract of *Coptis chinensis* exhibits a 100-fold stronger AChE inhibitory activity than the already known and widely sold AChE inhibitor galantamine, which might be due to the synergistic interaction of the individual alkaloids in this extract.

So far, no data is available about the physiological absorption rate of alkaloids contained in these extracts and it remains unclear if they can pass the blood-brain border. In vivo tests should be carried out to confirm these promising in vitro results in a mouse or rat model of Alzheimer's Disease.

These findings suggest that TCM plants represent an important source of natural compounds that affect the activity of AChE. Apart from isolating pure compounds as lead structures for novel drugs it might also be possible to administer TCM plant extracts as nutriceuticals. Furthermore, these extracts could be used as cheap alternative to other drugs in third world countries for the treatment of Alzheimer's Disease.

4. Materials and Methods

4.1. TCM Plants

All TCM plants were kindly provided by Prof. Thomas Efferth, Johannes Gutenberg University Mainz, Germany and were obtained commercially in China. Identity of the TCM plants was authenticated via DNA barcoding. All samples have accession numbers and voucher specimens were deposited at the IPMB, Department of Biology, Heidelberg University, Germany.

4.2. Chemicals

DMEM (Dulbecco's Modified Eagle's Medium) media, supplements, fetal bovine serum (FBS), trypsin-EDTA and dimethyl sulphoxide (DMSO) were purchased from Gibco Invitrogen (Karlsruhe, Germany). Berberine, coptisine, galantamine, physostigmine and palmatine were obtained from Fluka/Sigma-Aldrich (Steinheim, Germany).

4.3. DNA Barcoding

TCM plants were chosen according to their traditional use. TCM plant samples were obtained commercially. In order to authenticate the plant species, DNA barcoding was carried out to identify the respective species. The plant DNA was isolated from tissue using phenol chloroform extraction protocol [41]. A 700 bp fragment of the chloroplast marker gene rbcL was amplified using PCR.

The PCR products were sequenced and the identity of the plant species was confirmed on either the genus or the species level by comparing the respective sequence with database (NCBI) entries of authentic species.

Clustal W was used to align the sequences [42]; the genetic distances were calculated using MEGA 4.0 following the Kimura 2-Parameter (K2P) model [43]. BLAST database search was performed as described previously [44]; neighbour-joining was used for the phylogenetic tree construction [45].

4.4. Preparation of TCM Extracts

50 g finely milled TCM drugs were boiled in reflux in 500 mL of the solvent of choice (methanol, dichloromethane or water) for 6 h. The extract was then filtered through a grade 603 filter. After this, the filtrate was evaporated in a Rotavapor R-200 (Büchi, Flawil, Switzerland). The residual material was resolved in DMSO to a concentration of 50 mg/mL and stored at −20 °C until use.

4.5. Cytotoxicity / MTT Assay

COS7 (African green monkey epithelial kidney cells) cells were maintained in DMEM complete media (L-glutamine supplemented with 10% heat-inactivated fetal bovine serum, 5% penicillin/streptomycin). Cells were grown at 37 °C in a humidified atmosphere of 5% CO_2. All experiments were performed with cells in the logarithmic growth phase. Cytotoxicity of TCM extracts in COS7 cells was determined using different concentrations of extracts. MTT [3-(4,5-dimethylthiazol-2-yl)-2,5-diphenyltetrazolium bromide] was used in a colorimetric assay to determine cell viability and assess cytotoxicity [46]. All experiments were carried out in triplicates and repeated three times. The viability of the cells was determined and data are presented as the percentage of viable cells compared to the control (cells in serum-free medium) in relation to the concentration of the extract.

4.6. AChE Assay

An adapted version of the Ellmann assay [47] in 96-well plates was used to measure AChE activity. A mastermix consisting of 25 µL acetylthiocholine iodide (ACTI, 15 mM in phosphate buffer pH 7), 125 µL dithionitrobenzoic acid (DTNB, 3 mM in phosphate buffer pH 8) and 50 µL phosphate buffer (50 mM, pH 8) was prepared and added to 5 µL of TCM crude plant extract (stock 50 mg/mL) or 5 µL essential oil per well. It turned out to be crucial to prepare all reaction solutions freshly for every set of experiments. Two known AChE inhibitors, physostigmine and galantamine (50 mg/mL in phosphate buffer pH 8), served as positive controls. As all crude extracts (water, methanol, dichloromethane) were evaporated and then resolved in DMSO beforehand, DMSO was used as negative control in all experiments.

After shaking for 20 s, measurements at time t = 0, 3, 6, and 9 min were recorded at 450 nm using the EL808 plate reader (BioTek, Winooski, VT 05404, United States) to avoid interference of results due to spontaneous activity. After 9 min reading, 25 µL of acetylcholinesterase (AChE from electric eel, 3 U/mL in phosphate buffer pH 8) were added to each well and the plate was left to incubate at room temperature for 3 min. After shaking for 20 s a final reading was recorded at 450 nm. The inhibitory activity was calculated in comparison to the negative control. Potential effects were expressed as the percentage of inhibition. The experiments were carried out three times and all samples were measured three times. For the most active *Coptis chinensis* samples the experiment was carried out nine times to corroborate that the findings were correct.

4.7. Phytochemical Analysis

The most active extracts were analysed phytochemically by high performance liquid chromatography (HPLC) and mass spectrometry (MS).

HPLC: A Merck Hitachi HPLC system (Merck, Darmstadt, Germany) composed of a binary L-6200A intelligent pump and an ERC-3215α degasser was used. The extracts, with a final concentration of 500 µg/mL in methanol, were injected in the HPLC system via a Rheodyne system with a 20 µL loop. Separation was achieved using a RP-C18e Lichrospher 100 (250 mm length, 4 mm diameter column, 5 µm particle size) (Merck, Darmstadt, Germany). The mobile phase consisted of: A: Water HPLC grade with 0.5% formic acid and ammonium acetate pH = 7; B: acetonitrile. The gradient program at a flow rate of 1 mL/min as following: 0% to 40% B in 15 min, then to 100% B in 10 min, then in 5 min. back to the initial condition. A mechanical split with 10% to the MS machine and 90% as waste was used after the separation column.

MS: A Quattro II system (Waters, Eschborn, Germany) from VG with an ESI interface was used in the positive ion mode under the following conditions: Drying and nebulizing gas: N_2, capillary temperature: 120 °C; capillary voltage: 3.50 kV; lens voltage: 0.5 kV; cone voltage: 30 V. Scan mode at range m/z 300–600. Chromatograms were processed using Waters MassLynx software (Version 4.0, Waters, Eschborn, Germany).

4.8. Evaluation of Synergistic Effects

After screening the TCM crude extracts and their chemical compounds it became clear that the distinctive inhibitory effect of some of the crude extracts must be based on synergism of individual isoquinoline alkaloids in the extracts. Therefore, synergism studies were carried out with isoquinoline alkaloids berberine, coptisine and palmatine. First the IC_{30} values for all samples were calculated. For "compound A" a serial dilution was prepared and seeded to the 96-well plate. "Compound B" was added to each well at a fixed concentration that corresponded to its IC_{30} value. After this the AChE inhibition assay was carried out as described before. All possible combinations of diluted "compound A" and fixed "compound B" were analysed.

Drug interaction was classified as either synergistic, additive indifferent or antagonistic based on the fractional inhibitory concentration (FIC) index. The fractional effect (FE) of two compounds is calculated from the effect caused by two compounds in combination in relation to the effect of one compound alone: $FEa = IC_{50}(a + b)/IC_{50}(a)$; $FEb = IC_{50}(a + b)/IC_{50}(b)$. By plotting these values against each other the isobologram showing the areas of synergy is obtained.

The FIC index is the sum of both FE indexes. According to Berenbaum [48], FIC $\leq$ 1.0 signifies synergy, FIC = 1.0 an additive effect and FIC $\geq$ 1.0 antagonism. Schelz [49] regards FIC $\leq$ 0.5 as synergy, FIC > 0.5 to 1.0 as additive, FIC = 1.0 to 4.0 as indifferent and FIC $\geq$ 4.0 as antagonism. We were following the second perspective.

4.9. Statistical Analysis

All experiments were carried out in triplicates and repeated at three individual days. All data are expressed as mean ± standard deviation ($n = 3$). The IC_{50} values were calculated using a four-parameter logistic curve (SigmaPlot® 11.0) representing 50% reduction of activity. Statistical analysis of the effects of increasing concentrations of samples on the viability of COS7 cells and activity of AChE was performed using Student's t-test in SigmaPlot® 11.0 (Systat, Erkrath, Germany) to determine significance of the difference between two data sets. The significance level of $p < 0.05$ denotes significance for all cytotoxicity and AChE experiments.

5. Conclusions

Various plant-derived compounds are already used for the treatments of Alzheimer's Disease indicating that nature is a valuable source of new bioactive agents. We tested various plants from Traditional Chinese Medicine for their potential inhibition of AChE activity. Based on our results it can be stated that some TCM plants inhibit AChE via synergistic interaction of their secondary metabolites. The possibility to isolate pure lead compounds from the crude extracts or to administer these as nutraceuticals or as cheap alternative to drugs in third world countries make TCM plants a versatile source of natural inhibitors of AChE.

Acknowledgments: This research received no specific grant from any funding agency in the public, commercial or not-for-profit sectors.

Author Contributions: D.K., A.T., F.H. and M.W. conceived and designed the experiments; D.K., A.K.D., A.T., and F.H. performed the experiments; D.K., A.K.D., A.T., and F.H. analyzed the data; D.K. wrote the paper.

References

1. Alzheimer's Disease International. *World Alzheimer Report 2015*. Available online: https://www.alz.co.uk/research/WorldAlzheimerReport2015.pdf (accessed on 10 August 2016).
2. Czech, C.; Tremp, G.; Pradier, L. Presenilins and Alzheimer's disease: Biological functions and pathogenic mechanisms. *Prog. Neurobiol.* **2000**, *60*, 363–384. [CrossRef]
3. Cummings, J.L. Cognitive and behavioral heterogeneity in Alzheimer's disease: Seeking the neurobiological basis. *Neurobiol. Aging* **2000**, *21*, 845–861. [CrossRef]
4. Bartus, R.T.; Dean, R.L., 3rd; Beer, B.; Lippa, A.S. The cholinergic hypothesis of geriatric memory dysfunction. *Science* **1982**, *217*, 408–414. [CrossRef] [PubMed]
5. Perry, E.K.; Perry, R.H.; Blessed, G.; Tomlinson, B.E. Changes in brain cholinesterases in senile dementia of Alzheimer type. *Neuropathol. Appl. Neurobiol.* **1978**, *4*, 273–277. [CrossRef] [PubMed]
6. Courtney, C.; Farrell, D.; Gray, R.; Hills, R.; Lynch, L.; Sellwood, E.; Edwards, S.; Hardyman, W.; Raftery, J.; Crome, P.; et al. Long-term donepezil treatment in 565 patients with Alzheimer's disease (AD2000): Randomised double-blind trial. *Lancet* **2004**, *363*, 2105–2115. [PubMed]
7. Giacobini, E. Modulation of brain acetylcholine levels with cholinesterase inhibitors as a treatment of Alzheimer disease. *Keio J. Med.* **1987**, *36*, 381–391. [CrossRef] [PubMed]
8. Munoz-Torrero, D. Acetylcholinesterase inhibitors as disease-modifying therapies for Alzheimer's disease. *Curr. Med. Chem.* **2008**, *15*, 2433–2455. [CrossRef] [PubMed]
9. Sabbagh, M.N.; Farlow, M.R.; Relkin, N.; Beach, T.G. Do cholinergic therapies have disease-modifying effects in Alzheimer's disease? *Alzheimer's Dement.* **2006**, *2*, 118–125. [CrossRef] [PubMed]
10. Zemek, F.; Drtinova, L.; Nepovimova, E.; Sepsova, V.; Korabecny, J.; Klimes, J.; Kuca, K. Outcomes of Alzheimer's disease therapy with acetylcholinesterase inhibitors and memantine. *Expert Opin. Drug Saf.* **2014**, *13*, 759–774. [PubMed]
11. Ehret, M.J.; Chamberlin, K.W. Current Practices in the Treatment of Alzheimer Disease: Where is the Evidence After the Phase III Trials? *Clin. Ther.* **2015**, *37*, 1604–1616. [CrossRef] [PubMed]

12. Adams, M.; Gmunder, F.; Hamburger, M. Plants traditionally used in age related brain disorders—A survey of ethnobotanical literature. *J. Ethnopharmacol.* **2007**, *113*, 363–381. [CrossRef] [PubMed]
13. Wollen, K.A. Alzheimer's disease: The pros and cons of pharmaceutical, nutritional, botanical, and stimulatory therapies, with a discussion of treatment strategies from the perspective of patients and practitioners. *Altern. Med. Rev.* **2010**, *15*, 223–244. [PubMed]
14. Hostettmann, K.; Borloz, A.; Urbain, A.; Marston, A. Natural product inhibitors of acetylcholinesterase. *Curr. Org. Chem.* **2006**, *10*, 825–847. [CrossRef]
15. Tundis, R.; Bonesi, M.; Menichini, F.; Loizzo, M.R. Recent Knowledge on Medicinal Plants as Source of Cholinesterase Inhibitors for the Treatment of Dementia. *Mini Rev. Med. Chem.* **2015**, *16*, 605–618. [CrossRef]
16. Kaufmann, D.; Kaur Dogra, A.; Wink, M. Myrtenal inhibits acetylcholinesterase, a known Alzheimer target. *J. Pharm. Pharmacol.* **2011**, *63*, 1368–1371. [CrossRef] [PubMed]
17. Wink, M. Evolutionary advantage and molecular modes of action of multi-component mixtures used in phytomedicine. *Curr. Drug Metab.* **2008**, *9*, 996–1009. [CrossRef] [PubMed]
18. Wink, M. Modes of Action of Herbal Medicines and Plant Secondary Metabolites. *Medicines* **2015**, *2*, 251–286. [CrossRef]
19. Main, A.R.; Hastings, F.L. Carbamylation and binding constants for the inhibition of acetylcholinesterase by physostigmine (eserine). *Science* **1966**, *154*, 400–402. [CrossRef] [PubMed]
20. Li, A.R.; Zhu, Y.; Li, X.N.; Tian, X.J. Antimicrobial activity of four species of Berberidaceae. *Fitoterapia* **2007**, *78*, 379–381. [CrossRef] [PubMed]
21. Zeng, X.; Dong, Y.; Sheng, G.; Dong, X.; Sun, X.; Fu, J. Isolation and structure determination of anti-influenza component from *Mahonia Bealei*. *J. Ethnopharmacol.* **2006**, *108*, 317–319. [CrossRef] [PubMed]
22. Jiang, Y.L.; Wang, X.L.; Xue, S.G. Extraction of berberine hydrochloride from *Mahonia bealei* (Fort.) Carr. *Zhongguo Zhong Yao Za Zhi* **1993**, *18*, 347–348. [PubMed]
23. Zhao, T.F.; Wang, X.K.; Rimando, A.M.; Che, C.T. Folkloric medicinal plants: *Tinospora sagittata var. cravaniana* and *Mahonia bealei*. *Planta Med.* **1991**, *57*, 505–505. [CrossRef] [PubMed]
24. Ji, X.; Li, Y.; Liu, H.; Yan, Y.; Li, J. Determination of the alkaloid content in different parts of some *Mahonia* plants by HPCE. *Pharm. Acta Helv.* **2000**, *74*, 387–391. [CrossRef]
25. Jung, H.A.; Min, B.S.; Yokozawa, T.; Lee, J.H.; Kim, Y.S.; Choi, J.S. Anti-Alzheimer and antioxidant activities of Coptidis Rhizoma alkaloids. *Biol. Pharm. Bull.* **2009**, *32*, 1433–1438. [CrossRef] [PubMed]
26. Jung, H.A.; Yoon, N.Y.; Bae, H.J.; Min, B.S.; Choi, J.S. Inhibitory activities of the alkaloids from Coptidis Rhizoma against aldose reductase. *Arch. Pharm. Res.* **2008**, *31*, 1405–1412. [CrossRef] [PubMed]
27. Ma, B.L.; Ma, Y.M.; Shi, R.; Wang, T.M.; Zhang, N.; Wang, C.H.; Yang, Y. Identification of the toxic constituents in Rhizoma Coptidis. *J. Ethnopharmacol.* **2010**, *128*, 357–364. [CrossRef] [PubMed]
28. Van Wyk, B.E.; Wink, M. The plants in alphabetical order. In *Medicinal Plants of the World*, 1st ed.; Timber Press: London, UK, 2004; p. 238.
29. Wink, M. Plant secondary metabolism: Diversity, function and its evolution. *Nat. Prod. Commun.* **2008**, *3*, 1205–1216.
30. Lemes, L.F.; de Andrade Ramos, G.; de Oliveira, A.S.; da Silva, F.M.; de Castro Couto, G.; da Silva Boni, M.; Guimaraes, M.J.; Souza, I.N.; Bartolini, M.; Andrisano, V.; et al. Cardanol-derived AChE inhibitors: Towards the development of dual binding derivatives for Alzheimer's disease. *Eur. J. Med. Chem.* **2016**, *108*, 687–700. [CrossRef] [PubMed]
31. Bukhari, S.N.; Jantan, I. Synthetic Curcumin Analogs as Inhibitors of beta-Amyloid Peptide Aggregation: Potential Therapeutic and Diagnostic Agents for Alzheimer's Disease. *Mini Rev. Med. Chem.* **2015**, *15*, 1110–1121. [CrossRef] [PubMed]
32. Hung, T.M.; Na, M.; Dat, N.T.; Ngoc, T.M.; Youn, U.; Kim, H.J.; Min, B.S.; Lee, J.; Bae, K. Cholinesterase inhibitory and anti-amnesic activity of alkaloids from *Corydalis turtschaninovii*. *J. Ethnopharmacol.* **2008**, *119*, 74–80. [CrossRef] [PubMed]
33. Jung, M.; Park, M. Acetylcholinesterase inhibition by flavonoids from *Agrimonia pilosa*. *Molecules* **2007**, *12*, 2130–2139. [CrossRef] [PubMed]
34. Houghton, P.J.; Ren, Y.; Howes, M.J. Acetylcholinesterase inhibitors from plants and fungi. *Nat. Prod. Rep.* **2006**, *23*, 181–199. [CrossRef] [PubMed]
35. Durairajan, S.S.; Liu, L.F.; Lu, J.H.; Chen, L.L.; Yuan, Q.; Chung, S.K.; Huang, L.; Li, X.S.; Huang, J.D.; Li, M. Berberine ameliorates beta-amyloid pathology, gliosis, and cognitive impairment in an Alzheimer's disease transgenic mouse model. *Neurobiol. Aging* **2012**, *33*, 2903–2919. [CrossRef] [PubMed]

36. Zhong, W.B.; Wang, C.Y.; Ho, K.J.; Lu, F.J.; Chang, T.C.; Lee, W.S. Magnolol induces apoptosis in human leukemia cells via cytochrome c release and caspase activation. *Anticancer Drugs* **2003**, *14*, 211–217. [CrossRef] [PubMed]
37. Lee, J.W.; Lee, Y.K.; Lee, B.J.; Nam, S.Y.; Lee, S.I.; Kim, Y.H.; Kim, K.H.; Oh, K.W.; Hong, J.T. Inhibitory effect of ethanol extract of *Magnolia officinalis* and 4-*O*-methylhonokiol on memory impairment and neuronal toxicity induced by beta-amyloid. *Pharmacol. Biochem. Behav.* **2010**, *95*, 31–40. [CrossRef] [PubMed]
38. Lee, Y.J.; Choi, D.Y.; Han, S.B.; Kim, Y.H.; Kim, K.H.; Hwang, B.Y.; Kang, J.K.; Lee, B.J.; Oh, K.W.; Hong, J.T. Inhibitory effect of ethanol extract of *Magnolia officinalis* on memory impairment and amyloidogenesis in a transgenic mouse model of Alzheimer's disease via regulating beta-secretase activity. *Phytother. Res.* **2012**, *26*, 1884–1892. [CrossRef] [PubMed]
39. Shimada, Y.; Goto, H.; Kogure, T.; Kohta, K.; Shintani, T.; Itoh, T.; Terasawa, K. Extract prepared from the bark of *Cinnamomum cassia* Blume prevents glutamate-induced neuronal death in cultured cerebellar granule cells. *Phytother. Res.* **2000**, *14*, 466–468. [CrossRef]
40. Schmeller, T.; Latz-Bruning, B.; Wink, M. Biochemical activities of berberine, palmatine and sanguinarine mediating chemical defence against microorganisms and herbivores. *Phytochemistry* **1997**, *44*, 257–266. [CrossRef]
41. Doyle, J.J.; Doyle, J.L. Isolation of plant DNA from fresh tissue. *Focus* **1990**, *12*, 13–15.
42. Thompson, J.D.; Higgins, D.G.; Gibson, T.J. CLUSTAL W: Improving the sensitivity of progressive multiple sequence alignment through sequence weighting, position-specific gap penalties and weight matrix choice. *Nucleic Acids Res.* **1994**, *22*, 4673–4680. [CrossRef] [PubMed]
43. Tamura, K.; Dudley, J.; Nei, M.; Kumar, S. MEGA4: Molecular Evolutionary Genetics Analysis (MEGA) software version 4.0. *Mol. Biol. Evol.* **2007**, *24*, 1596–1599. [CrossRef] [PubMed]
44. Altschul, S.F.; Gish, W.; Miller, W.; Myers, E.W.; Lipman, D.J. Basic local alignment search tool. *J. Mol. Biol.* **1990**, *215*, 403–410. [CrossRef]
45. Saitou, N.; Nei, M. The neighbor-joining method: A new method for reconstructing phylogenetic trees. *Mol. Biol. Evol.* **1987**, *4*, 406–425. [PubMed]
46. Mosmann, T. Rapid colorimetric assay for cellular growth and survival: Application to proliferation and cytotoxicity assays. *J. Immunol. Methods* **1983**, *65*, 55–63. [CrossRef]
47. Ellman, G.L.; Courtney, K.D.; Andres, V., Jr.; Feather-Stone, R.M. A new and rapid colorimetric determination of acetylcholinesterase activity. *Biochem. Pharmacol.* **1961**, *7*, 88–95. [CrossRef]
48. Berenbaum, M.C. What is synergy? *Pharmacol. Rev.* **1989**, *41*, 93–141. [PubMed]
49. Schelz, Z.; Molnar, J.; Hohmann, J. Antimicrobial and antiplasmid activities of essential oils. *Fitoterapia* **2006**, *77*, 279–285. [CrossRef] [PubMed]

5

The Suppressive Effects of Cinnamomi Cortex and its Phytocompound Coumarin on Oxaliplatin-Induced Neuropathic Cold Allodynia in Rats

Changmin Kim [1,†], Ji Hwan Lee [2,†], Woojin Kim [1], Dongxing Li [3], Yangseok Kim [1], Kyungjin Lee [4,*] and Sun Kwang Kim [1,2,*]

1 Department of Physiology, College of Korean Medicine, Kyung Hee University, 26 Kyunghee-daero, Dongdamoon-gu, Seoul 02447, Korea; ckdals4302@naver.com (C.K.); thasnow@gmail.com (W.K.); yskim1158@khu.ac.kr (Y.K.)

2 Department of Science in Korean Medicine, Graduate School, Kyung Hee University, 26 Kyunghee-daero, Dongdamoon-gu, Seoul 02447, Korea; mibdna@gmail.com

3 Department of Anesthesiology, Renji Hospital, School of Medicine, Shanghai Jiaotong University, 573 Xujiahui Rd., Dapiqiao, Huangpu Qu, Shanghai 200025, China; leedongxing@naver.com

4 Department of Herbology, College of Korean Medicine, Kyung Hee University, 26 Kyunghee-daero, Dongdamoon-gu, Seoul 02447, Korea

* Correspondence: niceday@khu.ac.kr (K.L.); skkim77@khu.ac.kr (S.K.K.)

† These authors contributed equally to this work.

Academic Editor: Luigia Trabace

Abstract: Oxaliplatin, a chemotherapy drug, induces acute peripheral neuropathy characterized by cold allodynia, spinal glial activation and increased levels of pro-inflammatory cytokines. Herein, we determined whether Cinnamomi Cortex (C. Cortex), a widely used medicinal herb in East Asia for cold-related diseases, could attenuate oxaliplatin-induced cold allodynia in rats and the mechanisms involved. A single oxaliplatin injection (6 mg/kg, i.p.) induced significant cold allodynia signs based on tail immersion tests using cold water (4 °C). Daily oral administration of water extract of C. Cortex (WECC) (100, 200, and 400 mg/kg) for five consecutive days following an oxaliplatin injection dose-dependently alleviated cold allodynia with only a slight difference in efficacies between the middle dose at 200 mg/kg and the highest dose at 400 mg/kg. WECC at 200 mg/kg significantly suppressed the activation of astrocytes and microglia and decreased the expression levels of IL-1β and TNF in the spinal cord after injection with oxaliplatin. Furthermore, oral administration of coumarin (10 mg/kg), a major phytocompound of C. Cortex, markedly reduced cold allodynia. These results indicate that C. Cortex has a potent anti-allodynic effect in oxaliplatin-injected rats through inhibiting spinal glial cells and pro-inflammatory cytokines. We also suggest that coumarin might play a role in the anti-allodynic effect of C. Cortex.

Keywords: Cinnamomi Cortex; cold allodynia; coumarin; glia; spinal cord; pro-inflammatory cytokines

---

1. Introduction

Oxaliplatin, a third-generation platinum-based chemotherapy drug, displays anti-tumor activity against a wide range of tumors, including ovarian, breast, lung, and advanced colorectal cancers [1–3]. Unlike other platinum compounds (e.g., cisplatin and carboplatin), oxaliplatin rarely exhibits nephrotoxicity or hematotoxicity [4]. However, even a single injection of oxaliplatin can cause peripheral neuropathy manifesting as paresthesia and dysesthesia in the extremities. This peripheral neuropathy can be triggered or enhanced by exposure to cold [5,6]. The accurate mechanism involved in oxaliplatin-induced peripheral neuropathy remains unclear. An effective treatment method for neuropathic allodynia needs to be developed [7].

Glial cells are known to play an important role in neuropathic pain [8,9]. Once damage in the periphery or the dorsal horn of the spinal cord occurs, glial cells such as microglia and astrocytes become activated [10,11] and proliferate in number [8,12]. Recently, some articles have demonstrated that pharmacological treatments can effectively reduce neuropathic pain by preventing glial cell activation [13,14]. In an oxaliplatin-induced neuropathic pain model, the decrease of augmented spinal astrocytes and microglia by fluorocitrate and minocycline has been reported to attenuate pain [10]. Glia cells contribute to neuropathic pain by releasing various nociceptive mediators including pro-inflammatory cytokines, such as IL-1β and TNF [15–17]. Moreover, in our previous experiment conducted with oxaliplatin-induced neuropathic pain in rats, increased activation of spinal astrocytes and microglia [18] as well as increased levels of spinal TNF were observed [19].

Cinnamomi Cortex (C. Cortex; *Cinnamomum cassia* Presl in family Lauraceae) is classified as a medicinal herb for treating various cold related diseases such as common cold and influenza in oriental medicine. Using various human and animal models, extracts of C. Cortex have been found to be able to effectively attenuate influenza virus [20], inflammations [21], human platelet aggregation and arachidonic acid metabolism [22]. In our previous study [18], Gyejigachulbu-tang (GBT), a decoction comprising seven different medicinal herbs (Cinnamomi Cortex, Paeoniae Radix, Atractylodis Rhizoma, Zizyphi Fructus, Glycyrrhizae Radix, Zingiberis Rhizoma, and Aconiti Tuber) could effectively attenuate oxaliplatin-induced neuropathic pain. GBT also suppressed the activation of spinal glia and the up-regulation of pro-inflammatory cytokines. However, which medicinal herb plays a major role in the analgesic effect of GBT has not yet been determined.

Accordingly, in this study, we investigated whether C. Cortex, when administered alone, could attenuate oxaliplatin-induced cold allodynia in rats. We also examined whether C. Cortex could modulate the activation of astrocytes and microglia in the spinal cord and suppress the upregulation of pro-inflammatory cytokines such as IL-1β and TNF after oxaliplatin injection. Finally, we assessed whether coumarin, a major phytocompound of C. Cortex, could alleviate oxaliplatin-induced neuropathic pain.

2. Results

2.1. Suppresive Effect of WECC on Oxaliplatin-Induced Cold Allodynia in Rats

A single injection of oxaliplatin (6 mg/kg, intraperitoneal; i.p.) induced cold allodynia in rats whereas vehicle control (5% glucose) did not. Cold allodynia was assessed using tail immersion test by measuring tail withdrawal latency (TWL) to cold water (4 °C) stimuli [23]. As shown in Figure 1, the TWL in oxaliplatin-injected rats was significantly decreased compared to that in vehicle-injected control rats from day 3 to day 5. To evaluate the suppressive effect of C. Cortex on oxaliplatin-induced cold allodynia, water extract of C. Cortex (WECC) at three different doses (100, 200, and 400 mg/kg) was orally administered every day for five consecutive days after the oxaliplatin injection. Behavioral tests were performed before oxaliplatin injection and every 24 h after the administration of WECC or phosphate-buffered saline (PBS). WECC dose-dependently attenuated oxaliplatin-induced cold allodynia. The lowest dose of WECC at 100 mg/kg showed a significant effect only at day 4, whereas WECC at 200 and 400 mg/kg had potent analgesic effects from three to five days after the oxaliplatin injection with only slight difference in efficacies between the two doses (Figure 1). In addition, WECC at 200 mg/kg showed a significant suppressive effect against mechanical allodynia at day 5 (Figure S1).

2.2. Inhibitory Effect of WECC Treatment on Activation of Spinal Astrocytes

At the end of behavioral experiments, spinal cord sections were obtained from animals in Vehicle + PBS, Vehicle + 200 mg/kg WECC, Oxaliplatin + PBS, and Oxaliplatin + 200 mg/kg WECC groups and processed for immunohistochemical analyses of astrocytic activation (Figure 2). Statistical differences in the number of astrocytes (GFAP positive cells) in the spinal dorsal horn laminae I–II were found between oxaliplatin-injected rats and vehicle-injected rats (Vehicle + PBS vs. Oxa + PBS; $p < 0.001$). WECC at 200 mg/kg failed to change the number of spinal astrocytes in vehicle-injected rats (Vehicle + PBS vs. Vehicle + 200 mg/kg WECC; $p > 0.05$). However, it significantly decreased the number of spinal astrocytes in oxaliplatin-injected rats (Oxa + PBS vs. Oxa + 200 mg/kg WECC; $p < 0.001$).

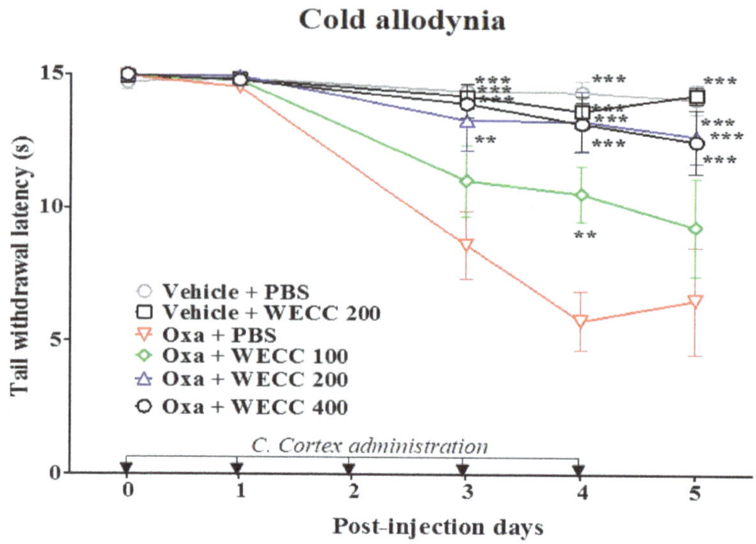

Figure 1. Effect of WECC in relieving oxaliplatin-induced cold allodynia in rats. Animals were randomly divided into five groups ($n = 6$ per group). Oxaliplatin (Oxa) or 5% glucose (Vehicle) was administered intraperitoneally at day 0. WECC (100, 200, and 400 mg/kg) or PBS was administered orally for five consecutive days after injection of oxaliplatin or vehicle control. Data are presented as mean ± S.E.M.; ** $p < 0.01$, *** $p < 0.001$ vs. Oxa + PBS by two-way ANOVA followed by Bonferroni's post-test.

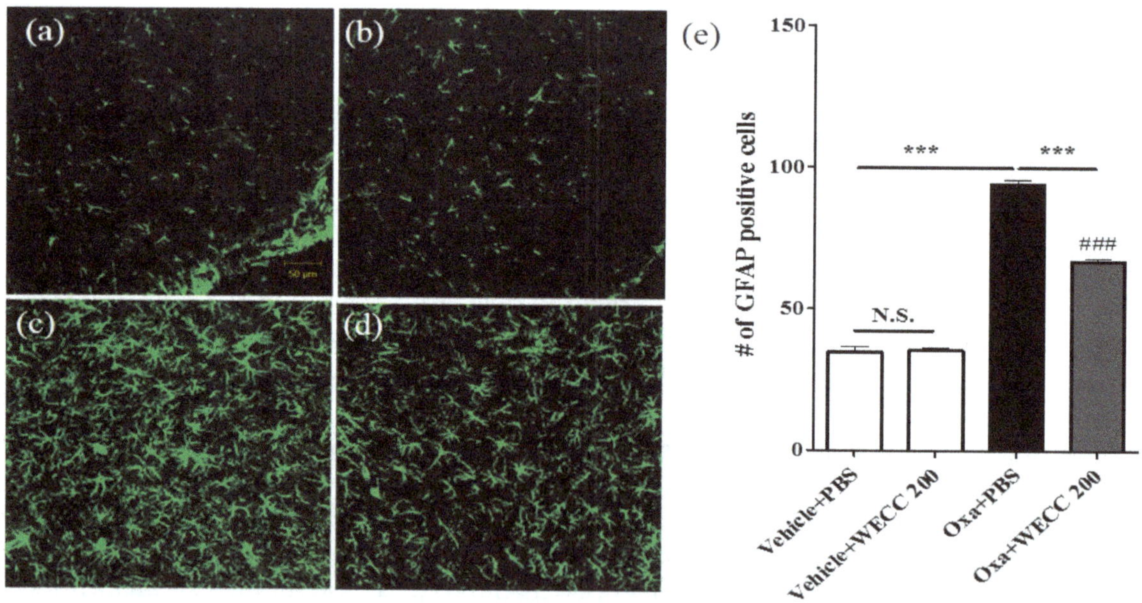

Figure 2. Immunohistochemical analyses of spinal astrocytes. Representative images of GFAP positive cells (astrocytes) in the spinal dorsal horn of Vehicle + PBS (**a**); Vehicle + 200 mg/kg WECC (**b**); Oxa + PBS (**c**); and Oxa + 200 mg/kg WECC (**d**) groups; (**e**) Quantification results of GFAP positive cells in the four groups. $n = 6$ per group. Data are presented as mean ± SEM. N.S.: non-significant; *** $p < 0.001$ vs. indicated group; ### $p < 0.001$ vs. Vehicle + PBS by one-way ANOVA followed by Bonferroni's post-test.

2.3. Inhibitory Effect of WECC Treatment on Spinal Microglia Activation

After the final assessment of cold allodynia, the spinal cord sections from animals in vehicle + PBS, vehicle + 200 mg/kg WECC, oxaliplatin + PBS, and oxaliplatin + 200 mg/kg WECC groups were obtained for histological examination (Figure 3). Statistical differences in the number of microglia (Iba-1 positive cells) in the spinal dorsal horn laminae I–II were found between oxaliplatin-injected rats and vehicle-injected rats (Vehicle + PBS vs. Oxa + PBS; $p < 0.001$). WECC failed to change the number of spinal microglia in vehicle-injected rats (Vehicle + PBS vs. Vehicle + 200 mg/kg WECC; $p > 0.05$). However, it significantly decreased the number of spinal microglia in oxaliplatin-injected rats (Oxa + PBS vs. Oxa + 200 mg/kg WECC; $p < 0.001$).

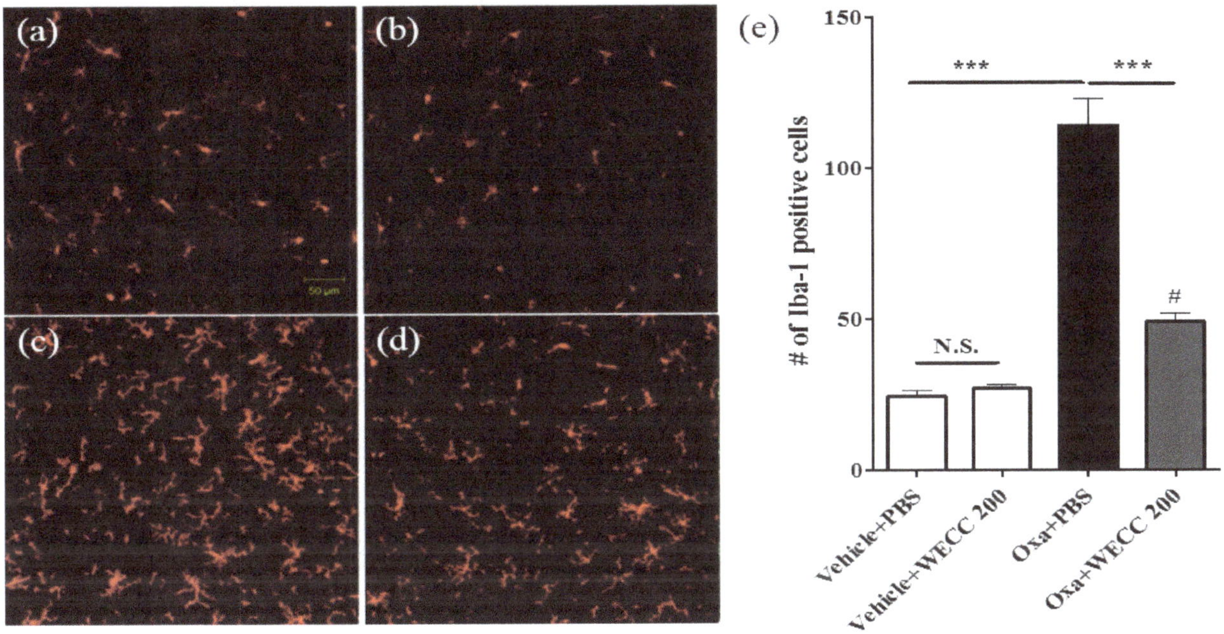

Figure 3. Immunohistochemical analyses of spinal microglia. Representative images of Iba-1 positive cells (microglia) in the spinal dorsal horn of Vehicle + PBS (**a**); Vehicle + 200 mg/kg WECC (**b**); Oxa + PBS (**c**); and Oxa + 200 mg/kg WECC (**d**) groups; (**e**) Quantification results of Iba-1 positive cells in the four groups. $n = 6$ per group. Data are presented as mean ± S.E.M. N.S.: non-significant; *** $p < 0.001$ vs. indicated group; # $p < 0.05$ vs. Vehicle + PBS by one-way ANOVA followed by Bonferroni's post-test.

2.4. Modulatory Effect of WECC on Pro-Inflammatory Cytokines IL-1β and TNF

To investigate whether C. Cortex could modulate pro-inflammatory cytokines IL-1β and TNF in the spinal cord, an enzyme-linked immunosorbent assay (ELISA) was used to measure the levels of cytokines IL-1β and TNF (Figure 4). A single oxaliplatin injection markedly increased spinal IL-1β levels compared to vehicle control injection (Figure 4a, Oxa + PBS vs. Vehicle + PBS; $p < 0.01$). Administration of WECC at 200 mg/kg significantly reduced spinal IL-1β levels compared to PBS administration in oxaliplatin-injected rats (Figure 4a, Oxa + PBS vs. Oxa + 200 mg/kg WECC; $p < 0.05$). Oxaliplatin also significantly increased spinal TNF levels compared to vehicle control (Figure 4b, Oxa + PBS vs. Vehicle + PBS; $p < 0.05$). The levels of TNF were significantly reduced by WECC at 200 mg/kg (Figure 4b, Oxa + PBS vs. Oxa + 200 mg/kg WECC; $p < 0.05$). WECC failed to significantly change the levels of spinal IL-1β or TNF in vehicle-injected rats (Figure 4a or Figure 4b, Vehicle + PBS vs. Vehicle + 200 mg/kg; $p > 0.05$). These results indicate that C. Cortex can reduce the levels of pro-inflammatory cytokines IL-1β and TNF in the spinal cord increased by injection of oxaliplatin.

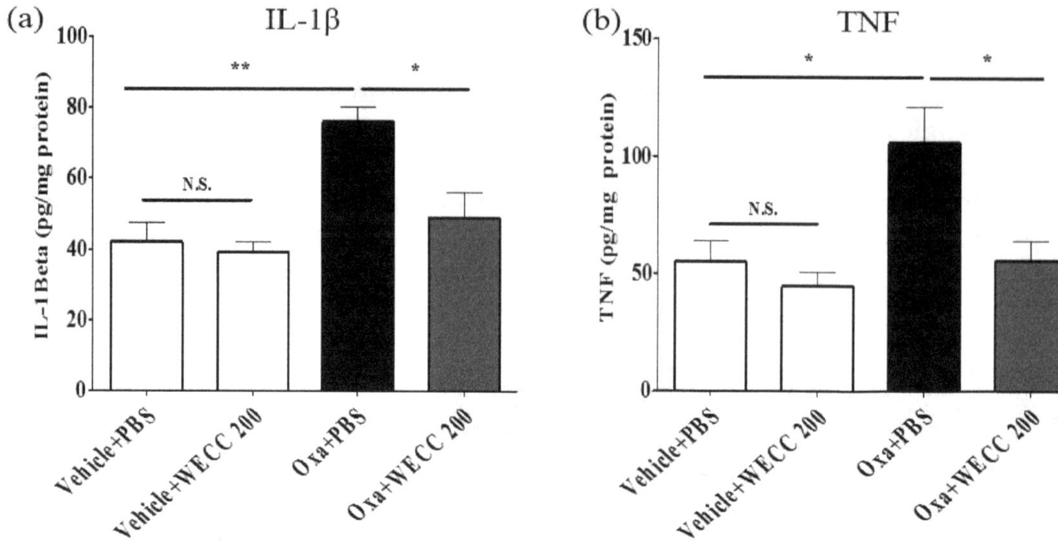

Figure 4. Inhibitory effect of WECC on spinal pro-inflammatory cytokines. Levels of IL-1β (**a**) and TNF (**b**) in the spinal cord were measured with ELISA. Vehicle and oxaliplatin were administered intraperitoneally. PBS and 200 mg/kg of WECC were administered orally. $n = 6$ per group. Data are presented as mean ± SEM. N.S.: non-significant; * $p < 0.05$; ** $p < 0.01$ by one-way ANOVA followed by Bonferroni's post-test.

2.5. *Qualitative and Quantitative Analysis of Three Chemicals in WECC*

The retention times of coumarin, cinnamic acid, and cinnamaldehyde in WECC were 2.430, 3.500, and 4.922 min, respectively (Figure 5a). The regression equation of the three compounds and their correlation coefficients (r^2) were estimated based on the plots of peak-area (y) versus concentration (x). For coumarin, the regression equation was $y = 0.0013x + 8.7147$ ($r^2 = 0.9987$). For cinnamic acid, it was $y = 0.0047x - 0.5087$ ($r^2 = 0.9992$). For cinnamaldehyde, it was $y = 0.0058x - 0.0110$ ($r^2 = 1.0000$). The contents of coumarin, cinnamic acid, and cinnamaldehyde in WECC were 1.468%, 0.226%, and 0.027%, respectively (Figure 5b).

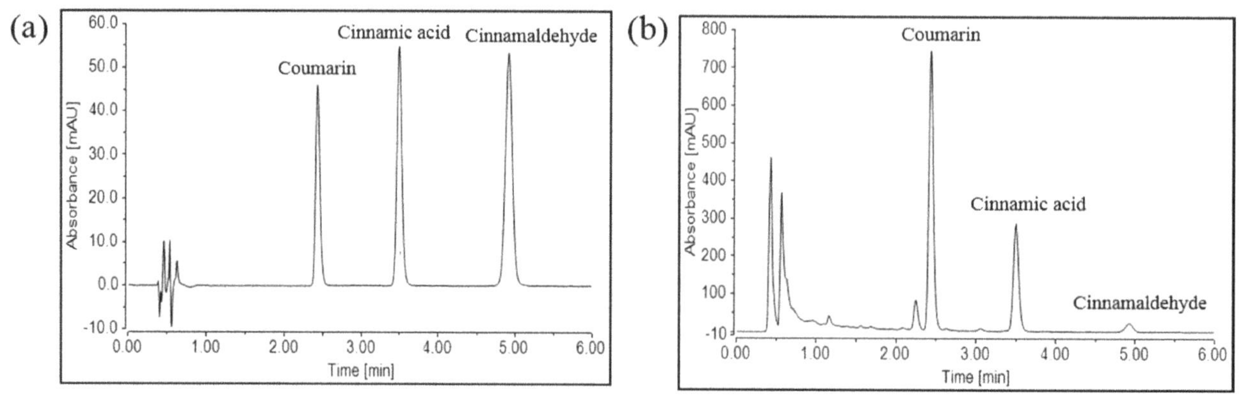

Figure 5. Quantification of chemicals in WECC using UHPLC. UHPLC chromatograms of three standards (**a**) and WECC (**b**). The three peaks represented coumarin (2.430 min, $y = 0.0013x + 8.7147$, $r^2 = 0.9987$), cinnamic acid (3.500 min, $y = 0.0047x - 0.5087$, $r^2 = 0.9992$), and cinnamaldehyde (4.922 min, $y = 0.0058x - 0.0110$, $r^2 = 1.0000$) sequentially.

2.6. *Anti-Allodynic Effect of Coumarin on Oxaliplatin-Induced Cold Allodynia in Rats*

A previous study [24] reported that coumarin at 10 mg/kg has the most effective antinociceptive action, as our preliminary study has confirmed in a rat model of oxaliplatin-induced cold allodynia.

In the present study, we thus tested the anti-allodynic effect of 10 mg/kg coumarin, a major chemical component of C. Cortex, by conducting tail immersion test. Results are shown in Figure 6. Coumarin (10 mg/kg) orally administered in vehicle (5% glucose) injected rats did not have any significant anti-allodynic effect (Vehicle + coumarin vs. Vehicle + PBS; $p > 0.05$). However, the same dose of coumarin significantly increased the TWL compared to PBS control in oxaliplatin-injected rats (Oxa + coumarin vs. Oxa + PBS; $p < 0.001$). The significant anti-allodynic effect of coumarin started at day 3 and lasted until day 5 after a single injection with oxaliplatin. In addition, coumarin slightly increased mechanical threshold in oxaliplatin-injected rats, although no significant difference was observed between the coumarin group and PBS control group (Figure S1).

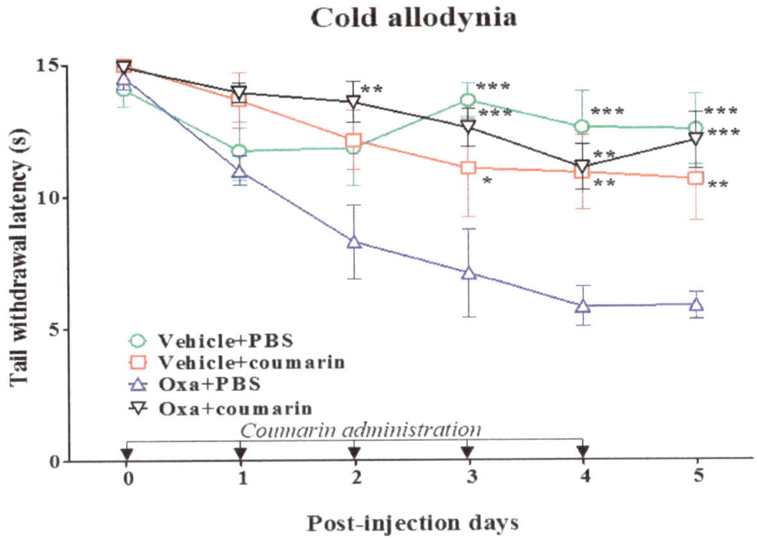

Figure 6. Anti-allodynic effect of coumarin on oxaliplatin-induced cold allodynia in rats. Animals were randomly divided into four groups ($n = 6$ per group). Oxaliplatin or vehicle (5% glucose) was administered intraperitoneally on day 0. Coumarin (10 mg/kg) or PBS was administered orally for five consecutive days after injection with oxaliplatin or vehicle control. Data are presented as mean ± S.E.M.; * $p < 0.05$, ** $p < 0.01$, *** $p < 0.001$ vs. Oxa + PBS by two-way ANOVA followed by Bonferroni's post-test.

3. Discussion

Oxaliplatin is a widely used chemotherapeutic agent. About 85% to 95% of oxaliplatin-treated patients rapidly develop significant pain without motor dysfunction, peaking at the first 24–48 h following the oxaliplatin injection [25,26]. This side effect can limit the use of this drug and lead to cessation of the treatment. However, the mechanism of oxaliplatin-induced peripheral neuropathy is not clearly understood yet. Analgesics currently used as first-line treatment also have side effects such as sedation, dizziness, and cardiac complications [27,28]. Thus, a novel treatment method is urgently needed.

Recently, deactivation of spinal astrocytes or microglia has been considered as a new pharmacological target for neuropathic pain relief [10,29]. In various models of neuropathic pain, glial activation has been reported to contribute to neuropathic pain by releasing pro-inflammatory cytokines [30]. Once activated after peripheral nerve injury, glia cells such as astrocytes and microglia can release a plethora of pro-inflammatory mediators such as IL-1β and TNF [31,32] involved in the process of nociceptor hypersensitivity [33]. In an injured sciatic nerve animal model, mRNA and protein levels of IL-1β and TNF are rapidly up-regulated, and mice lacking both IL-1 type 1 receptor and TNF type 1 receptor have lower nociceptive sensitivity compared to wild-type littermates after injury [34]. IL-1β up-regulation following nerve injury contributes to pain hypersensitivity through mediating the induction of Cox-2 in the central nervous system (CNS) [35]. TNF, a major pro-inflammatory cytokine, has been associated with both immediate and ongoing stages of neuropathic pain. TNF applications are associated with induction of thermal hyperalgesia and mechanical allodynia [36,37]. Moreover, intrathecal injection of minocycline or fluorocitrate that decreases the activation of microglia or astrocytes effectively attenuates oxaliplatin-induced neuropathic pain [10].

In our previous articles [18,19], we have shown that spinal glia and pro-inflammatory cytokines are up-regulated after a single injection with oxaliplatin. We also demonstrated that GBT, a mixture comprising seven different medicinal herbs including C. Cortex based on the *Sang Han Lun* and later modified in Japan [38], could alleviate neuropathic pain induced by oxaliplatin injection through suppressing the activation of spinal astrocytes and microglia and decreasing the levels of spinal TNF. However, a traditional formula of GBT contains Cinnamomi ramulus (C. Ramulus) instead of C. Cortex. Both C. Cortex and C. Ramulus originate from cinnamon. They are commonly used as traditional medicine for treating dyspepsia, gastritis, blood circulation issues, and inflammatory disease [39]. C. Ramulus is the twig of cinnamon while C. Cortex is the bark of cinnamon. Although the analgesic efficacies of C. Cortex and C. Ramulus for pain have been reported in several articles [40–42], we found that C. Ramulus did not significantly attenuate cold allodynia induced by oxaliplatin injection (Figure S2). In oriental medicine, different parts of the same plant are considered as distinct medicinal herbs having separate characteristics [43].

In this study, we clearly demonstrated that C. Cortex, one traditional medicinal herb generally used to treat cold related diseases such as common cold and influenza, could alleviate cold allodynia induced by a single injection of oxaliplatin in rats. Five consecutive oral administrations of WECC dose-dependently attenuated cold allodynia, suppressed the activation of spinal astrocytes and microglia, and inhibited the up-regulation of spinal pro-inflammatory cytokines IL-1β and TNF in oxaliplatin-injected rats. These results suggest that C. Cortex might play an important role in the inhibitory effect of GBT on oxaliplatin-induced cold allodynia via suppressing spinal glia and pro-inflammatory cytokines. C. Cortex contains various phytocompounds such as coumarin, cinnamic acid, and cinnamaldehyde [44]. Since previously published articles have reported that coumarin can exert anti-nociceptive action in different types of pain [24,45,46], we assessed the efficacy of coumarin on oxaliplatin-induced cold allodynia. Our results revealed that coumarin could effectively attenuate oxaliplatin-induced cold allodynia, suggesting that coumarin might play a role in the anti-allodynic effect of C. Cortex in a rat model of oxaliplatin-induced neuropathic cold allodynia.

Although some articles have reported that activation of spinal glial cells occurred throughout the spinal cord, in our study [47], we focused on glial activation in lamina I and II because it is well known that this area is important for pain sensation as the primary afferent nociceptive neurons form synapses to the secondary afferent ones in this area. Furthermore, other studies have also observed the activation of microglia and astrocytes in this area to assess whether their compound or drug could modulate the sensory transmission by decreasing the activation of spinal glial cells in neuropathic pain rats [48]. Because we used tail immersion tests for evaluating neuropathic cold allodynia, we assessed glial activation not only in the lumbar spinal cord (Figures 2 and 3), but also in the sacral spinal cord at the S1/S2 level that mainly innervates the tail (Figures S3 and S4). In these supplementary data, activation of astrocytes and microglia in the sacral spinal cord after oxaliplatin injection did not differ from that in the lumbar spinal cord. We confirmed that WECC at 200 mg/kg markedly suppressed oxaliplatin-induced activation of astrocytes and microglia in the sacral spinal cord. Coumarin also significantly inhibited such glial activation in the sacral spinal cord.

In conclusion, our results demonstrate that C. Cortex could be an effective medicinal herb to attenuate oxaliplatin-induced cold allodynia, by suppressing the activation of spinal astrocytes and microglia and inhibiting the increase of spinal levels of IL-1β and TNF. Our data also showed that coumarin, a major phytocompund of C. Cortex, might play a role in the anti-allodynic effect of C. Cortex. Additional animal studies using different neuropathic pain models, such as peripheral nerve injury and diabetic neuropathy, and clinical trials may be required to expand the therapeutic use of C. Cortex and/or coumarin.

4. Materials and Methods

4.1. Animals

Young adult male Sprague-Dawley rats (200–250 g, 7 weeks old) (Daehan Biolink, Chungbuk, Korea) were housed in cages (3–4 rats per cage) with water and food available *ad libitum*. The room was maintained with a 12 h-light/dark cycle (light cycle: 08:00–20:00, dark cycle: 20:00–08:00) and kept at 23 $\pm$ 2 °C. All animals were acclimated in their cages for one week prior to any experiment. All procedures involving animals were approved by the Institutional Animal Care and Use Committee of Kyung Hee University (KHUASP(SE)-15-088) and were conducted in accordance with the guidelines of the International Association for the Study of Pain [49].

4.2. Oxaliplatin Administration

As described previously [50], oxaliplatin (Sigma, St. Louis, MO, USA) was dissolved in a 5% glucose (Sigma) solution at a concentration of 2 mg/mL. It was intraperitoneally administered at 6 mg/kg [51]. The same volume of 5% glucose solution was intraperitoneally injected as vehicle control.

4.3. Behavior Test

To determine whether cold allodynia was induced, tail immersion test was carried out as described previously [23]. Briefly, each animal was immobilized in a plastic holder and its tail was drooped for proper application of cold water stimuli. Rats were adapted for one hour in the holder for two days before starting the behavioral tests. The tail was immersed in 4 °C water, and tail withdrawal latency (TWL) was measured with a cut-off time of 15 s. The cold immersion test was repeated six times at five minutes intervals. The average latency was taken as a measure for the severity of cold allodynia. A shorter TWL was interpreted as more severe allodynia. Our previous studies [18,23] showed that a significant allodynic behavior was induced from three days which lasted up to seven days after a single injection with oxaliplatin (6 mg/kg, i.p.). The behavior test was performed in blind condition.

4.4. Experimental Schedule and Grouping and Treatment of WECC

In this study, dried C. Cortex (500 g) was extracted with distilled water at 100 °C for 1 h. After filtration, the water extracts were evaporated using a rotary evaporator at 60 °C and lyophilized to yield 25.319 g of crude extract. Rats were orally injected with water extract of C. Cortex (WECC) diluted in PBS at 100, 200, or 400 mg/kg/day for five days after oxaliplatin injection. The doses of WECC used in this study were similar to those of other herbal formula used in our previous study [18,52] and those of Aconiti tuber in other's study [48]. Rats were randomly divided into the following six groups (n = 6 per group for cold): (1) Vehicle + PBS (i.p. injection of 5% glucose solution + daily oral administration of PBS); (2) Vehicle + 200 mg/kg WECC (i.p. injection of 5% glucose solution + daily oral administration of 200 mg/kg WECC); (3) Oxa + PBS (i.p. injection of oxaliplatin + daily oral administration of PBS); (4) Oxa + 100 mg/kg WECC (i.p. injection of oxaliplatin + daily oral administration of 100 mg/kg WECC); (5) Oxa + 200 mg/kg WECC (i.p. injection of oxaliplatin + daily oral administration of 200 mg/kg WECC); and (6) Oxa + 400 mg/kg WECC (oxaliplatin injection + daily oral administration of 400 mg/kg WECC). On day 0, tail immersion test was performed at 10:00–12:00 and then oxaliplatin (6 mg/kg) or vehicle (5% glucose solution) was intraperitoneally injected followed by oral administration of WECC or PBS at 12:00–13:00. From day 1 to day 4, WECC or PBS administration was daily performed at 12:00–13:00 after behavioral test was conducted at 10:00–12:00. On day 5, only behavior test was performed at 10:00–12:00.

4.5. Immunohistochemistry

The animals anesthetized with isoflurane were transcardially perfused with 0.1 M PBS and fixed with a freshly prepared solution consisting of 4% paraformaldehyde (PFA) in 0.1 M phosphate buffer (pH 7.4). The lumbar spinal cord segment at the L4/L5 level and the sacral spinal cord segment at the S1/S2 level were extracted and post-fixed overnight in 4% PFA and transferred into 30% sucrose. Post-fixed lumbar segments were embedded in optimal cutting temperature (OCT) compound (Sakura Finetek, Tokyo, Japan) and kept in a box filled with dry ice. Samples of lumbar spinal cord segments were sectioned at 20 μm thickness using cryostat (Microm HM 505N; Thermo Fisher Scientific, Waltham, MA, USA). These sections were collected in 0.1 M PBS at 4 °C, mounted onto glass slides (Matsunami, Osaka, Japan), and incubated in 0.2% Triton X-100 in 0.5% bovine serum albumin (BSA; BOVOGEN biologics, East Keilor, Australia) solution at room temperature for 1 h. After rinsing the glass slides with 0.5% BSA solution, double immunostaining using primary antibodies raised in different species was performed. These sections were incubated overnight at 4 °C with mixed primary antibodies: mouse anti-glial fibrillary acidic protein (GFAP 1:500; Millipore, Ramona, CA, USA) and rabbit anti-Iba 1 (1:500; Wako, Osaka, Japan). After 0.5% BSA solution rinses, these sections were incubated with secondary antibodies: anti-mouse and anti-rabbit-immunoglobulin G (IgG) labeled with Alexa Fluor 488 and Alexa Fluor 546 (1:200; Invitrogen, Carlsbad, CA, USA) at room temperature in dark for 1 h. Confocal laser microscope (LSM 5 Pascal, Zeiss, Oberkochen, Germany) was used to obtain immunohistochemical images. To determine the efficacy of WECC on oxaliplatin-induced spinal glial activation, the number of GFAP and Iba-1 positive cells were manually counted and averaged in both sides of the spinal dorsal horn laminae I and II. Six spinal cord sections from each animal were used. Cell counting procedure was performed in blind condition.

4.6. ELISA

To determine whether WECC administration decreased the levels of TNF or IL-1β in the spinal cord, the levels of each cytokine were measured by enzyme linked immunosorbent assay (ELISA). Isoflurane anesthetized animal were transcardially perfused with 0.1 M PBS, the L4/L5 segments of the spinal cord were exposed from the vertebral column via laminectomy and identified by tracing the dorsal roots from their respective dorsal root ganglia (DRG). Collected tissues were stored in 1 mL RIPA buffer (Thermo Scientific) containing protease inhibitor cocktail (Roche, Basel, Switzerland). Samples were assayed using a commercial rat TNF ELISA kit (BD OptEIA Set Rat TNF, BD biosciences, San Jose, CA, USA) and mouse IL-1β ELISA kit (BD OptEIA Set mouse IL-1β, BD biosciences) following the manufacturer's protocols. Optical density (O.D.) was measured at 450 nm with λ correction of 570 nm using a microplate reader (Tecan). Total amounts of protein in samples were measured using Bio-Rad protein assay kit (Bio-Rad, Hercules, CA, USA). Samples and standards were run in duplicate. All results were normalized to the total amount of protein in each sample.

4.7. Ultra High-Performance Liquid Chromatography (UHPLC) Analysis

Chromatographic analysis was performed using a Thermo Scientific Vanquish UHPLC system (Thermo Fisher Scientific) with Zorbax Eclipse Plus C18 (2.1 × 100 mm, 1.8 μm) column (Agilent Technology, Santa Clara, CA, USA). Mobile phase A (0.005% FA in water (*v*/*v*)) and mobile phase B (100% ACN) were operated with a gradient elution at a flow rate of 0.5 mL/min as follows: 25% B (0–6 min) → 100% B (6–6.5 min) → 100% B (6.5–9.5 min) → 25% B (9.5–10 min) → 25% B (10–13 min). The column temperature was set at 40 °C. Cinnamic acid (1 mg/mL), coumarin (1 mg/mL), and cinnamaldehyde (1 mg/mL) were dissolved in methanol and used as standards for the qualitative and quantitative analysis of WECC (2 mg/mL). Sample injection volume was 2 μL. Absorbance of column eluent was monitored with a UV spectrometer at wavelength of 280 nm.

4.8. Statistical Analysis

All data are presented as mean ± S.E.M (standard error of the mean). Statistical analysis and graphic works were done with Prism 5.0 (Graph Pad Software, La Jolla, CA, USA). The sample size was determined based on our previously conducted experiments [18,23]. One-way or two-way analysis of variance (ANOVA) followed by Bonferroni's post hoc test was used for comparisons between groups. In all cases, $p < 0.05$ was considered as statistically significant.

Acknowledgments: This work was supported by an undergraduate research program grant (KHKM-URP 2015) from Kyung Hee University College of Korean Medicine and a grant (HI14C0738) from the Korea Health Technology R&D Project through the Korea Health Industry Development Institute (KHIDI) funded by the Ministry of Health & Welfare, Republic of Korea.

Author Contributions: K.L. and S.K.K. conceived and designed the experiments; C.K., W.K., D.L. and J.H.L. performed the experiments; C.K., J.H.L., D.L., Y.K., K.L. and S.K.K. analyzed the data; C.K., J.H.L., W.K., K.L. and S.K.K. wrote the paper. All authors read and approved the final manuscript.

References

1. Baker, D. Oxaliplatin: A new drug for the treatment of metastatic carcinoma of the colon or rectum. *Rev. Gastroenterol. Disord.* **2002**, *3*, 31–38.
2. Argyriou, A.; Briani, C.; Cavaletti, G.; Bruna, J.; Alberti, P.; Velasco, R.; Lonardi, S.; Cortinovis, D.; Cazzaniga, M.; Campagnolo, M. Advanced age and liability to oxaliplatin-induced peripheral neuropathy: Post hoc analysis of a prospective study. *Eur. J. Neurol.* **2013**, *20*, 788–794. [CrossRef] [PubMed]
3. Petit, T.; Benider, A.; Yovine, A.; Bougnoux, P.; Spaeth, D.; Maindrault-Goebel, F.; Serin, D.; Tigaud, J.-D.; Eymard, J.C.; Simon, H. Phase II study of an oxaliplatin/vinorelbine combination in patients with anthracycline-and taxane-pre-treated metastatic breast cancer. *Anticancer Drugs* **2006**, *17*, 337–343. [CrossRef] [PubMed]
4. Desoize, B.; Madoulet, C. Particular aspects of platinum compounds used at present in cancer treatment. *Crit. Rev. Oncol. Hematol.* **2002**, *42*, 317–325. [CrossRef]
5. Cassidy, J.; Misset, J.-L. Oxaliplatin-related side effects: Characteristics and management. *Semin. Oncol.* **2002**, *29*, 11–20. [CrossRef] [PubMed]
6. Shidahara, Y.; Ogawa, S.; Nakamura, M.; Nemoto, S.; Awaga, Y.; Takashima, M.; Hama, A.; Matsuda, A.; Takamatsu, H. Pharmacological comparison of a nonhuman primate and a rat model of oxaliplatin-induced neuropathic cold hypersensitivity. *Pharmacol. Res. Perspect.* **2016**, *4*, e00216. [CrossRef] [PubMed]
7. Wolf, S.; Barton, D.; Kottschade, L.; Grothey, A.; Loprinzi, C. Chemotherapy-induced peripheral neuropathy: Prevention and treatment strategies. *Eur. J. Cancer* **2008**, *44*, 1507–1515. [CrossRef] [PubMed]
8. Inoue, K.; Tsuda, M.; Tozaki-Saitoh, H. Role of the glia in neuropathic pain caused by peripheral nerve injury. *Brain Nerve* **2012**, *64*, 1233–1239. (In Japanese) [PubMed]
9. Old, E.A.; Clark, A.K.; Malcangio, M. The role of glia in the spinal cord in neuropathic and inflammatory pain. In *Pain Control*; Springer: Berlin, Germany, 2015; pp. 145–170.
10. Mannelli, L.D.C.; Pacini, A.; Micheli, L.; Tani, A.; Zanardelli, M.; Ghelardini, C. Glial role in oxaliplatin-induced neuropathic pain. *Exp. Neurol.* **2014**, *261*, 22–33. [CrossRef] [PubMed]
11. Luongo, L.; Guida, F.; Boccella, S.; Bellini, G.; Gatta, L.; Rossi, F.; de Novellis, V.; Maione, S. Palmitoylethanolamide reduces formalin-induced neuropathic-like behaviour through spinal glial/ microglial phenotypical changes in mice. *CNS Neurol. Disord. Drug Targets* **2013**, *12*, 45–54. [CrossRef] [PubMed]
12. Old, E.A.; Malcangio, M. Chemokine mediated neuron–glia communication and aberrant signalling in neuropathic pain states. *Curr. Opin. Pharmacol.* **2012**, *12*, 67–73. [CrossRef] [PubMed]
13. Ledeboer, A.; Sloane, E.M.; Milligan, E.D.; Frank, M.G.; Mahony, J.H.; Maier, S.F.; Watkins, L.R. Minocycline attenuates mechanical allodynia and proinflammatory cytokine expression in rat models of pain facilitation. *Pain* **2005**, *115*, 71–83. [CrossRef] [PubMed]
14. Zhang, T.; Zhang, J.; Shi, J.; Feng, Y.; Sun, Z.S.; Li, H. Antinociceptive synergistic effect of spinal mglur2/3 antagonist and glial cells inhibitor on peripheral inflammation-induced mechanical hypersensitivity. *Brain Res. Bull.* **2009**, *79*, 219–223. [CrossRef] [PubMed]
15. Scholz, J.; Woolf, C.J. The neuropathic pain triad: Neurons, immune cells and glia. *Nat. Neurosci.* **2007**, *10*, 1361–1368. [CrossRef] [PubMed]
16. Miyoshi, K.; Obata, K.; Kondo, T.; Okamura, H.; Noguchi, K. Interleukin-18-mediated microglia/astrocyte interaction in the spinal cord enhances neuropathic pain processing after nerve injury. *J. Neurosci.* **2008**, *28*, 12775–12787. [CrossRef] [PubMed]

17. Sommer, C.; Kress, M. Recent findings on how proinflammatory cytokines cause pain: Peripheral mechanisms in inflammatory and neuropathic hyperalgesia. *Neurosci. Lett.* **2004**, *361*, 184–187. [CrossRef] [PubMed]
18. Ahn, B.-S.; Kim, S.-K.; Kim, H.N.; Lee, J.-H.; Lee, J.-H.; Hwang, D.S.; Bae, H.; Min, B.-I.; Kim, S.K. Gyejigachulbu-tang relieves oxaliplatin-induced neuropathic cold and mechanical hypersensitivity in rats via the suppression of spinal glial activation. *Evid. Based Complement. Altern. Med.* **2014**, *2014*, 436482. [CrossRef] [PubMed]
19. Kim, H.N. Gyejigachulbu-Tang Suppresses Oxaliplatin-Induced Neuropathic Mechanical Allodynia in Rats via Modulating Spinal tnf-α. Ph.D. Thesis, Kyung Hee University, Seoul, Korea, 2015.
20. Hayashi, K.; Imanishi, N.; Kashiwayama, Y.; Kawano, A.; Terasawa, K.; Shimada, Y.; Ochiai, H. Inhibitory effect of cinnamaldehyde, derived from Cinnamomi Cortex, on the growth of influenza A/PR/8 virus in vitro and in vivo. *Antivir. Res.* **2007**, *74*, 1–8. [CrossRef] [PubMed]
21. Kubo, M.; Ma, S.; Wu, J.; Matsuda, H. Anti-inflammatory activities of 70% methanolic extract from Cinnamomi Cortex. *Biol. Pharm. Bull.* **1996**, *19*, 1041–1045. [CrossRef] [PubMed]
22. Takenaga, M.; Hirai, A.; Terano, T.; Tamura, Y.; Kitagawa, H.; Yoshida, S. In vitro effect of cinnamic aldehyde, a main component of Cinnamomi Cortex, on human platelet aggregation and arachidonic acid metabolism. *J. Pharm. Dyn.* **1987**, *10*, 201–208. [CrossRef]
23. Moon, H.J.; Lim, B.-S.; Lee, D.-I.; Ye, M.S.; Lee, G.; Min, B.-I.; Bae, H.; Na, H.S.; Kim, S.K. Effects of electroacupuncture on oxaliplatin-induced neuropathic cold hypersensitivity in rats. *J. Physiol. Sci.* **2014**, *64*, 151–156. [CrossRef] [PubMed]
24. Park, S.-H.; Sim, Y.-B.; Kang, Y.-J.; Kim, S.-S.; Kim, C.-H.; Kim, S.-J.; Lim, S.-M.; Suh, H.-W. Antinociceptive profiles and mechanisms of orally administered coumarin in mice. *Biol. Pharm. Bull.* **2013**, *36*, 925–930. [CrossRef] [PubMed]
25. Lehky, T.; Leonard, G.; Wilson, R.; Grem, J.L.; Floeter, M. Oxaliplatin-induced neurotoxicity: Acute hyperexcitability and chronic neuropathy. *Muscle Nerve* **2004**, *29*, 387–392. [CrossRef] [PubMed]
26. Pasetto, L.M.; D'Andrea, M.R.; Rossi, E.; Monfardini, S. Oxaliplatin-related neurotoxicity: How and why? *Crit. Rev. Oncol. Hematol.* **2006**, *59*, 159–168. [CrossRef] [PubMed]
27. Ormseth, M.J.; Scholz, B.A.; Boomershine, C.S. Duloxetine in the management of diabetic peripheral neuropathic pain. *Patient Prefer Adherence* **2011**, *5*, 343–356. [PubMed]
28. Serpell, M.; Neuropathic pain study group. Gabapentin in neuropathic pain syndromes: A randomised, double-blind, placebo-controlled trial. *Pain* **2002**, *99*, 557–566. [CrossRef]
29. Sweitzer, S.; Martin, D.; DeLeo, J. Intrathecal interleukin-1 receptor antagonist in combination with soluble tumor necrosis factor receptor exhibits an anti-allodynic action in a rat model of neuropathic pain. *Neuroscience* **2001**, *103*, 529–539. [CrossRef]
30. Austin, P.J.; Moalem-Taylor, G. The neuro-immune balance in neuropathic pain: Involvement of inflammatory immune cells, immune-like glial cells and cytokines. *J. Neuroimmunol.* **2010**, *229*, 26–50. [CrossRef] [PubMed]
31. Chauvet, N.; Palin, K.; Verrier, D.; Poole, S.; Dantzer, R.; Lestage, J. Rat microglial cells secrete predominantly the precursor of interleukin-1β in response to lipopolysaccharide. *Eur. J. Neurosci.* **2001**, *14*, 609–617. [CrossRef] [PubMed]
32. Shigemoto-Mogami, Y.; Koizumi, S.; Tsuda, M.; Ohsawa, K.; Kohsaka, S.; Inoue, K. Mechanisms underlying extracellular ATP-evoked interleukin-6 release in mouse microglial cell line, MG-5. *J. Neurochem.* **2001**, *78*, 1339–1349. [CrossRef] [PubMed]
33. Sachs, D.; Cunha, F.Q.; Poole, S.; Ferreira, S.H. Tumour necrosis factor-α, interleukin-1β and interleukin-8 induce persistent mechanical nociceptor hypersensitivity. *Pain* **2002**, *96*, 89–97. [CrossRef]
34. Nadeau, S.; Filali, M.; Zhang, J.; Kerr, B.J.; Rivest, S.; Soulet, D.; Iwakura, Y.; de Rivero Vaccari, J.P.; Keane, R.W.; Lacroix, S. Functional recovery after peripheral nerve injury is dependent on the pro-inflammatory cytokines IL-1β and TNF: Implications for neuropathic pain. *J. Neurosci.* **2011**, *31*, 12533–12542. [CrossRef] [PubMed]
35. Shamash, S.; Reichert, F.; Rotshenker, S. The cytokine network of wallerian degeneration: Tumor necrosis factor-α, interleukin-1α, and interleukin-1β. *J. Neurosci.* **2002**, *22*, 3052–3060. [PubMed]
36. Homma, Y.; Brull, S.J.; Zhang, J.-M. A comparison of chronic pain behavior following local application of tumor necrosis factor α to the normal and mechanically compressed lumbar ganglia in the rat. *Pain* **2002**, *95*, 239–246. [CrossRef]

37. Murata, Y.; Onda, A.; Rydevik, B.; Takahashi, I.; Takahashi, K.; Olmarker, K. Changes in pain behavior and histologic changes caused by application of tumor necrosis factor-alpha to the dorsal root ganglion in rats. *Spine* **2006**, *31*, 530–535. [CrossRef] [PubMed]
38. Schroder, S.; Beckmann, K.; Franconi, G.; Meyer-Hamme, G.; Friedemann, T.; Greten, H.J.; Rostock, M.; Efferth, T. Can medical herbs stimulate regeneration or neuroprotection and treat neuropathic pain in chemotherapy-induced peripheral neuropathy? *Evid. Based Complement. Altern. Med.* **2013**, *2013*, 423713. [CrossRef] [PubMed]
39. Ding, Y.; Wu, E.Q.; Liang, C.; Chen, J.; Tran, M.N.; Hong, C.H.; Jang, Y.; Park, K.L.; Bae, K.; Kim, Y.H. Discrimination of cinnamon bark and cinnamon twig samples sourced from various countries using hplc-based fingerprint analysis. *Food Chem.* **2011**, *127*, 755–760. [CrossRef] [PubMed]
40. Li, X.; Yang, J.; Ma, D.; Lin, H.; Xu, X.; Jiang, Y.H. Effects of different compatibilities of ramulus cinnamomi and peony in guizhi decoction on diabetic cardiac autonomic neuropathy. *Zhongguo Zhong Xi Yi Jie He Za Zhi* **2015**, *35*, 741. (In Chinese) [PubMed]
41. Zhao, N.; Li, J.; Li, L.; Niu, X.-Y.; Jiang, M.; He, X.-J.; Bian, Z.-X.; Zhang, G.; Lu, A.-P. Molecular network-based analysis of guizhi-shaoyao-zhimu decoction, a TCM herbal formula, for treatment of diabetic peripheral neuropathy. *Acta Pharmacol. Sin.* **2015**, *36*, 716–723. [CrossRef] [PubMed]
42. Zhiling, Y.; Guangqin, Z.; Dai Yue, K.J.; Changgui, D.; Ruijian, L. Pharmacological study on compatibility of cortex cinnamomi with halloysitum rubrum. *China J. Chin. Mater. Med.* **1997**, *22*, 309–312.
43. Saghir, S.; Sadikun, A.; Al-Suede, F.; Abdul, M.A.; Murugaiyah, V. Antihyperlipidemic, antioxidant and cytotoxic activities of methanolic and aqueous extracts of different parts of star fruit. *Curr. Pharm. Biotechnol.* **2016**, *17*, 915–925. [CrossRef] [PubMed]
44. Wang, Y.H.; Avula, B.; Nanayakkara, N.P.; Zhao, J.; Khan, I.A. Cassia cinnamon as a source of coumarin in cinnamon-flavored food and food supplements in the united states. *J. Agric. Food Chem.* **2013**, *61*, 4470–4476. [CrossRef] [PubMed]
45. Meotti, F.C.; Missau, F.C.; Ferreira, J.; Pizzolatti, M.G.; Mizuzaki, C.; Nogueira, C.W.; Santos, A.R. Anti-allodynic property of flavonoid myricitrin in models of persistent inflammatory and neuropathic pain in mice. *Biochem. Pharmacol.* **2006**, *72*, 1707–1713. [CrossRef] [PubMed]
46. De Lima, F.O.; Nonato, F.R.; Couto, R.D.; Barbosa Filho, J.M.; Nunes, X.P.; Ribeiro dos Santos, R.; Soares, M.B.P.; Villarreal, C.F. Mechanisms involved in the antinociceptive effects of 7-hydroxycoumarin. *J. Nat. Prod.* **2011**, *74*, 596–602. [CrossRef] [PubMed]
47. Hashizume, H.; DeLeo, J.A.; Colburn, R.W.; Weinstein, J.N. Spinal glial activation and cytokine expression after lumbar root injury in the rat. *Spine* **2000**, *25*, 1206–1217. [CrossRef] [PubMed]
48. Shibata, K.; Sugawara, T.; Fujishita, K.; Shinozaki, Y.; Matsukawa, T.; Suzuki, T.; Koizumi, S. The astrocyte-targeted therapy by bushi for the neuropathic pain in mice. *PLoS ONE* **2011**, *6*, e23510. [CrossRef] [PubMed]
49. Zimmermann, M. Ethical guidelines for investigations of experimental pain in conscious animals. *Pain* **1983**, *16*, 109–110. [CrossRef]
50. Ling, B.; Coudoré-Civiale, M.-A.; Balayssac, D.; Eschalier, A.; Coudoré, F.; Authier, N. Behavioral and immunohistological assessment of painful neuropathy induced by a single oxaliplatin injection in the rat. *Toxicology* **2007**, *234*, 176–184. [CrossRef] [PubMed]
51. Ling, B.; Coudoré, F.; Decalonne, L.; Eschalier, A.; Authier, N. Comparative antiallodynic activity of morphine, pregabalin and lidocaine in a rat model of neuropathic pain produced by one oxaliplatin injection. *Neuropharmacology* **2008**, *55*, 724–728. [CrossRef] [PubMed]
52. Park, S.; Sohn, S.-H.; Jung, K.-H.; Lee, K.-Y.; Yeom, Y.R.; Kim, G.-E.; Jung, S.; Jung, H.; Bae, H. The effects of maekmoondong-tang on cockroach extract-induced allergic asthma. *Evid.-Based Complement. Altern. Med.* **2014**, *2014*, 958965. [CrossRef] [PubMed]

6

Antidepressant Potential of Chlorogenic Acid-Enriched Extract from *Eucommia ulmoides* Oliver Bark with Neuron Protection and Promotion of Serotonin Release through Enhancing Synapsin I Expression

Jianming Wu [1,*,†], Haixia Chen [1,†], Hua Li [1], Yong Tang [1], Le Yang [2], Shousong Cao [1] and Dalian Qin [1,*]

1. Department of Pharmacology, School of Pharmacy, Sichuan Medical University, Luzhou 86646-000, Sichuan, China; chx@lzmc.edu.cn (H.C.); lihua@lzmc.edu.cn (H.L.); tangy1989@yeah.net (Y.T.); shousongc@gmail.com (S.C.)
2. Chengdu Analytical Applications Center, Shimadzu (China) Co. Ltd., Chengdu 86610-063, Sichuan, China; sscyl@shimadzu.com.cn

* Correspondence: jianmingwu@lzmc.edu.cn (J.W.); dalianqin@lzmc.edu.cn (D.Q.)

† These authors contributed equally to this work.

Academic Editor: Luigia Trabace

Abstract: *Eucommia ulmoides* Oliver (*E. ulmoides*) is a traditional Chinese medicine with many beneficial effects, used as a tonic medicine in China and other countries. Chlorogenic acid (CGA) is an important compound in *E. ulmoides* with neuroprotective, cognition improvement and other pharmacological effects. However, it is unknown whether chlorogenic acid-enriched *Eucommia ulmoides* Oliver bark has antidepressant potential through neuron protection, serotonin release promotion and penetration of blood-cerebrospinal fluid barrier. In the present study, we demonstrated that CGA could stimulate axon and dendrite growth and promote serotonin release through enhancing synapsin I expression in the cells of fetal rat raphe neurons *in vitro*. More importantly, CGA-enriched extract of *E. ulmoides* (EUWE) at 200 and 400 mg/kg/day orally administered for 7 days showed antidepressant-like effects in the tail suspension test of KM mice. Furthermore, we also found CGA could be detected in the the cerebrospinal fluid of the rats orally treated with EUWE and reach the level of pharmacological effect for neuroprotection by UHPLC-ESI-MS/MS. The findings indicate CGA is able to cross the blood-cerebrospinal fluid barrier to exhibit its neuron protection and promotion of serotonin release through enhancing synapsin I expression. This is the first report of the effect of CGA on promoting 5-HT release through enhancing synapsin I expression and CGA-enriched EUWE has antidepressant-like effect *in vivo*. EUWE may be developed as the natural drugs for the treatment of depression.

Keywords: chlorogenic acid; *Eucommia ulmoides* Oliver; cerebrospinal fluid; UHPLC-ESI-MS/MS; antidepressant; raphe neurons; serotonin; synapsin I

1. Introduction

Eucommia ulmoides Oliver (*E. ulmoides*) known as Du-zhong (in Chinese) or Tuchong (in Japanese), is a traditional Chinese medicine (TCM) used as a tonic medicine in China, Japan, Korea, and other countries for a long time [1,2]. *E. ulmoides* has been widely used to tonify the liver and kidney, and strengthen tendons and bones according to the theory of TCM [3]. Pharmacological studies have shown that *E. ulmoides* exhibits many beneficial effects, including neuroprotection [4], bone loss prevention [5], learning and memory improvement [6,7], ameliorating insulin resistance [8], antihypertension [9], antibacterial [10], lipid-lowering and anti-obesity [11,12], treatment of osteoarthritis [2] and so on. Meanwhile, phytochemical studies have displayed the component complexity of *E. ulmoides*, from which 112 compounds have been isolated and identified, including 28 lignans, 24 iridoids, 27 phenolics, six steroids, five terpenoids, 13 flavonoids and nine others [1]. Among them, chlorogenic acid (CGA, 3-*O*-caffeoylquinic acid), a flavonoid with neuroprotection [13,14], cognition improvement, and other pharmacological effects [15–17], has been frequently used as the quality control marker for *E. ulmoides* and its preparations. Therefore, CGA, as the mainly active compound of *E. ulmoides* may be used in treatment of various diseases of central nervous system (CNS). Usually, as the most important feature for the agents used in treatment of CNS diseases, the penetration ability of crossing the blood-cerebrospinal fluid barrier (BLB) and blood-brain barrier (BBB) is critical for their therapeutic effect in the CNS [18]. However, CGA does not seem to be beneficial for crossing BLB and BBB due to its good aqueous solubility [19]. Previous study has clearly demonstrated that CGA from *E. ulmoides* has CNS pharmacological therapeutic activities, but it is unknown whether it can penetrate the BLB and BBB or not. A study by Park *et al.* showed that CGA isolated from *Artemisia capillaris* Thunb exhibited a potent antidepressant effect in a mouse model (30 mg/kg/day for 14 day oral administration) [20]. The study supports the idea that CGA may be able to cross the BLB and BBB of mice to display its therapeutical effects.

Depression is a state of affective disorder that can cause deficits in learning, memory and cognition and a major burden on society. These depression-related pathophysiological changes could be induced by excessive exposure to glucocorticoids, whose secretion is regulated by negative feedback loop in response to short-span mild stress [21]. However, this feedback regulation is lost when exposed to major or prolonged stress, causing a significant rise of glucocorticoid levels [22]. A main and potent glucocorticoid, corticosterone (Cort) could decrease serotonin (5-HT or 5-hydroxytryptamine) release and lead to neurodegeneration when chronic exposure to stress levels of Cort [23], which provided a basis for understanding the impairment of 5-HT decrease in depressive illness. Furthermore, clinical studies found that the hippocampal volume and the level of 5-HT were decreased in the patients with major depression [24]. Meanwhile, agents with enhancing 5-HT concentration at the synapse could alleviate the symptoms of depression [25]. Actually, 5-HT is an important monoamine neurotransmitter and can be found in neurons, platelets, mast cells, and enterochromaffin cells. Because 5-HT cannot cross the BBB, the brain synthesizes its own 5-HT which accounts for 1%–2% of the whole 5-HT supply of body, which is exclusively expressed in the dorsal and median raphe of the rostral brain, a heterogeneous region located between the periaquaduct and fourth ventricle of the midbrain [26]. However, numerous evidence indicates that the expression level of synapsin I, a presynaptic phosphoprotein that anchors synaptic vesicles containing neurotransmitters to the actin cytoskeleton in the distal pool, is positively associated with the maturation of 5-HT release mechanisms [27] and structural maintenance of presynaptic terminals [28], as well as neuronal differentiation, axonal outgrowth and synaptogenesis [29]. Those revelations indicate that 5-HT release via synapsin I plays the key role in the depression. As mentioned above, CGA from the extract of *E. ulmoides* is involved various CNS pharmacological and therapeutic activities, but the mode of action and associated mechanism(s) are still unclear. In the present study, we investigate whether CGA can protect neurons from Cort-induced injury and promote 5-HT release through enhancing synapsin I expression in the cultured cells of fetal rat raphe neurons *in vitro* and CGA-enriched water extract from *E. ulmoides* (EUWE) can cross BLB of rats and exhibit antidepressant-like effect in mice *in vivo*.

2. Results

2.1. CGA Promotes the Cell Growth of Fetal Rat Raphe Neurons in Vitro

In order to study the protective effect of CGA on Cort-induced cell injury of fetal rat raphe neurons, cell-proliferative assay was performed *in vitro* with cultured cells of raphe neurons treated with 10 μM Cort and 0.001–10.0 μM CGA alone or in combination. As shown in Figure 1, treatment with 10 μM Cort decreased the cell growth of raphe neurons, whereas CGA reversed the Cort-induced decrease of raphe neurons in a dose-dependent (Figure 1A) and time-dependent (Figure 1B) manner. Furthermore, although CGA alone does not affect the cell growth of neurons as similar to the cells of control morphologically (Figure 1C,D), we demonstrate that the inhibition of cell growth by Cort (10 μM) is involved in neuron damage including cell body atrophy, axon and dendrite loss (Figure 1E). Whereas CGA (1 nM) prevents Cort-induced cell damage of raphe neurons by stimulating new axon and dendrite growth (Figure 1F), suggesting the pharmacological effect of CGA on protection of Cort-induced neuron damage is likely to be associated with neurogenesis, which has been proved to be an important factor for antidepressant efficacy [30,31].

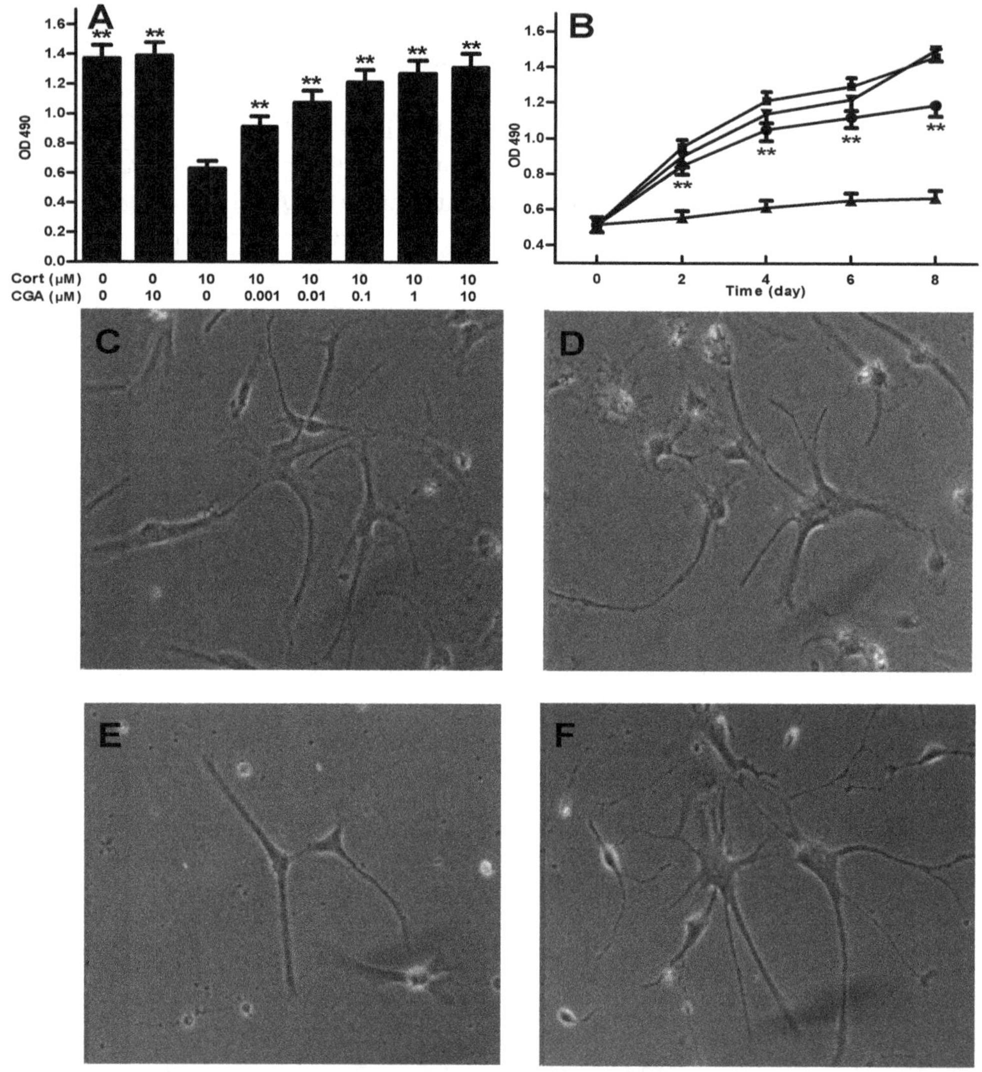

Figure 1. The effects of CGA ± Cort on the cell growth of fetal rat raphe neurons *in vitro*. (**A**) CGA dose response in protection of Cort-induced cell inhibition, CGA 0.001–10 μM and Cort 10 μM; (**B**) Time response curve of CGA in protection of Cort-induced cell inhibition; ■ Control; ▼ CGA 1 nM; ▲ Cort 10 μM; and ● CGA 1 nM + Cort 10 μM; (**C**) A representative image of control showing normal neurons; (**D**) A representative image of CGA (1 nM) treatment showing no neurons damage; (**E**) A representative image of Cort (10 μM) treatment showing Cort-induced neurons damage including cell body atrophy, axon and dendrite loss; (**F**) A representative image of co-treatment of CGA (1 nM) and Cort (10 μM) showing prevention of Cort-induced neurons damage by CGA. The control cells were treated with culture medium with 0.1% DMSO. The results are representative of at least three independent experiments run in triplicate and expressed as the mean ± SD. ** $p < 0.01$ *vs.* Cort treatment.

2.2. *Effect of CGA on 5-HT Release in the Cells of Fetal Rat Raphe Neurons in Vitro*

In order to study the effect of CGA on 5-HT release, Enzyme-linked immunosorbent assay (ELISA) was applied to examine the concentrations of 5-HT in the cultured cells of fetal rat raphe neurons after the cells were treated with 10 μM Cort alone or in combination with CGA at 0.5 nM or 1.0 nM. As shown in Figure 2, the level of 5-HT in culture supernatant is significantly reduced after treatment with 10 μM Cort compared to that of the control ($p < 0.01$), however, the reduction induced by Cort is remarkably averted by co-treatment with 0.5 and 1 nM CGA ($p < 0.01$). These results suggest that CGA may promote 5-HT release in the cells of fetal rat raphe neurons.

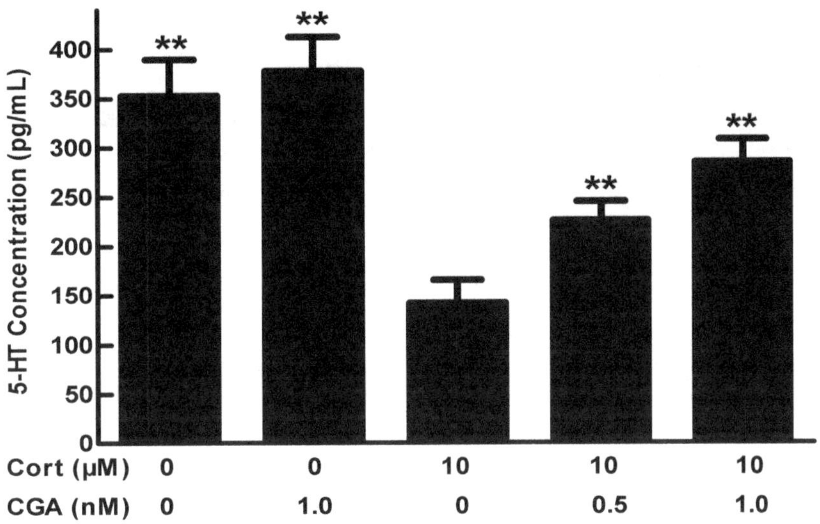

Figure 2. The effects of CGA ± Cort on 5-HT release from the cells of fetal rat raphe neurons *in vitro*. The results are representative of at least three independent experiments run in triplicate and expressed as the mean ± SD. ** $p < 0.01$ *vs*. Cort-treated group. The control cells were treated with culture medium with 0.1% DMSO.

2.3. *CGA Enhances the Expression of Synapsin I of the Cells of Fetal Rat Raphe Neurons in Vitro*

Synapsin I is an abundant synaptic vesicle-related protein that plays a critical role in the regulation of neurotransmitter release [32]. We hypothesized that synapsin I may involve in the neurotransmitter release in neurons. For this purpose, we used anti-synapsin I to examine the location and expression of synapsin I in cultured cells of fetal rat raphe neurons. The fluorescence images shown in Figure 3 illustrate 14-day-old cells of fetal rat raphe neurons, at which point synapsin I distributes to presynaptic terminals in a punctuate manner, concurrent with the formation of synaptic network in normal neurons (Figure 3A). CGA at 1.0 nM has no significant effect on the cells of neurons (Figure 3B). However, the loss of synapsin I puncta and the synaptic network is obvious in the cells of neurons treated with Cort at the concentration of 10 μM (Figure 3C). In contrast to Cort-treated cells of neurons, the loss of synapsin I puncta and the synaptic network are prevented by the co-treatment with CGA at the concentration of 1 nM (Figure 3D). Western blot analysis shows that synapsin I expression levels are significantly down-regulated in Cort-treated cells of neurons compared to that of normal control ($p < 0.01$), while it is significantly up-regulated in Cort plus CGA-treated group compared to that of Cort-treated group ($p < 0.01$), even much higher than that of control, quantified by densitometric analysis (Figure 4). These results indicate that the neurotransmitter release caused by CGA is associated with the expression of synapsin I, suggesting a possible mechanism involved in presynaptic vesicle-related proteins and related signaling pathways.

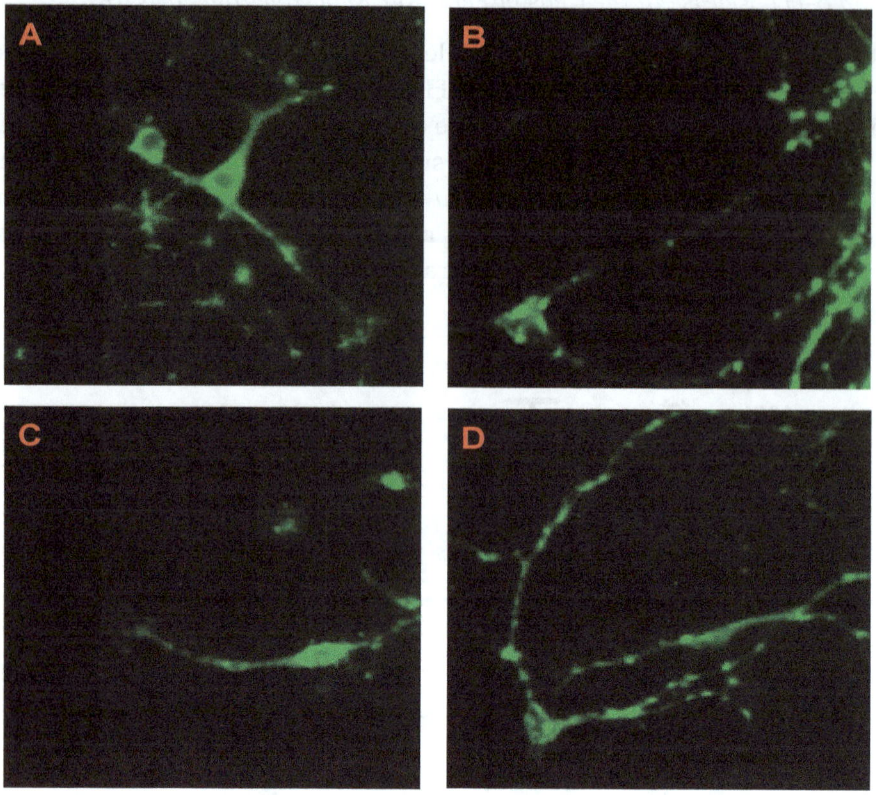

Figure 3. The effects of CGA ± Cort on the expression of synapsin I in the cells of fetal rat raphe neurons. (**A**) Control; (**B**) CGA treatment; (**C**) Cort treatment; and (**D**) Cort + CGA treatment. Notes: Fluorescence microscopy shows the representative images of neurons stained by FITC. The cells were treated with culture medium with 0.1% DMSO (control), or 1 nM CGA ± 10 μM Cort. The results are representative of at least three independent experiments.

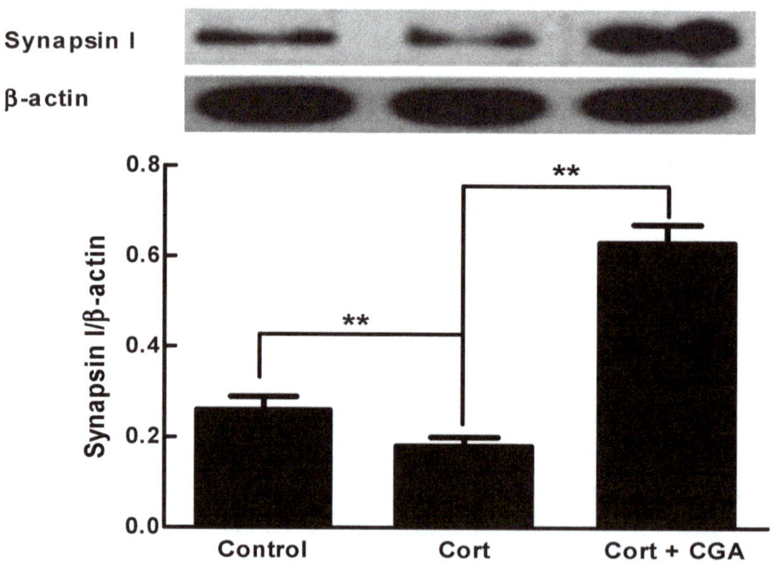

Figure 4. CGA up-regulates protein expression of synapsin I in the cells of fetal rat raphe neurons treated with Cort by western blotting. The cells were treated with culture medium with 0.1% DMSO (control), or 10 μM Cort, or 10 μM Cort + 1 nM CGA. Beta-actin was used as the loading control. The band intensities were quantified by densitometric analysis. The results are representative of at least three independent experiments run in triplicate and expressed as the mean ± SD. ** $p < 0.01$ *vs.* Cort-treated group.

2.4. *EUWE Shows Antidepressant-like Effect in the Tail Suspension Test of KM Mice in Vivo*

The tail suspension test is widely used for screening potential antidepressants. The immobility behavior displays in rodents when subjected to an unavoidable and inescapable stress has been hypothesized to reflect behavioral despair which in turn to reflect similar depressive disorders in human. There is, indeed, a significant correlation between clinical potency and effectiveness of antidepressants [20]. In proof-of- principle study for antidepressant effect of EUWE, we performed the tail suspension test in KM mice with EUWE at 200 and 400 mg/kg/day daily for 7 days, while same volume of distilled water as vehicle control and fluoxetine at 8 mg/kg/day as positive control. As the data shown in Figure 5, the duration of immobility is highest in the distilled water-treated group (control, 130.3 $\pm$ 15.9 s), however, it is significantly lessened in fluoxetine (109.1 $\pm$ 17.8 s) or EUWE-treated (115.2 $\pm$ 16.0 and 109.8 $\pm$ 21.9 s, respectively) groups compared to that of control group ($p < 0.05$), indicating EUWE may have antidepressant effects *in vivo*.

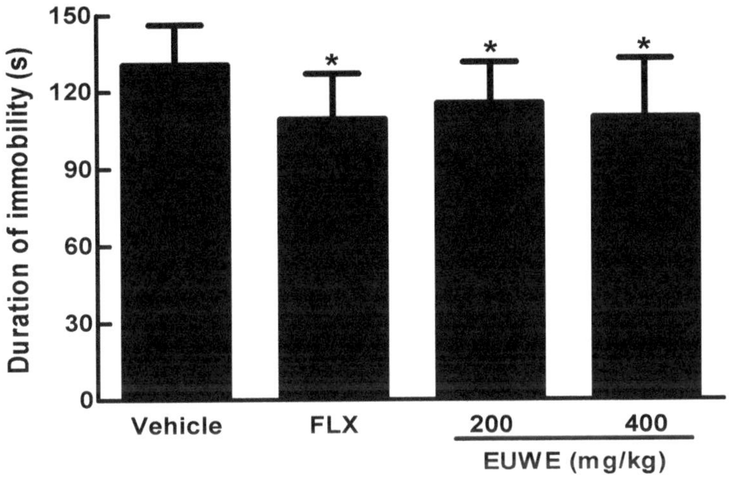

Figure 5. Antidepressant effect of water extract of *E. ulmoides* of (EUWE) in the tail suspension test of mice *in vivo*. The mice were treated orally with EUWE at 200 or 400 mg/kg/day, fluoxetine (FLX) at 8 mg/kg/day and distilled water as vehicle control daily for 7 days. The bars indicate the mean $\pm$ SD. The number of mice used for each group was 12. * $p < 0.05$ compared with distilled water (vehicle) group.

2.5. *Qualitative Analysis of CGA in the CSF of the Rats Treated with CGA-Enriched Water Extract of E. ulmoides*

After we demonstrated the pharmacological effects of CGA on the cells of fetal rat raphe neurons, next, we investigate whether CGA can be absorbed into the CSF of the rats treated with CGA-Enriched water extract of *E. ulmoides* (EUWE). In order to qualitative analysis of CGA in the CSF of rat, ultra high performance liquid chromatography coupled to tandem mass spectrometry (UHPLC-ESI-MS/MS) was employed in positive and negative scan modes to optimize conditions of mass spectrum (Figure 6A,B). Then MS/MS spectrum of m/z 353.10 in the negative ion mode was acquired (Figure 6C), and MRM mode was used to monitor both quasimolecular and fragment ions. Therefore, MRM chromatogram of m/z 353.10 > m/z 191.15 and m/z 353.10 > m/z 179.00 for CGA and CSF samples in the rats treated with EUWE were obtained, respectively (Figure 6D,E). The MRM negative mode was selected due to high sensitivity. As shown in Figure 7, the retention time and mass spectra of the CSF samples in the rats treated with EUWE are similar to that of CGA, indicating the CSF samples may contain CGA.

To further identify whether the CSF of the rats treated with EUWE contains CGA, UHPLC-ESI-MS/MS with both positive and negative ion modes were employed to study the fragmentation behaviors of authentic standard of CGA in ESI-MS/MS at first in order to facilitate the structure characterization of the marker constituent. The marker constituent are identified according to their fragmentation data and comparison with the authentic standard from previous studies [33,34]. The ion fragmentations and structure of marker constituent are shown in Figure 7 and Scheme 1. The quasi-molecular ions $[M + H]^+$ and $[M - H]^-$ of marker constituent are observed at m/z 355.15 and m/z 353.10 in MS spectrum. In the MS^2 spectrum, the precursor ion $[M - H]^-$ at m/z 353.10 ($C_{16}H_{17}O_9$) fragmented into product ions at m/z 191.15 ($C_7H_{11}O_6$, $[M - H - C_9H_6O_3]^-$) and m/z 179.00 ($C_9H_7O_4$, $[M - H - C_7H_{10}O_5]^-$). The ion at m/z 191.15 $[C_7H_{11}O_6]^-$ and m/z 179.00 $[C_9H_7O_4]^-$ are characteristic fragment ions for identifying the structures of caffeoyl and quinic acid from previous reports [35–37], which are also observed in the MS spectrum of the authentic standard. Therefore, the data demonstrate that the CSF of the rats treated with EUWE contains CGA and CGA-enriched EUWE can be absorbed into CSF of rats, indicating that CGA can cross the BLB of rats.

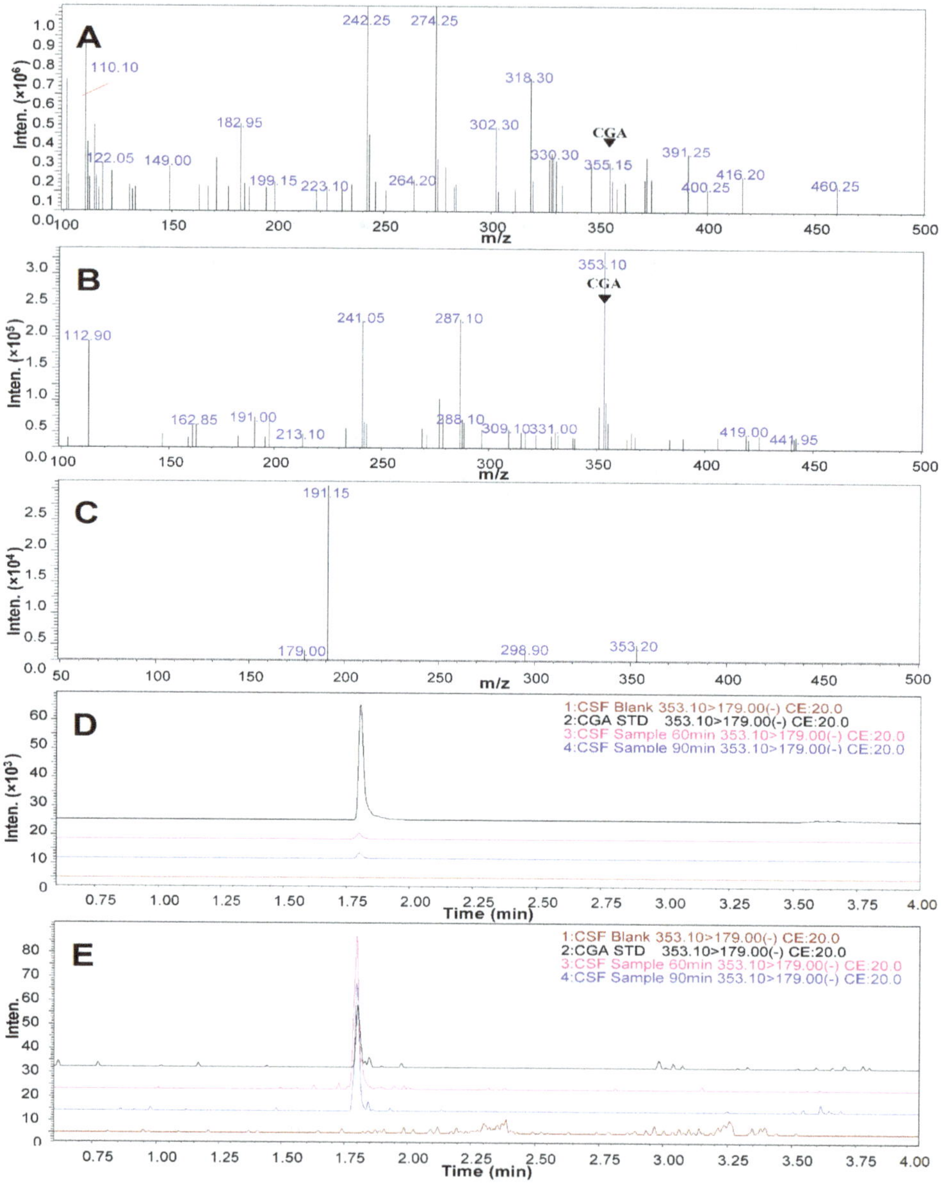

Figure 6. Analysis of CGA and CSF samples in the rats treated with water extract of *E. ulmoides* (EUWE) by UHPLC-ESI-MS/MS chromatogram. (**A**) Positive Scan m/z 100–500 of CGA; (**B**) Negative Scan m/z 100–500 of CGA; (**C**) MS/MS spectrum of m/z 353.10 of CGA in the negative ion mode; (**D**) MRM of channels ESI$^-$ 353.10/191.15 for CGA and CSF samples in rat treated with EUWE; (**E**) MRM of channels ESI$^-$ 353.10/179.00 for CGA and CSF samples in the rat treated with EUWE. Notes: chromatographic conditions are provided in the Experimental Section. The rats were treated with EUWE at 4.0 g/kg.

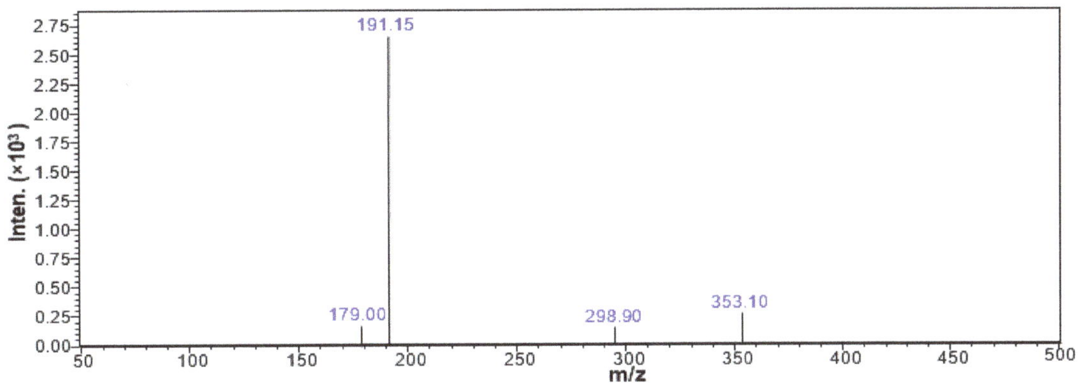

Figure 7. Marker constituents in the CSF of the rats treated with EUWE (4.0 g/kg) identified by ESI-MS/MS spectra in the negative ion mode.

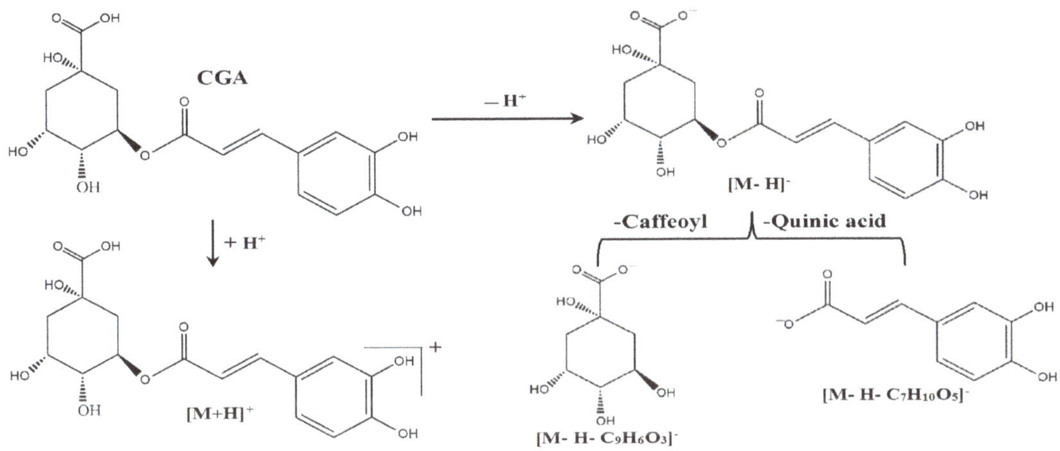

Scheme 1. The chemical structures and metabolic pathway of CGA fragmentations identified in the CSF of the rats treated with EUWE (4.0 g/kg).

2.6. *Quantitative Measurement of CGA in the CSF of Rat*

In order to achieve a better MS condition, both CGA and toosendanin (TSN, as the internal standard) were examined by negative scan in the MS or MS/MS scan mode (Figure 8A–D). Then MRM mode was used to monitor both quasimolecular and fragment ions, in which channel ESI$^-$ m/z 353.10 > m/z 191.15 was selected for CGA and channel ESI$^-$ m/z 573.15 > m/z 531.15 was selected for TSN. Notably, no endogenous interfering peaks are observed at or near the retention times of CGA and TSN by comparing with blank CSF, and TSN doesn't contribute to CGA signal (Figure 8E–H), indicating that CGA doesn't contribute to TSN response and endogenous interfering. Consequently, these results suggest the method has high selectivity for the measurement of CGA.

The calibration curve of CGA in the CSF of rat was constructed by plotting peak area ratios of CGA using the weight (1/C) linear regression. The method shows good linearity over the range from 0.5 to 200 ng/mL with a correlation coefficient r >0.999. The typical calibration curve is presented in Figure 9. The lower limit of quantitation is 0.5 ng/mL. The intra-day accuracy is 111.3% and the relative standard deviation (RSD) of intra-day precision is 7.11% at the concentration of 0.5 ng/mL. In addition, the matrix effect of CGA is 106.15%. Therefore, the method was proved to be sensitive for the measurement of CGA in the CSF of rat.

The established UHPLC-ESI-MS/MS analytical method was subsequently used to determine the CGA concentration in the CSF of the rats treated with EUWE at the dose of 4.0 g/kg and the mean CGA concentrations are 0.41954 ng/mL (1.184 nM) and 0.56224 ng/mL (1.588 nM) for 60 min and 90 min, respectively.

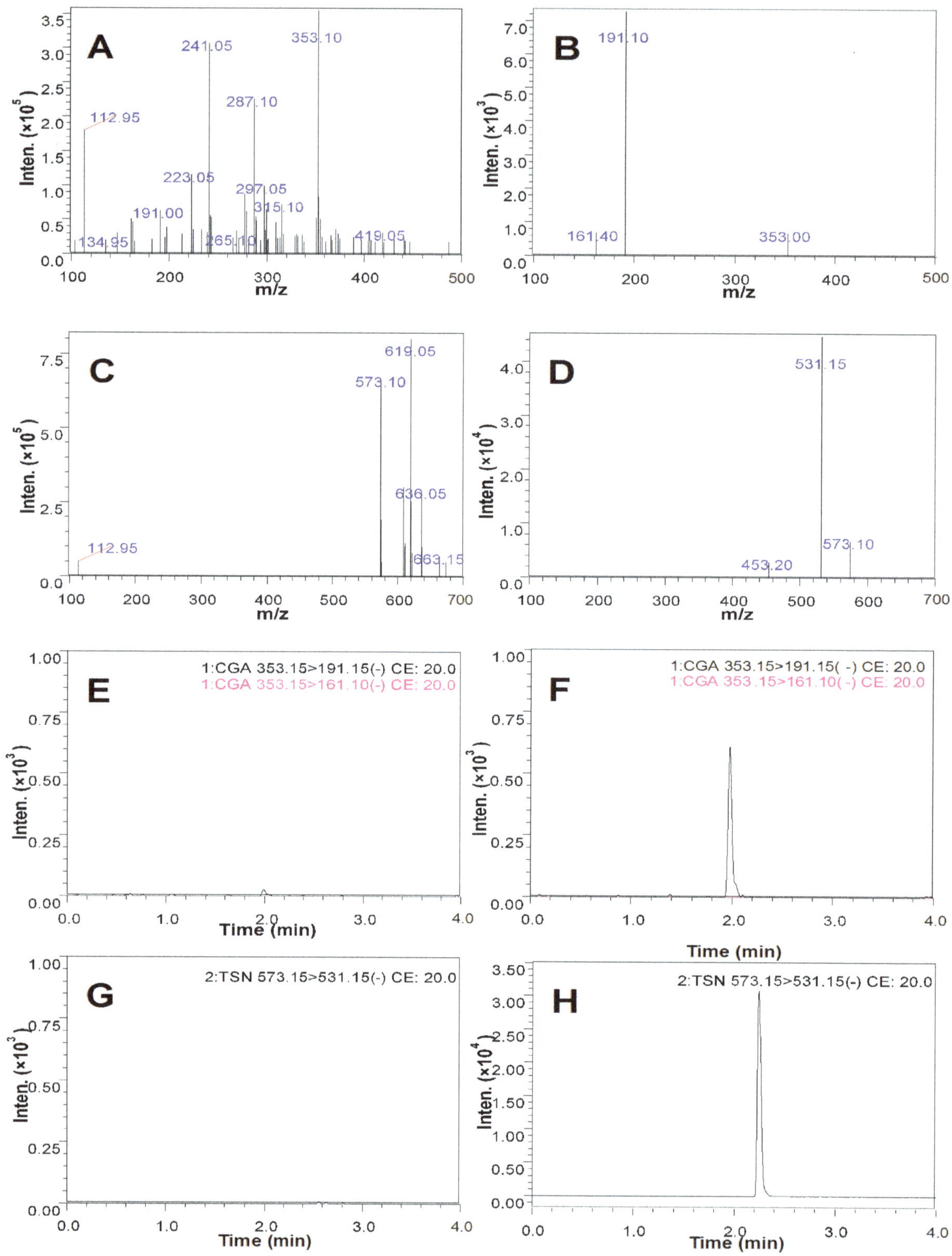

Figure 8. UHPLC-ESI-MS/MS chromatogram of CGA and toosendanin (TSN). (**A**) Negative Scan m/z 100–500 of CGA; (**B**) MS/MS spectrum of m/z 353.10 in the negative ion mode; (**C**) Negative Scan m/z 100–700 of TSN; (**D**) MS/MS spectrum of m/z 573.10 in the negative ion mode; (**E**) MRM of channels ESI^- 353.10/191.15 and 353.10/161.10 for blank CSF sample; (**F**) MRM of channels ESI^- 353.10/191.15 and 353.10/161.10 for CSF spiked with CGA; (**G**) MRM of channels ESI^- 573.15/531.15 for blank CSF sample; (**H**) MRM of channels ESI^- 573.15/531.15 for CSF spiked with TSN. Notes: Chromatographic conditions are provided in the Experimental Section.

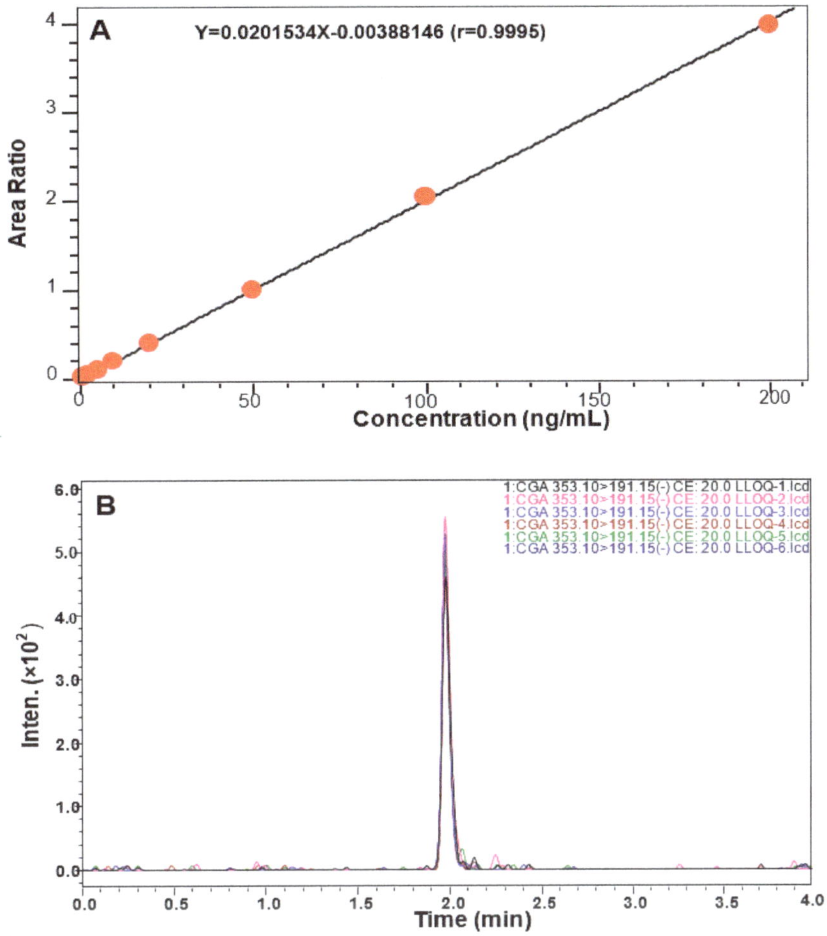

Figure 9. Linear regression calibration curves of CGA (**A**) and the six consecutive MRM of blank CSF spiked with 0.5 ng/mL CGA (**B**) in the CSF of rats.

3. Discussion

The present study aimed to explore whether CGA can protect from Cort-induced damage and promote 5-HT release through synapsin I expressionin in the cells of fetal rat raphe neurons *in vitro* and cross BLB of the rats orally treated with CGA-enriched EUWE *in vivo*. Our results indicate that CGA can indeed stimulate axon and dendrite growth, promote 5-HT release and enhance synapsin I expression in the cultured cells of fetal rat raphe neurons evidenced by immunofluorescence staining and western blots analysis. More important, our study of *in vivo* antidepressant like effect in the tail suspension test of mice demonstrated that CGA-enriched EUWE exhibited antidepressant effect (Figure 5). Furthermore, our results also show that CGA could be detected in the CSF of the rats orally treated with CGA-enriched EUWE at 4.0 g/kg and reach to the level of pharmacological effect for neuroprotection, indicating CGA can pass through the BLB of the rats treated with EUWE. Therefore, our findings suggest that CGA and CGA-enriched EUWE may have the potential to become the natural drugs for the treatment of depression. However, their action mode and associated mechanism(s) with anti-depression are still unclear and need to be further investigated.

Synapsin I is a presynaptic phosphoprotein that anchors synaptic vesicles containing neurotransmitters to the actin cytoskeleton in the distal pool [37]. The striking evidence indicates that the expression level of synapsin I is positively associated with the maturation of neurotransmitter release mechanisms [27]. In the present study, we found CGA significantly promoted 5-HT release and stimulated synapsin I expression in the cells of fetal rat raphe neurons *in vitro*, which may provide valuable information for the applications of CGA and CGA-enriched EUWE in potential treatment of depressive disorders in clinic.

However, synapsin I controls the fraction of synaptic vesicles available for release and thereby regulates the efficiency of neurotransmitter release by changing its phosphorylation state [38]. The phosphorylation of synapsin I is mediated by multiple protein kinases involved in various signaling pathways, including extracellular signal-regulated kinase (ERK) in mitogen-associated protein kinase (MAPK)/ERK pathway that modulates presynaptic plasticity and learning [39], protein kinase A (PKA) in cAMP-dependent pathway that modulates synaptic vesicle exocytosis [40], and Ca^{2+}/calmodulin-dependent protein kinase II (CaMK II) that modulates neurotransmitter release and synaptic plasticity [41]. Therefore, our further investigation into the molecular mechanisms associated with the anti-depression effects of CGA and CGA-enriched EUWE should include the study of phosphorylation of the respective site-specific kinases ERK, PKA and CaMK II in MAPK/ERK, cAMP/PKA, and Ca^{2+}/CaMK II pathways, which are upstream of synapsin I.

As we all know, several brain regions including hippocampus have been involved in depression. The hippocampus is an important region of the brain that is in charge of numerous cognitive and behavioral functions and related to the systems of 5-HT and glutamate, which are involved in the mechanism of action of antidepressants so the hippocampus is a key region in which to study depression [42,43]. Moreover, 5-HT has been shown to regulate synaptic neurotransmission in the hippocampus [44]. However, 5-HT is exclusively expressed in the dorsal and median raphe in the brain [26]. Then in order to study the effect of CGA and CGA-enriched EUWE on 5-HT release and its effects in hippocampus simultaneously, the method with a neuronal raphe/hippocampal co-culture *in vitro* should be developed to perform electrophysiological experiments as literature reported [25].

A most important feature for development of antidepressant is the ability to cross BLB and BBB *in vivo* to display its therapeutic efficacy [18]. In the present study, our data demonstrate that CGA-enriched EUWE at 200 and 400 mg/kg/day for 7 days showed antidepressant-like effect in the tail suspension test of mice and CGA from the rats orally treated with CGA-enriched EUWE can be detected in the CSF of rats by UHPLC-ESI-MS/MS analyses, indicating that CGA from EUWE can cross the BLB of the rats. This is the basic for further development of CGA and CGA-enriched EUWE as the antidepressants.

4. Experimental Section

4.1. Materials

CGA (Lot: 110753-200413) was purchased from National Institutes for Food and Drug Control (Beijing, China). The CGA structure was confirmed on a LCMS-8040 triple quadrupole mass spectrometer (Shimadzu Corporation, Kyoto, Japan). The CSF samples were analyzed by an ultrahigh performance liquid chromatography (UHPLC) system (LC-20 AD, Shimadzu Corporation) coupled to LCMS-8040 triple quadrupole mass spectrometer (Shimadzu Corporation). Acetonitrile (MS grade) and formic acid (MS grade) were purchased from Sigma-Aldrich (St. Louis, MO, USA). Deionized water was prepared using a Milli-Q water purification system (Millipore, Molsheim, France).

Dulbecco's modified Eagle's medium (DMEM), neurobasal medium, fetal bovine serum (FBS) and B-27 supplement were purchased from GIBCO Invitrogen (Carlsbad, CA, USA). Polylysine and Cort were purchased from Sigma-Aldrich. Anti-synapsin Ia/b antibody (H-170) was purchased from Santa Cruz Biotechnology (Dallas, TX, USA). Rat 5-HT ELISA kit was purchased from Cusabio Biotech (Newark, DE, USA).

4.2. Plant Material and Extraction

The bark of *E. ulmoides* used in this study was purchased from Taiji Group Limited Company (Chongqing, China), and were authenticated by Professor Can Tang at the Sichuan Medical University (Luzhou, Sichuan, China). The dry bark of *E. ulmoides* (100 g) was extracted three times with 1 L distilled water at 100 °C for 60 min each. Then the total extract was concentrated to dryness using a rotary vacuum evaporator and yielded 10.26 g dried extract. This crude EUWE was used for the experiments.

4.3. Animals and Sample Collection

Eight-to-ten-week old (body weight 250–300 g), and pregnant (16–20 weeks old and body weight 300–350 g, for primary raphe neuron study) Sprague Dawley rats (SPF Grade, Certificate No. SCXK2013-24) and Six-to-eight-week old (body weight 20–25 g) KM mice (for tail suspension test, SPF Grade, Certificate No. SCXK2013-24) were purchased from Experimental Animal Centre, Sichuan Provincial Academy of Medical Sciences in China (Chengdu, Sichuan, China). All animal experiments were performed in accordance with institutional guidelines and were approved by the Committee on Use and Care of Animals, Sichuan, China (Permit number: SYXK2013-065). All animals were housed under standard environmental conditions and fed with standard diet and water *ad libitum*. The adult rats in the EUWE group were administrated orally with a single dose of 4.0 g/kg EUWE and in the control group with same volume of deionized water before the CSF samples were collected. According to literature [45], rats were anesthetized by 40 mg/kg pentobarbitone, then the atlanto-occipital membrane was exposed by blunt dissection. CSF was collected by lowering a 25-gauge needle attached to polyethylene tubing into the cisterna magna. The pregnant Sprague Dawley rats on embryonic day 15 were used for preparing primary raphe neurons as literature reported [25].

4.4. Cell Culture and Treatment

The cells of primary raphe neurons were prepared from pregnant Sprague Dawley rats on embryonic day 15 as previously reported with slight modification [25]. Briefly, cells were gently dissociated with a pasteur pipette after digestion with 0.125% trypsin for 15 min at 37 °C, plated at a final density of 1×10^6 cells/well on polylysine-coated 6-well plates and cultured at 37 °C in a 5% CO_2 humidified incubator. After 24 h culture, the DMEM medium (with 10% FBS) was replaced by neurobasal medium containing 2% B-27 supplement. For cell proliferative assay, the cells of neurons were seeded into 96-well plates at a density of 3×10^4 cells/well and treated with 10 μM Cort for 24 h, then CGA was applied with different concentrations (0.001, 0.01, 0.1, 1 and 10 μM) or same volume of culture medium containing 0.1% DMSO as control. The assays were performed on the 2nd, 4th, 6th, 8th day using the Dojindo Cell Counting kit-8 according to the instruction supplied by the manufacturer. Absorbance values (490 nm) were recorded in triplicate using M5 Microplate Reader (Molecular Devices, Sunnyvale, CA, USA).

4.5. Neurotransmitter Detection

CGA was applied to Cort-pretreated cells of neurons for 5 days. Then the cells were washed 3 times and incubated in KPH buffer (130 mM NaCl, 5 mM KCl, 1.2 mM NaH_2PO_4, 1.8 mM $CaCl_2$′ 10 mM glucose, 1% BSA, 25 mM HEPES, pH 7.4) for 10 min at 37 °C, and subjected to 0.5 nM or 1.0 nM CGA, all treatments were brought up to final concentration in neurobasal medium containing 2% B-27 supplement. After 10 days, the supernatants were concentrated 10-fold using a nitrogen evaporator and the levels of 5-HT were determined using a rat 5-HT ELISA kit.

4.6. Immunofluorescence Staining

CGA (1 nM) was applied to Cort-pretreated cells of neurons for 8 days. The cells were fixed with 4% paraformaldehyde containing 0.05% Triton X-100 for 20 min and rinsed with PBS. After blocked with 4% BSA, the cells were incubated overnight at 4 °C with anti-synapsin I antibody (1:50). Afterward, fluorescein isothiocyanate (FITC) conjugated secondary antibodies (1:100) were applied at room temperature for 1 h. Immunoreactivity was observed with an IX51 fluorescence microscope (Olympus, Tokyo, Japan).

4.7. Western Blot Analysis

Neurons were harvested after 7 days CGA (1 nM), and/or Cort (10 μM) or medium with 0.1% DMSO (control) treatment and disrupted in cell RIPA buffer (0.5% NP-40, 50 mM Tris-HCl, 120 mM NaCl, 1 mM EDTA, 0.1mM Na_3VO_4, 1 mM NaF, 1 mM PMSF, 1 μg/mL leupeptin, pH 7.5), and then lysates were centrifuged at 12,000 rpm for 15 min at 4°C. The protein concentration was determined using the BCA method, after which equal amounts of protein (30 μg) were electrophoresedon 10% density SDS-acrylamide gels. Following electrophoresis, the proteins were transferred from the gel to a nitrocellulose membrane using an electric transfer system. Non-specific binding was blocked with 5% skim milk in TBST buffer (5 mM Tris-HCl, pH 7.6, 136 mM NaCl and 0.1% Tween-20) for 1 h. The blots were incubated with antibodies against synapsin I (1:200) overnight at 4 °C and were washed three times with 1 × TBST. Then, the blots were incubated for 1 h at room temperature with a 1:5000 dilution of horseradish peroxidase-labeled anti-rabbit or anti-mouse IgG and washed three times with 1 × TBST, the membranes were developed by incubation within the ECL western detection reagents.

4.8. Tail Suspension Test of Mice

The experiments were performed according to the method of Park *et al.* [20]. Briefly, forty-eight male KM mice were divided into four groups, and the mice were treated orally with distilled water (vehicle control), fluoxetine (FLX) at 8 mg/kg (as positive control), or EUWE at 200 and 400 mg/kg/day with a volume of 0.2 mL/20 g of body weight once a day for 7 days. One hour after the last administration of vehicle, FLX or EUWE, the mice were suspended by the tail to a horizontal ring stand bar (distance from floor 25 cm) using adhesive tape (distance from tip of tail 2 cm). Then the duration of immobility was recorded for the last 4 min during 6-min test session. There are 12 mice for each experimental group.

4.9. UHPLC-ESI-MS/MS Analysis

The UHPLC-ESI-MS/MS analyses were performed on a Shimadzu LCMS-8040 UHPLC system comprised of two LC-30AD pumps, a SIL-30AC autosampler with a CTO-30AC column oven, a DGU-20A$_5$ degasser, a Shimadzu CBM-20A system controller, a Labsolution LCMS Ver.5.75 workstation, an ESI ion source and a LCMS-8040 mass spectrometer. Chromatographic analyses were achieved at 45 °C with an InertSustain C18 column (GL Science, 2.0 μM particle size, 50 mm × 2.1 mm), using water-formic acid (100:0.05, *v*/*v*) and acetonitrile as the mobile phase A and phase B, respectively. The mobile phase was delivered at a rate of 0.35 mL/min. The injection volume was 10 μL. For the gradient separation, the gradient program was as follows: 5%–5% B at 0–0.8 min, 5%–100% B at 0.8–1.3 min, 100%–100% B at 1.3–2.5 min, 100%–5% B at 2.5–3.0 min, 5%–5% B at 3.0–4.0 min. For mass detection, the mass spectrometer was programmed to carry out a full scan over m/z 100–500 (MS^1) and the secondary mass spectrum data were collected by dependence pattern (MS^2) in positive ion and negative ion detection modes with a spray capillary voltage of 3.0 kV. The detector voltage was 2.04 kV. The desolvation line was heated to 250 °C and the heat block was heated to 450 °C. Nebulizing gas was introduced at 2.5 L/min, and the drying gas was set to 10.0 L/min. Collision-induced dissociation gas pressure was set to 230 kPa. The data analysis was performed using LabSolutions software (version 5.75, Shimadzu).

4.10. Statistical Analysis

All data were presented as means ± SD. The statistical significance of the data was analyzed by one-way analysis of variance (ANOVA), and values of $p < 0.05$ were considered statistically significant.

5. Conclusions

In the present study, we demonstrated that CGA plays an important role in neuron protection, promotion of 5-HT release and enhancement of synapsin I expression in the cultured cells of fetal rat raphe neurons. Furthermore, using UHPLC-ESI-MS/MS we also detected and identified CGA in the CSF of the rats after oral administration of CGA-enriched EUWE, indicating CGA could pass through the BLB of rats treated with EUWE *in vivo*. These results may provide important insights into potential discovery and development of CGA and CGA-enriched EUWE as the new antidepressants clinically. However, more studies are needed to further investigate the action mode and associated mechanism(s) of CGA and EUWE as the novel antidepressants. In addition, the *in vivo* antidepressant efficacy of CGA and EUWE should be tested in animal models of depression to validate the results.

Acknowledgments: This work is supported by the PhD research startup foundation of Sichuan Medical University (2014-0083). We thank Professor Can Tang (Sichuan Medical University) for identifying the plant specimens.

Author Contributions: Jianming Wu and Dalian Qin conceived and designed the experiments; Jianming Wu, Haixia Chen, Hua Li, Yong Tang and Le Yang performed the experiments; Jianming Wu and Haixia Chen analyzed the data; Dalian Qin contributed new reagents and analysis tools; Jianming Wu, Shousong Cao and Haixia Chen wrote the paper.

Abbreviations

E. ulmoides	*Eucommia ulmoides* Oliver
TCM	Traditional Chinese Medicine
CGA	Chlorogenic acid
BLB	Blood-cerebrospinal fluid barrier
BBB	Blood-brain barrier
Cort	Corticosterone
5-HT	5-hydroxytryptamine or serotonin
ELISA	Enzyme-linked immunosorbent assay
EUWE	Water extract of *E. ulmoides*
FLX	Fluoxetine
TSN	Toosendanin
RSD	Relative standard deviation
ERK	Extracellular signal-regulated kinase
MAPK	Mitogen-associated protein kinase
PKA	Protein kinase A
CaMK	Calmodulin-dependent protein kinase
UHPLC	Ultrahigh performance liquid chromatography
DMEM	Dulbecco's modified Eagle's medium
FBS	Fetal bovine serum

References

1. He, X.; Wang, J.; Li, M.; Hao, D.; Yang, Y.; Zhang, C.; He, R.; Tao, R. *Eucommia ulmoides* Oliv.: Ethnopharmacology, phytochemistry and pharmacology of an important traditional Chinese medicine. *J. Ethnopharmacol.* **2014**, *151*, 78–92. [CrossRef] [PubMed]
2. Xie, G.P.; Jiang, N.; Wang, S.N.; Qi, R.Z.; Wang, L.; Zhao, P.R.; Liang, L.; Yu, B. *Eucommia ulmoides* Oliv. bark aqueous extract inhibits osteoarthritis in a rat model of osteoarthritis. *J. Ethnopharmacol.* **2015**, *162*, 148–154. [CrossRef] [PubMed]
3. Kwon, S.H.; Ma, S.X.; Hong, S.I.; Kim, S.Y.; Lee, S.Y.; Jang, C.G. *Eucommia ulmoides* Oliv. bark. attenuates 6-hydroxydopamine-induced neuronal cell death through inhibition of oxidative stress in SH-SY5Y cells. *J. Ethnopharmacol.* **2014**, *152*, 173–182. [CrossRef] [PubMed]
4. Guo, H.; Shi, F.; Li, M.; Liu, Q.; Yu, B.; Hu, L. Neuroprotective effects of *Eucommia ulmoides* Oliv. and its bioactive constituent work via ameliorating the ubiquitin-proteasome system. *BMC Complement. Altern. Med.* **2015**, *15*, 151. [CrossRef] [PubMed]

5. Zhang, R.; Pan, Y.L.; Hu, S.J.; Kong, X.H.; Juan, W.; Mei, Q.B. Effects of total lignans from *Eucommia ulmoides* barks prevent bone loss *in vivo* and *in vitro*. *J. Ethnopharmacol.* **2014**, *155*, 104–112. [CrossRef] [PubMed]
6. Kwon, S.H.; Lee, H.K.; Kim, J.A.; Hong, S.I.; Kim, S.Y.; Jo, T.H.; Park, Y.I.; Lee, C.K.; Kim, Y.B.; Lee, S.Y.; *et al.* Neuroprotective effects of *Eucommia ulmoides* Oliv. Bark on amyloid beta-induced learning and memory impairments in mice. *Neurosci Lett.* **2011**, *487*, 123–127. [CrossRef] [PubMed]
7. Kwon, S.H.; Ma, S.X.; Joo, H.J.; Lee, S.Y.; Jang, C.G. Inhibitory Effects of *Eucommia ulmoides* Oliv. Bark on Scopolamine-Induced Learning and Memory Deficits in Mice. *Biomol. Ther.* **2013**, *21*, 462–469. [CrossRef] [PubMed]
8. Jin, X.; Amitani, K.; Zamami, Y.; Takatori, S.; Hobara, N.; Kawamura, N.; Hirata, T.; Wada, A.; Kitamura, Y.; Kawasaki, H. Ameliorative effect of *Eucommia ulmoides* Oliv. leaves extract (ELE) on insulin resistance and abnormal perivascular innervation in fructose-drinking rats. *J. Ethnopharmacol.* **2010**, *128*, 672–678. [CrossRef] [PubMed]
9. Yongsheng, L.; Shumei, L.; Guodong, W. Studies on resin purification process optimization of *Eucommia ulmoides* Oliver and its antihypertensive effect mechanism. *Afr. J. Tradit. Complement Altern. Med.* **2014**, *11*, 475–480. [CrossRef] [PubMed]
10. Peng, W.; Ge, S.; Li, D.; Mo, B.; Daochun, Q.; Ohkoshi, M. Report: Molecular basis of antibacterial activities in extracts of *Eucommia ulmoides* wood. *Pak. J. Pharm. Sci.* **2014**, *27*, 2133–2138. [PubMed]
11. Hao, S.; Xiao, Y.; Lin, Y.; Mo, Z.; Chen, Y.; Peng, X.; Xiang, C.; Li, Y.; Li, W. Chlorogenic acid-enriched extract from *Eucommia ulmoides* leaves inhibits hepatic lipid accumulation through regulation of cholesterol metabolism in $HepG_2$ cells. *Pharm. Biol.* **2016**, *54*, 251–259. [CrossRef] [PubMed]
12. Fujikawa, T.; Hirata, T.; Hosoo, S.; Nakajima, K.; Wada, A.; Yurugi, Y.; Soya, H.; Matsui, T.; Yamaguchi, A.; Ogata, M.; *et al.* Asperuloside stimulates metabolic function in rats across several organs under high-fat diet conditions, acting like the major ingredient of *Eucommi*a leaves with anti-obesity activity. *J. Nutr. Sci.* **2012**, *1*, e10. [CrossRef] [PubMed]
13. Kim, J.; Lee, S.; Shim, J.; Kim, H.W.; Kim, J.; Jang, Y.J.; Yang, H.; Park, J.; Choi, S.H.; Yoon, J.H.; *et al.* Caffeinated coffee, decaffeinated coffee, and the phenolic phytochemical chlorogenic acid up-regulate NQO1 expression and prevent H_2O_2-induced apoptosis in primary cortical neurons. *Neurochem. Int.* **2012**, *60*, 466–474. [CrossRef] [PubMed]
14. Shen, W.; Qi, R.; Zhang, J.; Wang, Z.; Wang, H.; Hu, C.; Zhao, Y.; Bie, M.; Wang, Y.; Fu, Y.; *et al.* Chlorogenic acid inhibits LPS-induced microglial activation and improves survival of dopaminergic neurons. *Brain Res. Bull.* **2012**, *88*, 487–494. [CrossRef] [PubMed]
15. Stefanello, N.; Schmatz, R.; Pereira, L.B.; Rubin, M.A.; da Rocha, J.B.; Facco, G.; Pereira, M.E.; Mazzanti, C.M.; Passamonti, S.; Rodrigues, M.V.; *et al.* Effects of chlorogenic acid, caffeine, and coffee on behavioral and biochemical parameters of diabetic rats. *Mol. Cell. Biochem.* **2014**, *388*, 277–286. [CrossRef] [PubMed]
16. Kwon, S.H.; Lee, H.K.; Kim, J.A.; Hong, S.I.; Kim, H.C.; Jo, T.H.; Park, Y.I.; Lee, C.K.; Kim, Y.B.; Lee, S.Y.; *et al.* Neuroprotective effects of chlorogenic acid on scopolamine-induced amnesia via anti-acetylcholinesterase and anti-oxidative activities in mice. *Eur. J. Pharmacol.* **2010**, *649*, 210–217. [CrossRef] [PubMed]
17. Oboh, G.; Agunloye, O.M.; Akinyemi, A.J.; Ademiluyi, A.O.; Adefegha, S.A. Comparative study on the inhibitory effect of caffeic and chlorogenic acids on key enzymes linked to Alzheimer's disease and some pro-oxidant induced oxidative stress in rats' brain-*in vitro*. *Neurochem. Res.* **2013**, *38*, 413–419. [CrossRef] [PubMed]
18. Uchida, M.; Katoh, T.; Mori, M.; Maeno, T.; Ohtake, K.; Kobayashi, J.; Morimoto, Y.; Natsume, H. Intranasal administration of milnacipran in rats: Evaluation of the transport of drugs to the systemic circulation and central nervous system and the pharmacological effect. *Biol. Pharm. Bull.* **2011**, *34*, 740–747. [CrossRef] [PubMed]
19. Chao, J.; Wang, H.; Zhao, W.; Zhang, M.; Zhang, L. Investigation of the inclusion behavior of chlorogenic acid with hydroxypropyl-ß-cyclodextrin. *Int. J. Biol. Macromol.* **2012**, *50*, 277–282. [CrossRef] [PubMed]
20. Park, S.H.; Sim, Y.B.; Han, P.L.; Lee, J.K.; Suh, H.W. Antidepressant-like effect of chlorogenic acid isolated from *Artemisia capillaris* Thunb. *Anim. Cells Syst.* **2010**, *4*, 253–259. [CrossRef]
21. Czéh, B.; Michaelis, T.; Watanabe, T.; Frahm, J.; de Biurrun, G.; van Kampen, M.; Bartolomucci, A.; Fuchs, E. Stress-induced changes in cerebral metabolites, hippocampal volume, and cell proliferation are prevented by antidepressant treatment with tianeptine. *Proc. Natl. Acad. Sci. USA* **2001**, *98*, 12796–12801. [CrossRef] [PubMed]

22. Pariante, C.M. The role of multi-drug resistance *p*-glycoprotein in glucocorticoid function: studies in animals and relevance in humans. *Eur. J. Pharmacol.* **2008**, *583*, 263–271. [CrossRef] [PubMed]
23. Orchinik, M.; Weiland, N.G.; McEwen, B.S. Chronic exposure to stress levels of corticosterone alters GABAA receptor subunit mRNA levels in rat hippocampus. *Brain Res. Mol. Brain Res.* **1995**, *34*, 29–37. [CrossRef]
24. Belmaker, R.H.; Agam, G. Major depressive disorder. *N. Engl. J. Med.* **2008**, *358*, 55–68. [CrossRef] [PubMed]
25. Ashimi, S.S. An *in Vitro* Characterization of the Raphe Nucleus and the Effects of SSRIs on Synaptic Neurotransmission. Ph.D. Thesis, The University of Texas Southwestern Medical Center, Dallas, TX, USA, 2010.
26. Smith, T.D.; Kuczenski, R.; George-Friedman, K.; Malley, J.D.; Foote, S.L. *In vivo* microdialysis assessment of extracellular serotonin and dopamine levels in awake monkeys during sustained fluoxetine administration. *Synapse* **2000**, *38*, 460–470. [CrossRef]
27. Valtorta, F.; Iezzi, N.; Benfenati, F.; Lu, B.; Poo, M.M.; Greengard, P. Accelerated structural maturation induced by synapsin I at developing neuromuscular synapses of *Xenopus laevis*. *Eur. J. Neurosci.* **1995**, *7*, 261–270. [CrossRef] [PubMed]
28. Takei, Y.; Harada, A.; Takeda, S.; Kobayashi, K.; Terada, S.; Noda, T.; Takahashi, T.; Hirokawa, N. Synapsin I deficiency results in the structural change in the presynaptic terminals in the murine nervous system. *J. Cell Biol.* **1995**, *131*, 1789–1800. [CrossRef] [PubMed]
29. Chin, L.S.; Li, L.; Ferreira, A.; Kosik, K.S.; Greengard, P. Impairment of axonal development and of synaptogenesis in hippocampal neurons of synapsin I-deficient mice. *Proc. Natl. Acad. Sci. USA* **1995**, *92*, 9230–9234. [CrossRef] [PubMed]
30. Petrik, D.; Lagace, D.C.; Eisch, A.J. The neurogenesis hypothesis of affective and anxiety disorders: Are we mistaking the scaffolding for the building? *Neuropharmacol.* **2012**, *62*, 21–34. [CrossRef] [PubMed]
31. Eisch, A.J.; Petrik, D. Depression and hippocampal neurogenesis: a road to remission? *Science.* **2012**, *338*, 72–75. [CrossRef] [PubMed]
32. Wu, L.M.; Han, H.; Wang, Q.N.; Hou, H.L.; Tong, H.; Yan, X.B.; Zhou, J.N. Mifepristone repairs region-dependent alteration of synapsin I in hippocampus in rat model of depression. *Neuropsychopharmacology* **2007**, *32*, 2500–2510. [CrossRef] [PubMed]
33. Zhu, C.S.; Zhang, B.; Lin, Z.J.; Wang, X.J.; Zhou, Y.; Sun, X.X.; Xiao, M.L. Relationship between high-performance liquid chromatography fingerprints and uric acid-lowering activities of *Cichorium intybus* L. *Molecules* **2015**, *20*, 9455–9467. [CrossRef] [PubMed]
34. Lopes-Lutz, D.; Dettmann, J.; Nimalaratne, C.; Schieber, A. Characterization and quantification of polyphenols in Amazon grape (*Pourouma cecropiifolia* Martius). *Molecules* **2010**, *15*, 8543–8552. [CrossRef] [PubMed]
35. Lech, K.; Witkoś, K.; Jarosz, M. HPLC-UV-ESI MS/MS identification of the color constituents of sawwort (*Serratula tinctoria* L.). *Anal. Bioanal. Chem.* **2014**, *406*, 3703–3708. [CrossRef] [PubMed]
36. Zhang, Q.; Zhagn, J.Y.; Sui, C.L.; Shi, X.Y.; Qiao, Y.J.; Lu, J.Q. Regularity of changes in chlorogenic acids in *Lonicera japonica* extracts by HPLC-DAD-ESI-MS/MS. *Zhongguo Zhong Yao Za Zhi (In Chinese)* **2012**, *37*, 3564–3568. [PubMed]
37. Pieribone, V.A.; Shupliakov, O.; Brodin, L.; Hilfiker-Rothenfluh, S.; Czernik, A.J.; Greengard, P. Distinct pools of synaptic vesicles in neurotransmitter release. *Nature* **1995**, *375*, 493–497. [CrossRef] [PubMed]
38. Greengard, P.; Valtorta, F.; Czernik, A.J.; Benfenati, F. Synaptic vesicle phosphoproteins and regulation of synaptic function. *Science.* **1993**, *259*, 780–785. [CrossRef] [PubMed]
39. Kushner, S.A.; Elgersma, Y.; Murphy, G.G.; Jaarsma, D.; van Woerden, G.M.; Hojjati, M.R.; Cui, Y.; LeBoutillier, J.C.; Marrone, D.F.; Choi, E.S.; *et al.* Modulation of presynaptic plasticity and learning by the H-ras/extracellular signal-regulated kinase/synapsin I signaling pathway. *J. Neurosci.* **2005**, *25*, 9721–9734. [CrossRef] [PubMed]
40. Menegon, A.; Bonanomi, D.; Albertinazzi, C.; Lotti, F.; Ferrari, G.; Kao, H.T.; Benfenati, F.; Baldelli, P.; Valtorta, F. Protein kinase A-mediated synapsin I phosphorylation is a central modulator of Ca^{2+}-dependent synaptic activity. *J. Neurosci.* **2006**, *26*, 11670–11681. [CrossRef] [PubMed]
41. Fiumara, F.; Onofri, F.; Benfenati, F.; Montarolo, P.G.; Ghirardi, M. Intracellular injection of synapsin I induces neurotransmitter release in C1 neurons of Helix pomatia contacting a wrong target. *Neuroscience* **2001**, *104*, 271–280. [CrossRef]

42. Pittaluga, A.; Raiteri, L.; Longordo, F.; Luccini, E.; Barbiero, V.S.; Racagni, G.; Popoli, M.; Raiteri, M. Antidepressant treatments and function of glutamate ionotropic receptors mediating amine release in hippocampus. *Neuropharmacology* **2007**, *53*, 27–36. [CrossRef] [PubMed]
43. Millan, M.J. The role of monoamines in the actions of established and "novel" antidepressant agents: A critical review. *Eur. J. Pharmacol.* **2004**, *500*, 371–384. [CrossRef] [PubMed]
44. Kobayashi, K.; Ikeda, Y.; Haneda, E.; Suzuki, H. Chronic fluoxetine bidirectionally modulates potentiating effects of serotonin on the hippocampal mossy fiber synaptic transmission. *J. Neurosci.* **2008**, *28*, 6272–6280. [CrossRef] [PubMed]
45. Svetlov, S.I.; Prima, V.; Kirk, D.R.; Gutierrez, H.; Curley, K.C.; Hayes, R.L.; Wang, K.K. Morphologic and biochemical characterization of brain injury in a model of controlled blast overpressure exposure. *J. Trauma* **2010**, *69*, 795–804. [CrossRef] [PubMed]

7

Neurodegenerative Diseases: Might *Citrus* Flavonoids Play a Protective Role?

Santa Cirmi [1], Nadia Ferlazzo [1], Giovanni E. Lombardo [2], Elvira Ventura-Spagnolo [3], Sebastiano Gangemi [4,5], Gioacchino Calapai [6] and Michele Navarra [1,*]

1 Department of Chemical, Biological, Pharmaceutical and Environmental Sciences, University of Messina, viale Annunziata, Messina I-98168, Italy; scirmi@unime.it (S.C.); nadiaferlazzo@email.it (N.F.)
2 Department of Health Sciences, University "Magna Graecia" of Catanzaro, Catanzaro I-88100, Italy; gelombardo@unicz.it
3 Department of Biotechnology and Legal Medicine, University of Palermo, Palermo I-90127, Italy; elvira.ventura@unipa.it
4 Department of Clinical and Experimental Medicine, University of Messina, Messina I-98125, Italy; gangemis@unime.it
5 Institute of Applied Sciences and Intelligent Systems (ISASI), National Research Council (CNR), Pozzuoli I-80078, Italy
6 Department of Biomedical and Dental Sciences and Morphofunctional Imaging, University of Messina, Messina I-98125, Italy; gcalapai@unime.it
* Correspondence: mnavarra@unime.it

Academic Editor: Luigia Trabace

Abstract: Neurodegenerative diseases (ND) result from the gradual and progressive degeneration of the structure and function of the central nervous system or the peripheral nervous system or both. They are characterized by deterioration of neurons and/or myelin sheath, disruption of sensory information transmission and loss of movement control. There is no effective treatment for ND, and the drugs currently marketed are symptom-oriented, albeit with several side effects. Within the past decades, several natural remedies have gained attention as potential neuroprotective drugs. Moreover, an increasing number of studies have suggested that dietary intake of vegetables and fruits can prevent or delay the onset of ND. These properties are mainly due to the presence of polyphenols, an important group of phytochemicals that are abundantly present in fruits, vegetables, cereals and beverages. The main class of polyphenols is flavonoids, abundant in *Citrus* fruits. Our review is an overview on the scientific literature concerning the neuroprotective effects of the *Citrus* flavonoids in the prevention or treatment of ND. This review may be used as scientific basis for the development of nutraceuticals, food supplements or complementary and alternative drugs to maintain and improve the neurophysiological status.

Keywords: *Citrus*; flavonoids; neurodegeneration; neurodegenerative disorders; nutraceutical

---

1. Introduction

The increase of the lifespan in populations of developed countries is leading to a rise in the incidence of age-related illnesses such as neurodegenerative diseases (ND). ND are a heterogeneous group of chronic and untreatable conditions that, in terms of human suffering and economic cost for society, represent the fourth highest source of overall disease burden in high-income countries. ND result from the gradual and progressive degeneration of the structure and function of both the central nervous system (CNS) and the peripheral nervous system (PNS), characterized by deterioration of neurons and/or myelin sheath, sensory information transmission disruption and movement control.

It is known that oxidative stress and chronic inflammation play an important role in ND. Free radicals represent a common denominator of many oxidative-based diseases, including ND, although they are normally and continuously produced in CNS, acting as important cellular messenger. However, excessive levels of reactive oxygen species (ROS) or reactive nitrogen species (RNS) are involved in numerous neuroinflammatory processes. In physiological conditions, the levels of free radicals are tightly regulated by a complex antioxidant defense system including both enzymatic and non-enzymatic antioxidants. Disruption of the delicate oxidant/antioxidant balance between the production and removal of oxidizing chemical species can lead to oxidative stress triggering cell damage. This may be due to an excessive production of ROS and RNS and/or at a reduced efficiency of the physiological antioxidant defense systems. Moreover, because of their high metabolic activities and low antioxidant defense capability, neural cells in brains are more vulnerable to oxidative stress, especially those of the aging brain. Furthermore, cytokines released by the activated glial cells amplify the free radicals-induced damage responsible for uncontrolled proteolysis, DNA mutagenesis, lipid peroxidation and cell death.

Currently there is no effective treatment for ND, and the marketed drugs are mainly symptom-oriented, albeit with many side effects, limited efficacy and partial capability to inhibit disease progression. Therefore, in order to develop novel preventive strategies or co-adjuvant therapy for ND, within the past decades, a great number of natural medicinal plants has gained attention as potential neuroprotective agents [1]. Moreover, an increasing number of studies have suggested that dietary intake of vegetables and fruits can prevent or delay the onset of ND [2,3]. These properties might be due to the presence of polyphenols, an important group of phytochemicals that are abundantly present in fruits, vegetables, cereals and beverages [4]. The main class of polyphenols is flavonoids which display a remarkable spectrum of biological activities, including antioxidant, free radical scavenger, metal ions chelating, vasoprotective, hepatoprotective, anti-inflammatory, anti-cancer and anti-infective [5,6]. Main dietary sources of flavonoids are fruits, especially *Citrus* fruits, vegetables, fruit juices, tea, coffee, and red wine [7]. Several lines of evidence have demonstrated the beneficial effects of *Citrus* fruits in the context of numerous pathologies, including ND, inflammation, cardiovascular diseases, dyslipidemia, diabetes, allergy, immune system diseases and cancer [8–24].

Our review is an overview on the scientific literature concerning the neuroprotective effects of the *Citrus* flavonoids in the prevention or treatment of ND.

2. Focus on Neurodegenerative Disorders

ND are incurable conditions due to the progressive nervous system dysfunction caused by degeneration and loss of nerve cells for reasons that have not yet been fully understood. Today, a growing number of people worldwide are affected by ND, characterized by deterioration in emotional control, social behavior and social communication. ND exist in many forms, such as Multiple Sclerosis, Alzheimer's, Parkinson's, Huntington's, human prion and motoneuron diseases.

Alzheimer's disease (AD) is a debilitating ND classified as the major subtype of dementia [25], and is characterized by progressive loss of memory. It results in decline in cognitive and behavioral functions like memory, thinking and language skills [26]. The hallmarks of AD are (i) the accumulation of amyloid-beta (Aβ) peptide in the brain; (ii) the presence of neurofibrillary tangles (NFTs) containing hyper-phosphorylated tau fragments and (iii) the loss of cortical neurons and synapses [27,28]. It is also known that the innate immune system activation plays a relevant role in the age-related ND, including AD. Microglia are innate immune cells in the CNS that mediate inflammatory responses to injury and pathogens by releasing pro-inflammatory cytokines that amplify and aggravate inflammation throughout the brain. These pro-inflammatory factors may induce degeneration of normal neurons through upregulation of nuclear factor kappa B (NF-κB), mitogen-activated protein kinase (MAPK), and c-Jun N-terminal kinase (JNK) [29].

Parkinson's disease (PD) is the second common neurodegenerative disorder and its incidence is increasing among people over the age of 60 years [30]. It is consistently higher in men than in women [31]. Pathologically, it is characterized by the progressive and diffuse loss of dopaminergic neurons in the substantia nigra and the accumulation of Lewy bodies (inclusions containing α-synuclein) in nerve cells. The major clinical symptoms are tremor at rest, rigidity, bradykinesia and postural instability. It has been suggested that activated microglia may be beneficial to the host in the early phase of neurodegeneration but excessive activation of microglia leads to the elevated expression of pro-inflammatory mediators such as tumor necrosis factor alpha (TNF-α), interleukin 1 beta (IL-1β), interleukin-6 (IL-6) and interferon gamma (IFN-γ) [32], that induce the degeneration of substantia nigra pars compacta dopaminergic neurons [29,33]. Furthermore, the release of these pro-inflammatory mediators can activate astrocytes that participate to the neuroinflammatory processes linked to PD [34].

Huntington's disease (HD) is a hereditary neurological disorder inherited as an autosomal dominant trait [35] caused by an expanded polyglutamine tract in the N-terminal region of mutant huntingtin [36]. HD usually occurs in early middle life even if there is an uncommon juvenile form [37]. It is an illness that recurs with abnormal movements together with psychiatric symptoms including psychosis, depression, and obsessive-compulsive disorder and progressive cognitive impairment [38–40]. In the early stage of disease, neuronal loss occur preferentially in the striatum, while in the later stages the extensive neurodegeneration happens in a variety of brain regions [36,41].

Human prion diseases are fatal neurodegenerative disorders which include Kuru, Creutzfeldt-Jakob disease, Gerstmann-Sträussler-Scheinker syndrome, and fatal familial insomnia [42]. Prion diseases result from the conformational conversion of a normal cellular prion protein (PrP^{C}) into an abnormal misfolded pathological form (PrP^{Sc}). Its accumulation in the CNS resulted in progressive neuronal degeneration and vacuolation [43].

Motor neuron disease (MND) is a neurodegenerative condition, among which the most common is the amyotrophic lateral sclerosis (ALS). MND affects both brain and spinal cord, and is due to the degeneration of motor neurons, that in turn causes muscle weakness. The major clinical symptoms include muscle weakness, wasting, cramps and stiffness of arms and/or legs, problems with speech and/or swallowing or, more rarely, with breathing problem [44]. The etiopathogenesis of MND is unknown and the aim of the cure is to maintain functional ability and enabling MND patients to live life as fully as possible [45].

Multiple sclerosis (MS) is a CNS chronic inflammatory disease that is caused by autoimmune-mediated loss of myelin and axonal damage. Its etiopathogenesis is poorly understood. MS is the most common neurological disorder affecting young adults, with a total of 2.5 million people in worldwide [46]. It causes a range of relapsing symptoms during the early phase of the disease, but becomes more persistent and less amenable to treatment at later stages. The research focused on identifying treatments that slow progression of neurodegeneration and also restore myelin of affected CNS regions [47].

3. *Citrus* Flavonoids

The genus *Citrus* belongs to the family Rutaceae, subfamily Aurantioideae, tribe Citreae, subtribe Citrinae. According to statistics of Food and Agriculture Organization of the United Nations (FAO), *Citrus* species are grown in more than 140 countries. China, Brazil, USA, India, Mexico, and Spain are the world's leading *Citrus* fruit-producing countries, representing close to two-thirds of global production (FAO STAT) [48].

The basic structural feature of flavonoid is 2-phenyl-benzo-γ-pyrane nucleus, contains a C6−C3−C6 heterocyclic skeleton, consisting of two benzene rings linked through a heterocyclic pyran ring. Based on the oxidization of the heterocyclic (C3) ring, *Citrus* flavonoids can be divided in flavanones, flavonols, flavones, and polymethoxiflavone (Figure 1). Anthocyanins are considered as metabolites of flavones and are present only in blood oranges. Structurally, they derived from pyran or flavan. Flavonoids are mainly present in plants as glycosides, while aglycones (the forms lacking sugar moieties) occur less frequently. Therefore, the large number of flavonoids is a result of many different combinations of aglycones and sugars, mainly D-glucose and L-rhamnose, bounded the hydroxyl group at the C-3 or C-7 position.

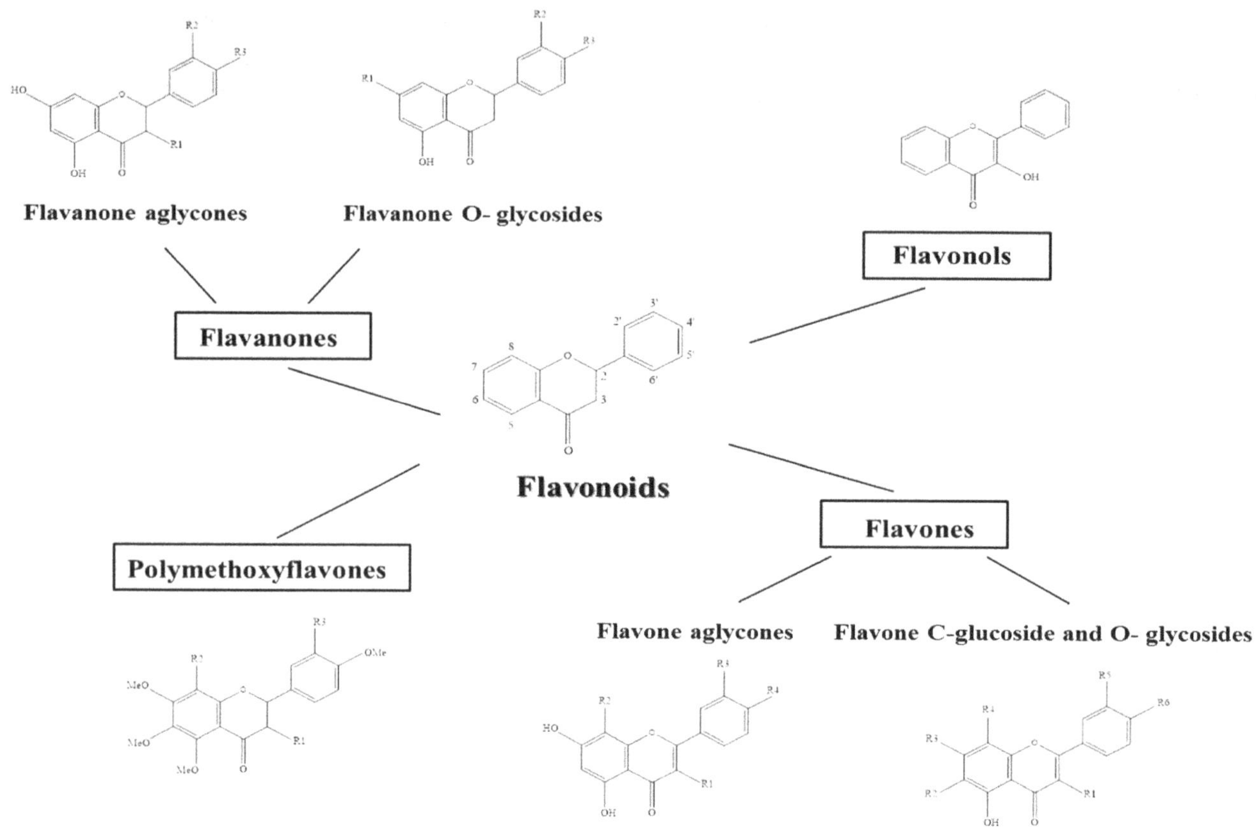

Figure 1. Chemical structure of *Citrus* flavonoids subclasses.

Flavanones comprise approximately 95% of the total flavonoids. Their concentration depends on the age of the plant, and the highest levels are detected in tissues, showing pronounced cell divisions [49]. They are present in both the glycoside and aglycone forms. Glycosylation occurs at position 7 either by rutinose or neohesperidose. The most important flavanones present in the aglycone forms are naringenin and hesperetin. Among flavanones with neohesperidose (rhamnosyl-α-1,2 glucose), naringin, neoeriocitrin, neohesperedin and poncirin are the most abundant. Hesperidin, narirutin, eriocitrin and didymin are the main flavanone with rutinose (rhamnosyl-α-1,6 glucose). Luteolin and diosmetin are the most present flavones in the aglycone form, while diosmin and neodismin represent the major flavones in the rutinosides and neohesperidosides forms, respectively [50]. Flavonols are the 3-hydroxy derivatives of flavones. Glycosylation occurs preferentially at the 3-hydroxyl group of the central ring. The most common flavonol aglycones are quercetin and kaempferol, while rutin and rutinosides are the main in the glycosidic form. Even if present in smaller quantities, the most common polymethoxiflavones are tangeretin and nobiletin. The chemical structures of *Citrus* flavonoids discussed in this review are presented in Figure 2.

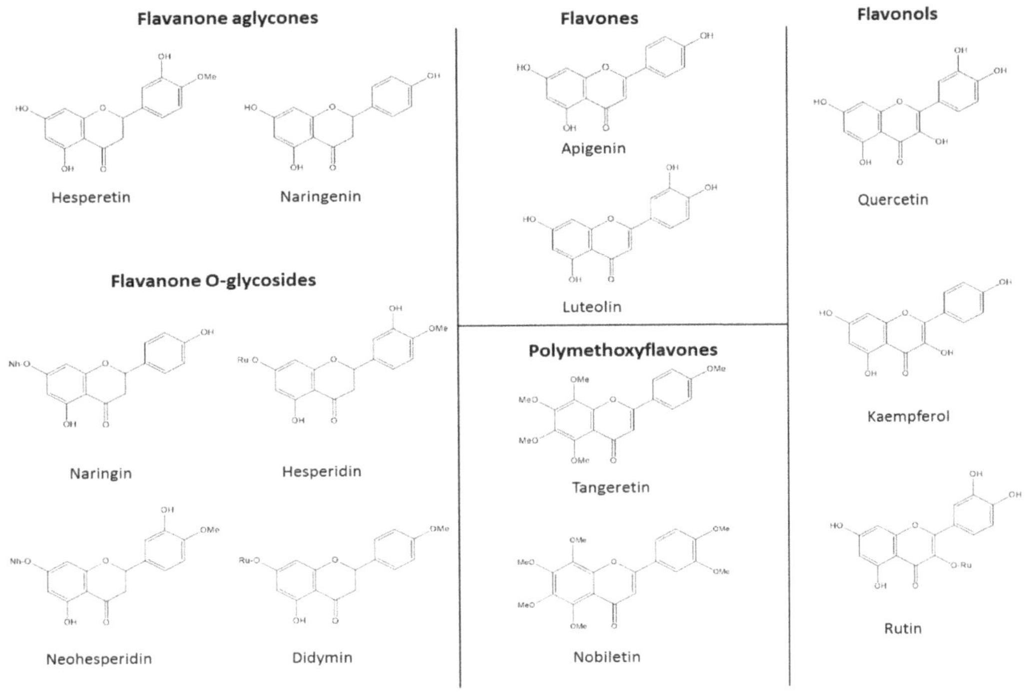

Figure 2. Molecular structure of *Citrus* flavonoids discussed in this review. Rutinose (Ru), neohesperidose (Nh), methoxy (Me).

3.1. Flavanones

In Table 1 are summarized the studies reporting the neuroprotective activity of *Citrus* flavanones.

3.1.1. Naringin

Naringin is a major flavanone glycoside in *Citrus* fruits and it is considered a neuroprotective agent mainly because its anti-apoptotic [75,76] and anti-oxidant activities [77], together with its capability to induce neurotrophic factors such as brain-derived neurotrophic factor (BDNF) and vascular endothelial growth factor (VEGF). Recently, Leem and coworkers (2014) evaluated the effect of naringin in a neurotoxic model of PD in vivo. They found that the flavanone could prevent the degeneration of the nigrostriatal dopaminergic (DA) projection by increasing the level of glia-derived neurotrophic factor (GDNF) in nigral DA neurons, with activation of mammalian target of rapamycin complex 1 (mTORC1). Furthermore, they observed that naringin could attenuate the rise of TNF-α induced by 1-methyl-4-phenylpyridinium (MPP^+) in microglia, indicating its anti-inflammatory activity in CNS [51]. Very recently, the same research group evaluated the effects of pre- or post-treatment with naringin in a 6-hydroxydopamine (OHDA)-treated mice [52], suggesting that it protected the nigrostriatal DA projection from 6-OHDA-induced neurotoxicity by both the activation of mTORC1 and the inhibition of microglial activation [51]. In 2012, Gopinath and Sudhandiran investigated on the neuroprotective effect of naringin on 3-nitropropionic acid (3-NP)-induced neurodegeneration [53]. The 3-NP is a natural environmental toxin that causes selective neuronal degeneration in the striatum, reproducing in animal models the brain lesions observed in HD patients [78]. The experimental protocol required that rats received naringin orally (80 mg/kg body weight/day) 1 h prior to the intraperitoneal injection of 3-NP (10 mg/kg body weight/day) for 2 weeks (the time to develop neurodegeneration). The Authors observed that naringin can mitigate 3-NP-induced neurodegeneration, through the enhancement of antioxidant enzyme gene expressions via nuclear factor E2-related factor 2 (Nrf2) activation, thus modulating oxidative stress and inflammatory responses.

Table 1. *Citrus* flavanones and experimental models of neurodegenerative diseases.

Flavanones	Model	Disease/Condition	References
naringin	In vivo	MPP^+-treated rats	Leem et al., 2014 [51]
	In vivo	6-OHDA-injected mice	Kim et al., 2016 [52]
	In vivo	3-NP-injected rats	Gopinath and Sudhandiran, 2012 [53]
	In vivo	aluminum-treated rats	Prakash et al., 2013 [54]
	In vivo	colchicine-treated rats	Kumar et al., 2010 [55]
hesperidin	In vivo	6-OHDA-injected mice	Antunes et al., 2014 [56]
	In vivo	3-NP-treated mice	Menze et al., 2012 [57]
	In vivo	APP/PS1–21 transgenic mice	Li et al., 2015 [58]
	In vivo	APPswe/PS1dE9 transgenic mice	Wang et al., 2014 [59]
	In vivo	ICV-STZ-injected mice	Javed et al., 2015 [60]
	In vivo	$AlCl_3$-injected rats	Thenmozhi et al., 2015 [61]
	In vivo	$AlCl_3$-injected rats	Thenmozhi et al., 2016 [62]
	In vivo	4-AP-treated rats KA-injected rat	Chang et al., 2015 [63]
hesperetin	In vivo	Mice	Choi and Ahn, 2008 [64]
	In vivo	6-OHDA-injected rats	Kiasalari et al., 2016 [65]
	In vitro	staurosporine-treated cortical neurons cultures	Rainey-Smith et al., 2008 [66]
	In vitro	H_2O_2-treated cortical neurons	Vauzour et al., 2007 [67]
neohesperidin	In vitro	H_2O_2-treated PC12 cells	Hwang et al., 2008 [68]
naringenin	In vivo	ICV-STZ-injected rats	Khan et al., 2012 [69]
	In vivo	ICV-STZ-injected rats	Baluchnejadmojarad and Roghani, 2006 [70]
	In vitro	Aβ-treated PC12 cells	Heo et al., 2004 [71]
	In vitro	microglial cells	Wu et al., 2016 [72]
	In vitro	LPS/IFN-γ exposed primary neuronal-glial cells	Vafeiadou et al., 2009 [73]
didymin	In vitro	H_2O_2-treated neuronal cells	Morelli et al, 2014 [74]

In the last decade, flavonoids have been used to reduce neurotoxic effects of aluminum (Al) chloride ($AlCl_3$) in rats. In this field, Prakash and collaborators (2013), explored the possible role of naringin against Al-induced cognitive dysfunction and oxidative damage in rats. The Authors observed that chronic administration of naringin (40 and 80 mg/kg) for six weeks significantly improved cognitive performance and attenuated mitochondria oxidative damage, acetyl cholinesterase activity, and Al concentration in Al-treated (100 mg/kg) rats [54]. The same authors showed that treatment with naringin (40 and 80 mg/kg/day) for 25 consecutive days beginning 4 days prior to colchicine (15 μg/5 μL) injected intracerebroventricularly significantly improved the cognitive performance and attenuated oxidative damage in colchicine-treated rats [55].

3.1.2. Hesperidin

Hesperidin, a flavonoid that is particularly abundant in oranges and lemons, exerts anticarcinogenic, antihypertensive, antiviral, antioxidant and antiinflammatory effects [79]. In addition, hesperidin can cross the blood-brain barrier [80] and can protect the neurons against various types of insult associated with neurodegenerative diseases, including AD, PD, and HD. A study performed by Antunes and collaborators (2014) was aimed to evaluate the role of hesperidin in an animal model of PD induced by 6-OHDA. The Authors demonstrated that hesperidin (50 mg/kg), administrated for 28 days after an intracerebroventricular injection of 6-OHDA, was effective in preventing memory impairment and depressive-like behavior in mice. Furthermore, in the striatum of aged mice, hesperidin attenuated the 6-OHDA-induced reduction in (i) glutathione peroxidase (GPx) and catalase (CAT) activity, (ii) the total reactive antioxidant potential and (iii) the dopamine levels. Finally, the flavanone mitigated both the increased levels of ROS and the activity of glutathione reductase induced by 6-OHDA [56].

The implications of nitric oxide (NO) in a variety of neurodegenerative diseases suggests a potential role of flavonoids in HD and other oxidative-based disorders. Menze et al., (2012) investigated the potential effect of hesperidin on 3-NP-induced behavioral, neurochemical, histopathological and cellular changes. They showed that pretreatment with hesperidin (100 mg/kg) ahead of 3-NP (20 mg/kg) for 5 days prevented any changes of locomotor activity or prepulse inhibition, slightly increased malondialdehyde (MDA) levels and reduced inducible nitric oxide synthase (iNOS) positive cells as well as CAT activity in cortex, striatum and hippocampus evoked by 3-NP [57].

One of the most distinctive neuropathological characteristics of AD, are the senile plaques of aggregates Aβ peptide. Moreover, besides the well-known Aβ aggregation, neuro-inflammation also plays a pivotal role in the etiopathogenesis of this multifactorial disorder [81]. Li and coworkers (2015), evaluated the potential therapeutic effect of hesperidin on behavioral dysfunction, Aβ deposition and neuro-inflammation in the transgenic APP/PS1 mouse, a useful model of cerebral amyloidosis for AD. Hesperidin (100 mg/kg body weight) was orally given to the mice for 10 days. It recovered deficits in non-cognitive nesting capability and social interaction and attenuated Aβ deposition, plaque associated amyloid precursor protein (APP) expression, microglial activation and TGF-β1 immunoreactivity in both cerebral cortex and hippocampus of APP/PS1 mice [58]. The same dose of hesperidin (100 mg/kg) administrated for 16 weeks to three-month-old APPswe/PS1dE9 transgenic mice reduced their learning and memory deficits, improved locomotor activity and increased glycogen synthase kinase-3β (GSK-3β) phosphorylation, anti-oxidative defense and mitochondrial complex I–IV enzymes activities [58]. However, there was not observed obvious change in Aβ deposition [59]. Hesperedin was effective also in the experimental model of intracerebroventricular streptozotocin (ICV-STZ)-induced sporadic dementia of Alzheimer's type (SDAT) [60]. Indeed, pretreatment with hesperidin (100 or 200 mg/kg/day orally for 15 days) improved memory consolidation process possibly through modulation of acetylcholine esterase activity (AChE) in mice injected bilaterally with single dose of ICV-STZ (2.57 mg/kg body weight each side). Moreover, hesperidin decreased neuronal cell death by reducing the overexpression of pro-inflammatory mediators like NF-κB, iNOS, cyclooxygenase-2 (COX-2) and attenuated astrogliosis [60].

One of the key factors in the progression of neurodegenerative diseases is the deregulation of metal ion homeostasis, such as Al, a major risk factor for the AD [82]. Thenmozhi and coworkers (2015) evaluated the protective effect of hesperidin on $AlCl_3$ induced neurobehavioral and pathological changes in Alzheimeric rats. Orally administration of hesperidin (100 mg/kg) along with $AlCl_3$ injection (100 mg/kg) for 60 days, significantly reduced the Al concentration in hippocampus and cortex, the acetylcholinesterase (AChE) activity, the APP expressions, the levels of both $A\beta_{1-42}$ and its synthesis-related molecules (β and γ secretases). Moreover, hesperidin significantly attenuated the behavioral impairments caused by $AlCl_3$ and preserved the normal histoarchitecture pattern of the hippocampus and cortex, as observed by histopathological studies [61]. Very recently, with the same experimental model Thenmozhi et al., (2016) showed that hesperidin prevented oxidative stress and apoptosis induced by $AlCl_3$ compared to control group [62].

Excitotoxicity is considered one of the constitutive components of the neurodegenerative diseases pathogenesis [83] caused by excessive release of aminoacids such as glutamate, a crucial excitatory neurotransmitter in the mammals CNS. This provokes the overstimulation of glutamate receptors which leads to an overload of intracellular Ca^{2+}, generation of free radicals and subsequent neuronal cell death [84]. Chang and coworkers (2015) evaluated the potential role of hesperidin in neurotoxicity induced by glutamate release in rat hippocampus. They observed that hesperidin (IC_{50} 20 μM) inhibited both the release of glutamate and the elevation of cytosolic free Ca^{2+} concentration evoked by 4-aminopyridine (4-AP) in rat hippocampal nerve terminals (synaptosomes). Furthermore, in hippocampal slice preparations, whole-cell patch clamp experiments showed that hesperidin reduced the frequency of spontaneous excitatory postsynaptic currents without affecting their amplitude, indicating the involvement of a presynaptic mechanism. In addition, the Authors observed that pre-treatment with hesperidin (10 or 50 mg/kg) attenuated the rise of extracellular glutamate and the neuronal loss in the hippocampal CA3 area caused by the intraperitoneal injection of kainic acid (KA; 15 mg/kg) [63].

3.1.3. Hesperetin

Hesperetin is a flavanone abundant in *Citrus* fruit and juice, and represents the major circulating aglycone metabolite of hesperidin. Hesperetin displays several biological properties, such as antioxidant, neuroprotective and anti-inflammatory activities.

Experiments performed in vitro showed that 1 μM hesperetin has neuroprotective effects against H_2O_2-induced cytotoxicity in PC12 cells [68], and that much lower concentrations both inhibit H_2O_2-induced apoptosis and counteract staurosporine-induced cell death in primary cortical neurons (0.01 μM/L and 300 nM, respectively) [66,67], suggesting its potential role in the intervention for neurodegenerative diseases.

In vivo, Choi and Ahn (2008) observed that hesperetin (10 or 50 mg/kg body weight) inhibited biomarkers of oxidative stress, such as the thiobarbituric acid-reactive substance (TBARS) and carbonyl, in the brains of mice, and activated both CAT and superoxide dismutase (SOD). Moreover, hesperetin increased the reduced glutathione (GSH)/oxidized glutathione (GSSG) ratio, the glutathione peroxidase (GSH-px) and the glutathione reductase (GR) activities [64]. Very recently, Kiasalari and coworkers (2016), evaluated the protective effect of hesperetin against 6-OHDA-induced striatal lesion and have explored some underlying mechanisms including apoptosis, inflammation and oxidative stress. They administrated hesperetin (50 mg/kg/day) for 1 week at intrastriatal 6-OHDA-lesioned rats. They observed that hesperetin reduced the rotational asymmetry induced by apomorphine, as well as the latency and the total time on the narrow beam task. It also decreased striatal malondialdehyde and increases both striatal CAT activity and GSH content. Moreover, hesperetin lowered striatal level of glial fibrillary acidic protein (GFAP) and increased Bcl_2 [65]. Finally, hesperetin treatment was also capable to mitigate nigral DNA fragmentation and to prevent loss of SNC dopaminergic neurons [65].

3.1.4. Neohesperidin

Neohesperidin is a flavanone glycoside found in *Citrus* fruits. Hwang and coworkers (2008) demonstrated the protective effects of pretreatments (6 h) with neohesperidin, hesperidin and hesperetin (0.8, 4, 20, and 50 μM) on H_2O_2-induced (400 μM, 16 h) neurotoxicity in PC12 cells by scavenging ROS, attenuating the elevation of intracellular free Ca^{2+}, preventing membrane damage and increasing CAT activity. Furthermore, neohesperidin attenuated both the decrease of mitochondrial membrane potential and the increase of caspase-3 activity evoked by H_2O_2 [68].

3.1.5. Naringenin

It is known that naringenin possesses various pharmacologic properties including antioxidant, free radical scavenger, anticancer, anti-inflammatory, immunomodulator and memory enhancer.

It's known that ICV-STZ administration at a sub-diabetogenic dose provided a relevant model for AD-type neurodegeneration with cognitive impairment (AD-TNDCI) [85,86]. In this field, Khan and collaborators (2012), investigated the effects of naringenin on cognitive dysfunction and, oxidative stress in a rat model of AD-TNDCI. The rats were orally pre-treated with naringin at 50 mg/kg for 2 weeks followed by ICV-STZ (3 mg/kg; 5 μL per site) injection bilaterally. The Authors observed that the imbalance of several markers of oxidative stress (enzymatic and non-enzymatic) with impairments in spatial learning and memory, loss of ChAT positive neuron and damage to hippocampal ones induced by ICV-STZ, were ameliorated by pre-treatment with naringenin [69]. The ability of naringenin to improve learning, memory and cognitive impairment was also confirmed by Baluchnejadmojarad and Roghani (2006) in an experimental model very similar to those described above [70].

Heo et al., (2004) examined the neuroprotective effect of naringenin found in *C. junos* against oxidative cell death induced by Aβ peptide in PC12 cells, and evaluated the anti-amnesic activity of naringenin using ICR mice with scopolamine-induced amnesia (1 mg/kg body weight). They showed that pretreatment with naringenin prevented the generation of Aβ-induced ROS and decreased Aβ toxicity in a concentration dependent manner. Furthermore, naringenin (4.5 mg/kg body weight), significantly ameliorated scopolamine-induced amnesia [71]. Vafeiadou and coworkers (2009) [73] demonstrated that naringenin (0.01–0.3 μmol/L) protected against LPS/IFN-gamma-induced neuronal death in a primary neuronal-glial co-culture system by inhibiting the p38 mitogen-activated protein kinase (MAPK) phosphorylation and downstream signal transducer and activator of transcription-1 (STAT-1).

More recently, Wu and coworkers (2016) demonstrated that naringenin inhibits the expression of cytokine signaling (SOCS)-3, iNOS and COX-2, as well as the release of NO and pro-inflammatory cytokines in microglial cells. These actions were modulated by adenosine monophosphate-activated protein kinase α (AMPKα) and protein kinase C δ (PKCδ) [72].

3.1.6. Didymin

Only one paper suggested a neuroprotective effect of didymin that was found to increase cell viability of neuronal cells injured by H_2O_2 by decreasing mitochondrial dysfunctions and levels of intracellular ROS, stimulating SOD, CAT and GPx activity [74]. The mechanism underlying the protective effects of didymin in differentiated-SH-SY5Y exposed to H_2O_2 might be related to the activation of antioxidant defense enzymes as well as to the inhibition of apoptotic features such as p-JNK and caspase-3 [74].

3.2. Flavones

3.2.1. Apigenin

Apigenin is a member of the flavone subclass of flavonoids present in fruits and vegetables. It has long been considered to have various biological activities such as antioxidant, antiinflammatory, anti-mutagenic and anti-tumorigenic properties. Apigenin has been shown to exert neuroprotective activity against endoplasmic reticulum stress-induced apoptosis in the HT22 murine hippocampal neuronal cells [87], in primary cultures of human neurons subjected to quinoloinic acid-induced excitotoxicity [88] and in glutamate-induced neurotoxicity in both murine cerebellar and cortical cell cultures [89].

Zhao et al. (2013) [90] reported the neuroprotective effects of the flavone in the amyloid precursor protein/presenilin 1 protein (APP/PS1) double transgenic AD mouse model. After feeding four month-old mice with apigenin (40 mg/kg) for 3 months, they observed both improvements in memory and learning deficits and reduction of fibrillar amyloid deposits. Additionally, the apigenin-treated mice showed restoration of the cortical extracellular signal-regulated protein kinase 1 (ERK)/cAMP response element-binding protein (CREB)/BDNF pathway that is known to be involved in learning and memory typically affected AD patients. Finally, apigenin enhances both SOD and GPx activities [90]. Likewise, in $A\beta_{25-35}$-induced amnesia mouse models, Liu et al. (2011) reported the capability of apigenin (20 mg/kg) to improve the spatial learning and memory and the neurovascular functionality [91]. Cognitive enhancing effects by apigenin (20 mg/kg, intraperitoneally) have been described also in an animal model in which the flavone delayed the long-term forgetting [92]. Another study performed by Taupin et al. (2009) highlighted that the administration of apigenin (25 mg/kg) for 10 days stimulated neurogenesis in the hippocampal region of the brain in 7-week old mice and resulted in improved performance in the Morris water maze [93]. Patil and its research group demonstrated that chronic intraperitoneally administration of apigenin (5–20 mg/kg) reversed cognitive deficits in aged and lipopolysaccharide (LPS)-intoxicated mice [94]. Additionally, apigenin improved motor skills and enhanced neurotrophic potential which has been reduced in

1-methyl-4-phenyl-1,2,3,6-tetrahydropyridine (MPTP)-induced Parkinsonism in mice [95]. Particularly, MPTP (25 mg/kg) was administrated for five consecutive days and then apigenin (10 and 20 mg/kg) was orally administrated for 26 days, including 5 days of pretreatment. After that, the Author performed behavioral study and biochemical estimation of oxidative stress biomarkers, observing (i) a reduced tyrosine hydroxylase (TH)-positive cells; (ii) a rise of BDNF amount and (iii) a decreased level of GFAP in the substantia nigra of MPTP-treated mice [95]. More recently, Liu et al. (2015) demonstrated that apigenin exerts a protective effect against MPP^+-induced neurotoxicity in neuronal like catecholaminergic PC12 cells. This effect is mediated through the inhibition of oxidative stress, the stabilization of mitochondrial function and the reduction of neuronal apoptosis via the mitochondrial pathway [96]. The cytoprotective effect of apigenin was also evaluated by Wu and coworkers (2015), showing that apigenin restored cell viability and repressed both caspase-3 and PARP-1 activation in 4-HNE-treated PC12 cells. Moreover, apigenin activated MAPK and Nrf2 signaling, which in turn evoked adaptive cellular stress response pathways, restored ER homeostasis altered by 4-HNE and inhibited cytotoxicity [97].

Table 2 reported the studies in which was evaluated apigenin as potential neuroprotective agent.

Table 2. Studies employed the *Citrus* flavones and their experimental models of neurodegeneration.

Flavones	Model	Disease/Condition	Reference
apigenin	In vitro	HT22 cells	Choi et al., 2010 [87]
	In vitro	QUIN-treated primary human neuron	Braidy et al., 2010 [88]
	In vitro	glutamate-treated cerebellar and cortical neurons	Losi et al., 2004 [89]
	In vivo	APP/PS1 double transgenic mouse	Zhao et al., 2013 [90]
	In vivo	$A\beta_{25-35}$-treated mouse	Liu et al., 2011 [91]
	In vivo	young male Wistar rats	Popovic et al., 2014 [92]
	In vivo	7-week old mice	Taupin et al., 2009 [93]
	In vivo	MPTP-treated mice	Patil et al., 2014 [95]
	In vitro	MPP^+-incubated PC12 cells	Liu et al., 2015 [96]
	In vitro	4-HNE-exposed PC12 cells	Wu et al., 2015 [97]
	In vivo	aged and LPS-intoxicated mice	Patil et al., 2003 [94]
luteolin	In vivo	chronic cerebral hypoperfusion in rats	Fu et al., 2014 [98]
	In vivo	chronic cerebral hypoperfusion in rats	Xu et al., 2010 [99]
	In vivo	obesity mice	Liu et al., 2014 [100]
	In vivo	ICV-STZ injected rat	Wang et al., 2016 [101]
	In vitro	6-OHDA-exposed PC12 cells	Hu et al., 2014 [102]
	In vivo	MPTP-treated mice	Patil et al., 2014 [95]
	In vitro	MPP^+-exposed PC12 and glial C6 cells	Wruck et al., 2007 [103]
	In vitro	IFN-γ-incubated N9 and microglia cells	Rezai-Zadeh et al., 2008 [104]
	In vitro	N2a cells transfected with SweAPP	Rezai-Zadeh et al., 2009 [105]
	In vitro	LPS/IFN-γ-treated rat primary microglia and BV-2 microglial cells	Kao et al., 2011 [106]
	In vitro	LPS-incubated microglia cells	Chen et al., 2008 [107]
	In vitro	LPS-exposed BV2 microglia	Zhu et al., 2011 [108]
	In vitro	SH-SY5Y cells co-cultured with LPS-stimulated BV2 microglia	Zhu et al., 2014 [109]
	In vitro	LPS-treated microglia cells	Dirscherl et al., 2010 [110]

3.2.2. Luteolin

In the last decades, several studies reported the neuroprotective properties of luteolin [111]. They are summarized in Table 2. In vivo studies showed that luteolin protected against cognitive dysfunction induced by chronic cerebral hypoperfusion in rats [98,99]. Luteolin also protected against high fat diet-induced cognitive defects in obesity mice [100]. Recently, Wang et al., (2016) demonstrated that the flavone significantly ameliorated the spatial learning and memory impairment and increased the thickness of CA1 pyramidal layer in STZ-treated animals [101]. Moreover, luteolin (20 μM) can attenuate 6-OHDA-caused oxidative stress, cytotoxicity, and caspase-3 activation in PC12 cells [102]. Another study displayed as luteolin (10 and 20 mg/kg) could improve locomotor and muscular alterations in mice exposed to MPTP, also decreasing the TH-positive cells, the neurotrophic factors, the GFAP, and the BDNF [95]. In addition, Wruck et al., (2007) demonstrated that luteolin protected rat neural PC12 and glial C6 cells from MPP^+-induced toxicity and activated Nrf2 [103]. The research group of Rezai-Zadeh (2008) demonstrated that treatment of both N9 and murine-derived primary microglia cell lines with luteolin significantly reduced both the IFN-γ-induced CD40 expression and the release of pro-inflammatory cytokines IL-6 and TNF-α through the inactivation of STAT1 [104]. One year later, the same authors showed that luteolin treatment of murine N2a cells transfected with SweAPP and primary neuronal cells derived from SweAPP overexpressing mice resulted in a significant reduction in Aβ generation. The mechanism seems to be involved in the selective inactivation of the GSK-3α isoform, which in turn increases the phosphorylation of PS1, the catalytic core of the γ secretase complex, thereby reducing PS1 APP interaction and Aβ generation [105].

Excessive production of NO and pro-inflammatory cytokines by activated microglia plays a pivotal role in the pathogenesis of ND. Kao and collaborators (2011) reported the inhibitory effect of luteolin on LPS/interferon γ (IFN-γ)-induced NO and cytokines production in rat primary microglia and BV-2 microglial cells. Particularly, luteolin concentration-dependently abolished LPS/IFN-γ-induced NO, TNF-α and IL-1β production as well as iNOS expression. Luteolin also exerted inhibitory effect on transcription factor activity including NF-κB, signal transducer and activator of transcription 1 (STAT1) and interferon regulatory factor 1 (IRF-1). These effects were accompanied by down-regulation of ERK, p38, JNK, protein kinase B (Akt) and Src [106].

Chen and coworkers (2008) demonstrated that luteolin may protect dopaminergic neurons from LPS-induced injury and its efficacy in inhibiting microglia activation [107]. Another research showed that luteolin inhibited the LPS-stimulated expression of inducible iNOS, COX-2, TNF-α and IL-1β as well as blocked the LPS-induced NF-κB activation [108]. A few years later, the same authors, demonstrated that luteolin inhibited the LPS-stimulated expression of TLR-4, blocked LPS-induced NF-κB, p38, JNK and Akt activation, but had no effect on ERK. In addition, pre-treatment with luteolin increased cell viability and reduced apoptosis of SH-SY5Y cells co-cultured with LPS-stimulated BV2 microglia [109]. To better understand the immuno-modulatory effects of luteolin, Dirscherl et al., (2010) carried out a genome-wide expression study in LPS-exposed BV-2 microglia cells treated with luteolin and performed a phenotypic and functional profile. They observed that luteolin suppressed pro-inflammatory marker expression in LPS-activated microglia and triggered global changes in the microglial transcriptome with more than 50 differentially expressed transcripts. Moreover, pro-inflammatory and pro-apoptotic gene expression was blocked by luteolin, while mRNA levels of genes involved into anti-oxidant metabolism, phagocytosis, ramification, and chemotaxis were significantly induced [110].

3.3. *Flavonols*

3.3.1. Kaempferol

There are few evidences for the neuroprotective effect of kaempferol (Table 3). LPS-activated microglial cells have been suggested to be a useful in vitro model to test the potential of drugs for neuroinflammatory disorders [112,113]. Park and coworkers (2011) demonstrated the activity of kaempferol against neuroinflammatory toxicity caused by LPS-activated microglia. Particularly, they showed that kaempferol inhibit the LPS-induced expression of iNOS, COX-2, matrix metalloproteinases (MMPs) and the subsequent production of ROS, TNF-α, NO, PGE2 and IL-1β in BV2 microglial cells, through the inhibition of TLR4, NF-κB, p38 MAPK, JNK and AKT activation [114]. Yang and collaborators (2014) demonstrated the neuroprotective effects of kaempferol in glutamate-treated hippocampal neuronal cells, suggesting that kaempferol may be a useful candidate for neurodegenerative diseases [115].

Table 3. *Citrus* flavonols kaempferol and rutin in models of neurodegenerations.

Flavonols	Model	Disease/Condition	Reference
kaempferol	In vitro	LPS-activated microglia	Park et al., 2011 [114]
	In vitro	glutamate-treated hippocampal neuronal	Yang et al., 2014 [115]
rutin	In vitro	6-OHDA-incubated PC-12 cells	Magalingam et al., 2013 [116]
	In vitro	ethanol-exposed HT22 cells	Song et al., 2014 [117]
	In vitro	amylin-treated SH-SY5Y cells	Yu et al., 2015 [118]
	In vitro	neuronal cells	Na et al., 2014 [119]
	In vivo	KA-injected BALB/c mice	Nasiri-Asl et al., 2013 [120]
	In vivo	6-OHDA-treated rats	Kham et al., 2012 [121]
	In vitro	Ab_{42}-incubated SH-SY5Y cells	Wang et al., 2012 [122]
	In vivo	APPswe/PS1dE9 transgenic mice	Xu et al., 2014 [123]
	In vivo	mice	Machawal and Kumar, 2014 [124]
	In vivo	Aβ-injected rats	Moghbelinejad et al., 2014 [125]

3.3.2. Rutin

Rutin is a multifunctional flavonoid glycoside acting on various cellular functions under pathological conditions such as ND, maybe due to its ability to cross the blood brain barrier (BBB) [126]. Table 3 summarizes the studies aimed to evaluate the effects of rutin in models of neurodegenerations. In an in vitro model of PD, it has been demonstrated that rutin reduced lipid peroxidation in 6-OHDA-treated PC-12 cells, activating antioxidant enzymes like SOD, CAT, GPx and GSH [116]. The neuroprotective effects of rutin against 6-OHDA were evaluated also in vivo. Rats was pre-treated with this flavonoids (25 mg/kg body weight, orally) for 3 weeks and then subjected to unilateral intrastriatal injection of 6-OHDA (10 μg in 0.1% ascorbic acid). Rutin prevented the deficits in locomotor activity and motor coordination, and protected neurons from deleterious effects of 6-OHDA in the substantia nigra, as suggested by histopathological and immunohistochemical assays [121].

Oxidative stress has been proposed to be a potential mechanism underlying ethanol-induced damage and may contribute to neuronal degeneration [127]. Song et al., (2014) investigated the antioxidant effect of rutin in hippocampal neuronal cells exposed to ethanol, and found that it prevented the ethanol-induced decrease in nerve growth factor expression, GDNF and BDNF in HT22 cells. Moreover, rutin significantly increased the level of the antioxidant glutathione, and the activities of SOD and CAT [117]. Oxidative stress may play a role also in hippocampal cell death associated with KA-induced neurotoxicity [128]. It has been reported that rutin (100 and 200 mg/kg, i.p. for 7 days) has potential anticonvulsant and antioxidative activities against oxidative stress in KA-induced (10 mg/kg, i.p.) seizures in mice [120].

Wang and coworkers (2012) showed that rutin can inhibit $A\beta_{42}$ fibrillization in concentration dependent manner and can attenuate $A\beta_{42}$-induced cytotoxicity in SH-SY5Y neuroblastoma cells [122]. More recently, the same authors demonstrated that orally administered rutin significantly attenuated memory deficits in APPswe/PS1dE9 transgenic mice, decreased oligomeric Aβ level, reduced oxidative stress, downregulated gliosis and diminished IL-1 and IL-6 levels in the brain [123]. Another study suggested a role for rutin in protecting against AD. Moghbelinejad and coworkers (2014) showed that rutin improved memory retrieval in rats injected with Aβ by increasing ERK1, CREB and BDNF [125].

Recently, Yu et al., (2015) showed that rutin inhibited amylin-induced neurocytotoxicity, decreasing the production of ROS, NO, glutathione disulfide (GSSG), MDA, TNF-α and IL-1β, thus attenuating mitochondrial damage and increasing the GSH/GSSG ratio. These protective effects could be derived by its ability to inhibit amylin aggregation, enhance the activity of SOD, CAT, and GPx, and reduce that of iNOS [118]. Machawal and Kumar (2014) suggested that the neuroprotective mechanism of rutin against immobilization stress-induced anxiety-like behavioral and oxidative damage in mice is mediated by a reduction of NO [124]. Finally, it has been proposed that rutin protects against the neurodegenerative effects of prion accumulation in vitro, by reducing levels of ROS and NO, increasing production of neurotropic factors and inhibiting mitochondrial apoptotic events leading to HT22 neuronal cell death [119].

3.3.3. Quercetin

Quercetin exhibits numerous pharmacological activities including anti-cancer, anti-inflammatory, anti-atherosclerotic, anti-thrombotic and anti-hypertensive effects, as well as benefits for human endurance exercise capacity. Several in vitro and in vivo studies have provided supportive evidence also for its neuroprotective effects in various models of neuronal injury and chronic neurodegenerative diseases (Table 4). In vitro studies have shown that low micromolar concentrations of quercetin inhibited cell toxicity induced by neurotoxic molecules known to be inducer of oxidative stress. In particular, several research employed H_2O_2 as stressor. Suematsu et al., (2011) demonstrated that quercetin suppressed the H_2O_2-caused cytotoxicity and inhibited apoptosis in human neuronal SH-SY5Y cells [129]. Quercetin also decreased H_2O_2-induced oxidative stress in SK-N-MC cells by reducing HIF-1a, Foxo-3a, NICD and pro-apoptotic mediators including p53 and Bax [130]. The anti-oxidative and anti-apoptotic role of quercetin was further supported by the study of Jazvinšćak Jembrek and coworkers (2012) [131]. Sajad et al., (2013) showed that pre-treatment with quercetin prevented protein nitration and glycolytic block of proliferation in cultured neuronal precursor cells (NPCs) [132].

Table 4. Studies employed quercetin in experimental models of neurodegeneration.

Flavonol	Model	Disease/Condition	Reference
	In vitro	H_2O_2-incubated SH-SY5Y cells	Suematsu et al., 2011 [129]
	In vitro	H_2O_2-exposed SK-N-MC cells	Roshanzamir and Yazdanparast, 2014 [130]
	In vitro	H_2O_2-treated NPCs cells	Sajad et al., 2013 [132]
	In vitro	H_2O_2-treated -P19 neurons	Jazvinšćak J et al., 2012 [131]
	In vitro	neuronal cells	Ansari et al., 2009 [133]
	In vivo	Aβ-injected mice	Zhang et al., 2016 [134]
	In vivo	MPTP-treated mice	Lv et al., 2012 [135]
	In vitro	LPS- and IFN-γ-treated BV-2 microglia	Chen et al., 2005 [136]
	In vitro	LPS-treated BV-2 microglia	Kang et al., 2013 [137]
	In vitro	high-glucose exposed PC12 cells	Bournival et al., 2012 [138]
quercetin	In vivo	high-fat diet in mice	Xia et al., 2015 [139]
	In vivo	high-cholesterol diet in mice	Lu et al., 2010 [140]
	In vivo	intracerebral hemorrhage in rats	Zhang et al., 2015 [141]
	In vivo	ischemia reperfusion injury in rats	Arikan et al., 2015 [142]
	In vivo	STZ-treated mice	Tota et al., 2010 [143]
	In vivo	scopolamine-treated zebrafish	Richetti et al., 2011 [144]
	In vivo	Pb-exposed rats	Hu et al., 2008 [145]
	In vivo	ethylmercury-exposed rats	Barcelos et al., 2011 [146]
	In vivo	tungsten-exposed rats	Sachdeva et al., 2015 [147]
	In vivo	Al-treated rats	Sharma et al., 2013 [148]
	In vivo	Al -treated rats	Sharma et al., 2015 [149]
	In vivo	Al -treated rats	Sharma et al., 2016 [150]
	In vivo	PCBs-treated rats	Bavithra et al., 2012 [151]
	In vivo	PCBs-treated rats	Selvakumar et al., 2013 [152]
	In vivo	ethidium bromide-treated rats	Beckmann et al., 2014 [153]

Protection of neuronal cells from the toxicity of Aβ peptide-induced toxicity has also been reported. Ansari et al., (2009) showed that low concentration of quercetin significantly attenuated protein oxidation, lipid peroxidation and apoptosis induced by $A\beta_{1-42}$ in neuronal cultures [133], while Zhang et al., (2016) demonstrated that quercetin enhanced brain apoE levels and decreased Aβ levels in the cortex of amyloid model mice [134]. Moreover, the orally administration of quercetin (50, 100 and 200 mg/kg body weight) markedly improves MPTP-induced dopamine depletion in the brain tissue, the motor balance and the coordination which is significantly altered following MPTP injection in an animal model of PD [135].

In 2005, Chen and collaborators, demonstrated that quercetin suppressed LPS- and IFN-γ-induced NO production and iNOS gene transcription and enhanced heme oxygenase-1 (HO-1) expression [136]. More recently, Kang and coworkers (2013) found that the suppression of NO system in BV2 microglial cell line is mediated by the inhibition of NF-κB and the induction of Nrf2/HO-1 [137]. Furthermore, quercetin protected neuronal PC12 cells from high-glucose-induced oxidation, nitrosative stress, and apoptosis [138], and antagonized cognitive impairment induced by feeding mice with a high fat [139] or high-cholesterol diet [140].

There is a lot of evidence showing that memory deficit is associated with impaired cerebral circulation and a decrease in the cholinergic system. It has been shown that quercetin protected the retina from apoptotic damage due to ischemia reperfusion injury in vivo [142] and was also neuroprotective in models of intracerebral hemorrhage in rats [141]. Tota et al., (2010) demonstrated that orally daily pre-treatment with quercetin (2.5, 5 and 10 mg/kg) showed a dose-dependent restoration of cerebral blood flow (CBF) and ATP content, significantly reduced by the administration of STZ (0.5 mg/kg) in mice. Further, quercetin prevented STZ-induced memory impairment and decreased AChE activity as well as oxidative and nitrosative stress, as evidenced by a significant decrease in MDA and nitrite, and increase in GSH levels [143]. Richetti et al., (2011) demonstrated the protective role of quercetin (single injection of 50 mg/kg concentration) against scopolamine-induced inhibitory avoidance memory deficits in zebrafish [144]. However, Nassiri-Asl (2013) observed that quercetin (50 mg/kg) could not be effective against oxidative stress in the hippocampus and cerebral cortex in kindled rats besides its anticonvulsant effects and protection against memory impairment [154].

Quercetin provided protection also against the neurotoxicity of several metals. Hu et al., (2008) evaluated the effect of quercetin on chronic lead (Pb) exposure-induced impairment of synaptic plasticity in dentate gyrus (DG) area of rat hippocampus. The results showed that quercetin significantly increase the depressed input/output (I/O) functions, paired-pulse reactions (PPR) and long-term potentiation (LTP) of Pb-exposed group. In addition, concentration of Pb in hippocampus was partially reduced after quercetin treatment [145]. Quercetin (0.5–50 mg/kg/bw/day) protected also against DNA damage caused by exposure to methylmercury [146] and tungsten [147]. Several lines of evidences suggested that Al has severe toxic manifestations on the CNS. The research group of Sharma, found that pre-treatment with quercetin (10 mg/kg/bw/day) before intragastrically administration of Al (10 mg/kg/bw/day) decreased ROS levels, mitochondrial DNA oxidation and citrate synthase activity in both hippocampus and corpus striatum regions, while increased MnSOD activity of rat brain. In addition, quercetin prevented Al-induced translocation of cytochrome c (cyt-c), up-regulated Bcl-2, and down-regulated Bax, p53 and caspase-3 activation. It also reduced DNA fragmentation and increased the mitochondrial DNA copy number and mitochondrial content in the regions of rat brain [148–150].

Polychlorinated biphenyls (PCBs) are very toxic environmental contaminants known to trigger neurochemical damages and behavioral disorders. Bavithra et al. (2012) showed that quercetin acted as scavenger of the PCBs-induced free radicals and protected dopaminergic receptors in the cerebellum of rat [151]. Another study carried out by Selvakumar and coworkers (2013), evidenced that quercetin (50 mg/kg) suppresses ROS, enhances both enzymatic antioxidants and neurotransmitter levels and improves the cognitive functions damned by PCBs (2 mg/kg) [152]. Moreover, quercetin prevented alterations on cholinergic neurotransmission and in the behavioral tests also in rats experimentally demyelinated by ethidium bromide [153].

3.4. *Polymethoxiflavones*

In Table 5 are summarized the studies reporting the neuroprotective activity of *Citrus* polymethoxiflavones.

Table 5. Studies and experimental models of neurodegenerative diseases in which tangeretin or nobiletin were used.

Polymethoxyflavones	Model	Disease/Condition	Reference
tangeretin	In vivo	6-OHDA-injected rat	Datla et al., 2001 [155]
	In vitro	LPS-stimulated microglia and BV-2 cells	Shu et al., 2014 [156]
nobiletin	In vitro	$A\beta_{1-42}$ or $A\beta_{1-40}$-exposed hippocampus neurons of rats	Matzukazi et al., 2006 [157]
	In vivo	$A\beta_{1-40}$-treated rats	
	In vivo	APP-SL 7-5 mice	Onozuka et al., 2008 [158]
	In vivo	SAMP8 mice	Nakajima et al., 2013 [159]
	In vivo	3XTg-AD mice	Nakajima et al., 2015 [160]
	In vivo	transgenic mice	Yamakuni et al., 2010 [161]
	In vivo	MPP^+- injected mice	Jeong et al., 2014 [162]
	In vitro	LPS-treated BV-2 microglia cell	Cui et al., 2010 [163]
	In vivo	cerebral ischemia inducted mice	Yamamoto et al., 2009 [164]
	In vivo	cerebral ischemia inducted rats	Zhang et al., 2016 [165]

3.4.1. Tangeretin

Tangeretin is a polymethoxyflavone present exclusively in *Citrus* fruit peels. Neuroprotective effects of tangeretin were elucidated in an animal model of PD. Sub-chronic treatment of rats with tangeretin (20 mg/kg/day) for 4 days before 6-OHDA injection markedly reduced the loss of both TH^+ cells and striatal dopamine content evoked by unilateral infusion of 6-OHDA (8 μg) onto medial forebrain bundle [155]. More recently, Shu and coworkers (2014) demonstrated that tangeretin suppressed microglial activation in the LPS-stimulated primary rat microglia and BV-2 cell culture [156] (Table 5).

3.4.2. Nobiletin

Nobiletin is a polymethoxylated flavone that is commonly presents in *Citrus* peels. Several papers reported the protective effect of nobiletin in different model of AD. Matsuzaki and coworkers (2006) observed that nobiletin (10 and 30 μM) reversed a reduction in the activity of CREB-phosphorylation by the sublethal concentration of $A\beta_{1-42}$ or $A\beta_{1-40}$ in cultured rat hippocampus neurons. Moreover, it ameliorated $A\beta_{1-40}$-induced impairment of memory in AD model rats [157].

Onozuka and collaborators (2008) demonstrated that daily administrated nobiletin (10 mg/kg, i.p.) for 4 months reduced Aβ plaque pathology and improved cognitive deficits in APP-SL 7–5 mice, a transgenic mouse model of AD [158]. More recently, the same authors showed that nobiletin (10–50 mg/kg/day, i.p.) improved age-related cognitive impairment of senescence-accelerated mouse prone 8 (SAMP8) mice, and reduced both the oxidative stress and tau phosphorylation in their brain [159]. Moreover, they showed that nobiletin (30 mg/kg) administered for 3 months counteracted the impairment of short-term memory and recognition memory in a triple transgenic mouse model of AD (3XTg-AD mice). In addition, nobiletin reduced the levels of both soluble $A\beta_{1-40}$ and ROS in the brain and in the hippocampus of 3XTg-AD mice, respectively [160]. Furthermore, daily administration of nobiletin for four months rescued the memory impairment in fear conditioning, and decreased hippocampal Aβ deposit in the transgenic mice [161].

The effect of nobiletin on neurological disorders was also evaluated in a neurotoxic model of PD. MPP^+ was unilaterally injected into the median forebrain bundle of rat brains with or without daily intraperitoneal injection of nobiletin (1, 10 and 20 mg/kg). The latter, at a dose of 10 mg/kg, but not at 1 or 20 mg/kg, significantly protected DA neurons in the substantia nigra of MPP^+-treated rats, also reducing microglial activation [162]. The capability of nobiletin to suppress microgliosis was demonstrated also by the results of the study performed by Cui et al. (2010) [163]. They found that the polymethoxiflavone suppressed the activation of NF-κB signaling pathway and the release of NO, TNF-α and IL-1β, as well as the phosphorylations of ERK, JNK and p-38 evoked by LPS in BV-2 microglia cells.

It is known that decreased cerebral blood flow causes cognitive impairments and neuronal injury in the progressive age-related neurodegenerative disorders such as AD and vascular dementia. Yamamoto et al., (2009) showed that treatment with 50 mg/kg of nobiletin (i.p.) for the consecutive 7 days before and after the induction of brain ischemia significantly inhibited delayed neuronal death in the hippocampal CA1 neurons and improved the contextual cerebral ischemia-induced memory deficits [164]. Very recently, Zhang et al. (2016) demonstrated that nobiletin (10 and 25 mg/kg/day; i.p.) administrated for 3 days prior to the experimental ischemia and immediately after surgery reduced brain edema and neurological deficit, as well as increased the expression of Nrf2, HO-1, SOD1 and GSH, while decreased the levels of NF-κB, MMP-9 and MDA [165].

4. Conclusion Remarks and Future Perspectives

During the last decades, several studies were performed to evaluate the neuroprotective effects of *Citrus* flavonoids and to identify their molecular targets. Literature data collected in our review support their protective activity in neuropathological conditions, especially in the presence of prooxidants or neurotoxins. These findings highlight the antioxidant nature of flavonoids, able to arrest free radical-induced oxidative damage, which is known to play a pivotal role in many degenerative diseases. Moreover, their neuroprotective action is mediated by the interaction with specific intracellular targets that are implicated in several signaling pathways important for maintaining the physiological status. In this way, *Citrus* flavonoids prevent the neuronal dysfunction due to both acute and chronic injuries in several in vivo experimental models. Nevertheless, the majority of studies on the beneficial effects of *Citrus* flavonoids have been performed in vitro and in vivo, without evidence from equivalent clinical trials. This means that in some cases, the experimental research on the neuroprotective effects of *Citrus* flavonoids does not take into account some aspects which are of great importance in clinical practice. For example, in some study, the pharmacological effect was observed at concentrations or dosages (in vitro and in vivo studies, respectively) of active substance which are unlikely to be reached in the clinical setting. Moreover, in some study it was used routes of administration that highly unlikely to be used by humans. Generally, a natural drug is orally administered (often as nutraceutical or dietary supplement), but bioavailability and presystemic elimination issues are often ignored by researchers. Consequently, the beneficial effects of orally administered flavonoids to improve or prevent CNS pathologies still remain an uncompleted debated topic. This because their poor absorption, rapid metabolism and selective permeability across the BBB limits their access to the CNS and, consequently, their neuroprotective efficacy. In other words, we do not know if the exciting preclinical results correspond to a real therapeutic success. This is the reason for their limited clinical application both alone and as an add-on therapy. Nevertheless, the development of novel natural compound-loaded delivery systems has improved the bioavailability of flavonoids together with their delivery to the brain, enhancing the potential of flavonoids as neuroprotective agents. Further studies are necessary to unravel more pharmacokinetics aspects of flavonoids, which in turn would be very important to stimulate well designed and well-controlled clinical trials confirming the excellent preclinical results.

Anyway, as suggested by this literature revision, we can consider *Citrus* flavonoids as key compounds for the development of a new generation of pharmacological agents effective in preventing and treating neurodegenerative diseases.

This review may be used as a starting point for novel nutraceuticals, food supplements or complementary and alternative drugs to maintain or improve the neurophysiological status.

Acknowledgments: This review has been written within the framework of the project "MEPRA" (PO FESR Sicilia 2007/2013, Linea d'Intervento 4.1.1.1, CUP G73F11000050004).

Author Contributions: Santa Cirmi performed the literature review and drafted the paper; Nadia Ferlazzo and Giovanni E. Lombardo and Elvira Ventura-Spagnolo helped in the collection of literature; Sebastiano Gangemi and Gioacchino Calapai revised the paper; Michele Navarra conceived and designed the study as well as assisted in writing the paper. All authors read and approved the manuscript.

References

1. Perez-Hernandez, J.; Zaldivar-Machorro, V.J.; Villanueva-Porras, D.; Vega-Avila, E.; Chavarria, A. A potential alternative against neurodegenerative diseases: Phytodrugs. *Oxid. Med. Cell. Longev.* **2016**, *2016*, 8378613. [CrossRef] [PubMed]
2. Solanki, L.; Parihar, P.; Mansuri, M.L.; Parihar, M.S. Flavonoid-based therapies in the early management of neurodegenerative diseases. *Adv. Nutr.* **2015**, *6*, 64–72. [CrossRef] [PubMed]
3. Hwang, S.L.; Shih, P.H.; Yen, G.C. Neuroprotective effects of *Citrus* flavonoids. *J. Agric. Food Chem.* **2012**, *60*, 877–885. [CrossRef] [PubMed]
4. Manach, C.; Scalbert, A.; Morand, C.; Remesy, C.; Jimenez, L. Polyphenols: Food sources and bioavailability. *Am. J. Clin. Nutr.* **2004**, *79*, 727–747. [PubMed]
5. Middleton, E., Jr.; Kandaswami, C.; Theoharides, T.C. The effects of plant flavonoids on mammalian cells: Implications for inflammation, heart disease, and cancer. *Pharmacol. Rev.* **2000**, *52*, 673–751. [PubMed]
6. Kumar, S.; Pandey, A.K. Chemistry and biological activities of flavonoids: An overview. *Sci. World J.* **2013**, *2013*, 162750. [CrossRef] [PubMed]
7. Yao, L.H.; Jiang, Y.M.; Shi, J.; Tomas-Barberan, F.A.; Datta, N.; Singanusong, R.; Chen, S.S. Flavonoids in food and their health benefits. *Plant Foods Hum. Nutr.* **2004**, *59*, 113–122. [CrossRef] [PubMed]
8. Benavente-Garcia, O.; Castillo, J. Update on uses and properties of *Citrus* flavonoids: New findings in anticancer, cardiovascular, and anti-inflammatory activity. *J. Agric. Food Chem.* **2008**, *56*, 6185–6205. [CrossRef] [PubMed]
9. Curro, M.; Risitano, R.; Ferlazzo, N.; Cirmi, S.; Gangemi, C.; Caccamo, D.; Ientile, R.; Navarra, M. *Citrus bergamia* juice extract attenuates β-amyloid-induced pro-inflammatory activation of thp-1 cells through mapk and ap-1 pathways. *Sci. Rep.* **2016**, *6*, 20809. [CrossRef] [PubMed]
10. Ferlazzo, N.; Visalli, G.; Smeriglio, A.; Cirmi, S.; Lombardo, G.E.; Campiglia, P.; Di Pietro, A.; Navarra, M. Flavonoid fraction of orange and bergamot juices protect human lung epithelial cells from hydrogen peroxide-induced oxidative stress. *Evid. Based Complement. Altern. Med.* **2015**, *2015*, 957031. [CrossRef] [PubMed]
11. Ferlazzo, N.; Cirmi, S.; Russo, M.; Trapasso, E.; Ursino, M.R.; Lombardo, G.E.; Gangemi, S.; Calapai, G.; Navarra, M. NF-κB mediates the antiproliferative and proapoptotic effects of bergamot juice in HepG2 cells. *Life Sci.* **2016**, *146*, 81–91. [CrossRef] [PubMed]
12. Ferlazzo, N.; Visalli, G.; Cirmi, S.; Lombardo, G.E.; Lagana, P.; di Pietro, A.; Navarra, M. Natural iron chelators: Protective role in A549 cells of flavonoids-rich extracts of *Citrus* juices in Fe^{3+}-induced oxidative stress. *Environ. Toxicol. Pharmacol.* **2016**, *43*, 248–256. [CrossRef] [PubMed]
13. Risitano, R.; Curro, M.; Cirmi, S.; Ferlazzo, N.; Campiglia, P.; Caccamo, D.; Ientile, R.; Navarra, M. Flavonoid fraction of bergamot juice reduces LPS-induced inflammatory response through SIRT1-mediated NF-κB inhibition in THP-1 monocytes. *PLoS ONE* **2014**, *9*, e107431. [CrossRef] [PubMed]
14. Visalli, G.; Ferlazzo, N.; Cirmi, S.; Campiglia, P.; Gangemi, S.; di Pietro, A.; Calapai, G.; Navarra, M. Bergamot juice extract inhibits proliferation by inducing apoptosis in human colon cancer cells. *Anti-Cancer Agents Med. Chem.* **2014**, *14*, 1402–1413. [CrossRef]
15. Delle Monache, S.; Sanita, P.; Trapasso, E.; Ursino, M.R.; Dugo, P.; Russo, M.; Ferlazzo, N.; Calapai, G.; Angelucci, A.; Navarra, M. Mechanisms underlying the anti-tumoral effects of *Citrus bergamia* juice. *PLoS ONE* **2013**, *8*, e61484. [CrossRef] [PubMed]

16. Filocamo, A.; Bisignano, C.; Ferlazzo, N.; Cirmi, S.; Mandalari, G.; Navarra, M. In vitro effect of bergamot (*Citrus bergamia*) juice against caga-positive and-negative clinical isolates of helicobacter pylori. *BMC Complement. Altern. Med.* **2015**, *15*, 256. [CrossRef] [PubMed]
17. Impellizzeri, D.; Bruschetta, G.; di Paola, R.; Ahmad, A.; Campolo, M.; Cuzzocrea, S.; Esposito, E.; Navarra, M. The anti-inflammatory and antioxidant effects of bergamot juice extract (BJe) in an experimental model of inflammatory bowel disease. *Clin. Nutr.* **2015**, *34*, 1146–1154. [CrossRef] [PubMed]
18. Navarra, M.; Ursino, M.R.; Ferlazzo, N.; Russo, M.; Schumacher, U.; Valentiner, U. Effect of *Citrus bergamia* juice on human neuroblastoma cells in vitro and in metastatic xenograft models. *Fitoterapia* **2014**, *95*, 83–92. [CrossRef] [PubMed]
19. Celano, M.; Maggisano, V.; de Rose, R.F.; Bulotta, S.; Maiuolo, J.; Navarra, M.; Russo, D. Flavonoid fraction of *Citrus reticulata* juice reduces proliferation and migration of anaplastic thyroid carcinoma cells. *Nutr. Cancer* **2015**, *67*, 1183–1190. [CrossRef] [PubMed]
20. Marino, A.; Paterniti, I.; Cordaro, M.; Morabito, R.; Campolo, M.; Navarra, M.; Esposito, E.; Cuzzocrea, S. Role of natural antioxidants and potential use of bergamot in treating rheumatoid arthritis. *PharmaNutrition* **2015**, *3*, 53–59. [CrossRef]
21. Cirmi, S.; Bisignano, C.; Mandalari, G.; Navarra, M. Anti-infective potential of *Citrus bergamia* Risso et Poiteau (bergamot) derivatives: A systematic review. *Phytother. Res.* **2016**, *30*, 1404–1411. [CrossRef] [PubMed]
22. Impellizzeri, D.; Cordaro, M.; Campolo, M.; Gugliandolo, E.; Esposito, E.; Benedetto, F.; Cuzzocrea, S.; Navarra, M. Anti-inflammatory and antioxidant effects of flavonoid-rich fraction of bergamot juice (BJe) in a mouse model of intestinal ischemia/reperfusion injury. *Front. Pharmacol.* **2016**, *30*. [CrossRef] [PubMed]
23. Ferlazzo, N.; Cirmi, S.; Calapai, G.; Ventura-Spagnolo, E.; Gangemi, S.; Navarra, M. Anti-inflammatory activity of *Citrus bergamia* derivatives: Where do we stand? *Molecules* **2016**, *21*, 1273. [CrossRef] [PubMed]
24. Citraro, R.; Navarra, M.; Leo, A.; Donato di Paola, E.; Santangelo, E.; Lippiello, P.; Aiello, R.; Russo, E.; de Sarro, G. The anticonvulsant activity of a flavonoid-rich extract from orange juice involves both NMDA and GABA-benzodiazepine receptor complexes. *Molecules* **2016**, *21*, 1261. [CrossRef] [PubMed]
25. Fratiglioni, L.; Launer, L.J.; Andersen, K.; Breteler, M.M.; Copeland, J.R.; Dartigues, J.F.; Lobo, A.; Martinez-Lage, J.; Soininen, H.; Hofman, A. Incidence of dementia and major subtypes in europe: A collaborative study of population-based cohorts. Neurologic diseases in the elderly research group. *Neurology* **2000**, *54*, S10–S15. [PubMed]
26. O'Brien, R.J.; Wong, P.C. Amyloid precursor protein processing and Alzheimer's disease. *Annu. Rev. Neurosci.* **2011**, *34*, 185–204. [CrossRef] [PubMed]
27. Sarkar, A.; Irwin, M.; Singh, A.; Riccetti, M.; Singh, A. Alzheimer's disease: The silver tsunami of the 21st century. *Neural. Regen. Res.* **2016**, *11*, 693–697. [PubMed]
28. Murphy, M.P.; LeVine, H., III. Alzheimer's disease and the amyloid-β peptide. *J. Alzheimers Dis.* **2010**, *19*, 311–323. [PubMed]
29. Hong, H.; Kim, B.S.; Im, H.I. Pathophysiological role of neuroinflammation in neurodegenerative diseases and psychiatric disorders. *Int. Neurourol. J.* **2016**, *20*, S2–S7. [CrossRef] [PubMed]
30. Reeve, A.; Simcox, E.; Turnbull, D. Ageing and Parkinson's disease: Why is advancing age the biggest risk factor? *Ageing Res. Rev.* **2014**, *14*, 19–30. [CrossRef] [PubMed]
31. Wirdefeldt, K.; Adami, H.O.; Cole, P.; Trichopoulos, D.; Mandel, J. Epidemiology and etiology of Parkinson's disease: A review of the evidence. *Eur. J. Epidemiol.* **2011**, *26*, S1–S58. [CrossRef] [PubMed]
32. Norden, D.M.; Muccigrosso, M.M.; Godbout, J.P. Microglial priming and enhanced reactivity to secondary insult in aging, and traumatic cns injury, and neurodegenerative disease. *Neuropharmacology* **2015**, *96*, 29–41. [CrossRef] [PubMed]
33. Cagnin, A.; Kassiou, M.; Meikle, S.R.; Banati, R.B. In vivo evidence for microglial activation in neurodegenerative dementia. *Acta Neurol. Scand. Suppl.* **2006**, *185*, 107–114. [CrossRef] [PubMed]
34. Ferrari, C.C.; Pott Godoy, M.C.; Tarelli, R.; Chertoff, M.; Depino, A.M.; Pitossi, F.J. Progressive neurodegeneration and motor disabilities induced by chronic expression of il-1β in the substantia nigra. *Neurobiol. Dis.* **2006**, *24*, 183–193. [CrossRef] [PubMed]
35. Novak, M.J.; Tabrizi, S.J. Huntington's disease. *BMJ* **2010**, *340*, c3109. [CrossRef] [PubMed]
36. Zhao, T.; Hong, Y.; Li, X.J.; Li, S.H. Subcellular clearance and accumulation of huntington disease protein: A mini-review. *Front. Mol. Neurosci.* **2016**, *9*, 27. [CrossRef] [PubMed]

37. Quarrell, O.; O'Donovan, K.L.; Bandmann, O.; Strong, M. The prevalence of juvenile huntington's disease: A review of the literature and meta-analysis. *PLoS Curr.* **2012**, *4*, e4f8606b742ef3. [CrossRef] [PubMed]
38. Rawlins, M.D.; Wexler, N.S.; Wexler, A.R.; Tabrizi, S.J.; Douglas, I.; Evans, S.J.; Smeeth, L. The prevalence of huntington's disease. *Neuroepidemiology* **2016**, *46*, 144–153. [CrossRef] [PubMed]
39. Wexler, N.S. Huntington's disease: Advocacy driving science. *Annu. Rev Med.* **2012**, *63*, 1–22. [CrossRef] [PubMed]
40. Hannan, A.J. Novel therapeutic targets for huntington's disease. *Expert. Opin. Ther. Targets* **2005**, *9*, 639–650. [CrossRef] [PubMed]
41. Ross, C.A.; Aylward, E.H.; Wild, E.J.; Langbehn, D.R.; Long, J.D.; Warner, J.H.; Scahill, R.I.; Leavitt, B.R.; Stout, J.C.; Paulsen, J.S.; et al. Huntington disease: Natural history, biomarkers and prospects for therapeutics. *Nat. Rev. Neurol.* **2014**, *10*, 204–216. [CrossRef] [PubMed]
42. Chen, C.; Dong, X.P. Epidemiological characteristics of human prion diseases. *Infect. Dis. Poverty* **2016**, *5*, 47. [CrossRef] [PubMed]
43. Prusiner, S.B. Prions. *Proc. Natl. Acad. Sci. USA* **1998**, *95*, 13363–13383. [CrossRef] [PubMed]
44. National Clinical Guideline Centre (UK). *Motor Neurone Disease: Assessment and Management*; National Institute for Health and Care Excellence (UK): London, UK, 2016; No. 42.
45. Balendra, R.; Patani, R. Quo vadis motor neuron disease? *World J. Methodol.* **2016**, *6*, 56–64. [CrossRef] [PubMed]
46. Madill, M.; Fitzgerald, D.; O'Connell, K.E.; Dev, K.K.; Shen, S.; FitzGerald, U. In vitro and ex vivo models of multiple sclerosis. *Drug Discov. Today* **2016**. [CrossRef] [PubMed]
47. Watad, A.; Azrielant, S.; Soriano, A.; Bracco, D.; Abu Much, A.; Amital, H. Association between seasonal factors and multiple sclerosis. *Eur. J. Epidemiol.* **2016**. [CrossRef] [PubMed]
48. Food and Agricultural Organization of the United Nations. Available online: http://www.fao.org/docrep/006/y5143e/y5143e12.htm (accessed on 28 September 2016).
49. Castillo, J.; Benavente, O.; Delrio, J.A. Naringin and neohesperidin levels during development of leaves, flower buds, and fruits of *Citrus*-aurantium. *Plant Physiol.* **1992**, *99*, 67–73. [CrossRef] [PubMed]
50. Jiang, N.; Doseff, A.I.; Grotewold, E. Flavones: From biosynthesis to health benefits. *Plants* **2016**, *5*, 27. [CrossRef] [PubMed]
51. Leem, E.; Nam, J.H.; Jeon, M.T.; Shin, W.H.; Won, S.Y.; Park, S.J.; Choi, M.S.; Jin, B.K.; Jung, U.J.; Kim, S.R. Naringin protects the nigrostriatal dopaminergic projection through induction of gdnf in a neurotoxin model of Parkinson's disease. *J. Nutr. Biochem.* **2014**, *25*, 801–806. [CrossRef] [PubMed]
52. Kim, H.D.; Jeong, K.H.; Jung, U.J.; Kim, S.R. Naringin treatment induces neuroprotective effects in a mouse model of Parkinson's disease in vivo, but not enough to restore the lesioned dopaminergic system. *J. Nutr. Biochem.* **2016**, *28*, 140–146. [CrossRef] [PubMed]
53. Gopinath, K.; Sudhandiran, G. Naringin modulates oxidative stress and inflammation in 3-nitropropionic acid-induced neurodegeneration through the activation of nuclear factor-erythroid 2-related factor-2 signalling pathway. *Neuroscience* **2012**, *227*, 134–143. [CrossRef] [PubMed]
54. Prakash, A.; Shur, B.; Kumar, A. Naringin protects memory impairment and mitochondrial oxidative damage against aluminum-induced neurotoxicity in rats. *Int. J. Neurosci.* **2013**, *123*, 636–645. [CrossRef] [PubMed]
55. Kumar, A.; Dogra, S.; Prakash, A. Protective effect of naringin, a *Citrus* flavonoid, against colchicine-induced cognitive dysfunction and oxidative damage in rats. *J. Med. Food* **2010**, *13*, 976–984. [CrossRef] [PubMed]
56. Antunes, M.S.; Goes, A.T.R.; Boeira, S.P.; Prigol, M.; Jesse, C.R. Protective effect of hesperidin in a model of Parkinson's disease induced by 6-hydroxydopamine in aged mice. *Nutrition* **2014**, *30*, 1415–1422. [CrossRef] [PubMed]
57. Menze, E.T.; Tadros, M.G.; Abdel-Tawab, A.M.; Khalifa, A.E. Potential neuroprotective effects of hesperidin on 3-nitropropionic acid-induced neurotoxicity in rats. *Neurotoxicology* **2012**, *33*, 1265–1275. [CrossRef] [PubMed]
58. Li, C.Y.; Zug, C.; Qu, H.C.; Schluesener, H.; Zhang, Z.Y. Hesperidin ameliorates behavioral impairments and neuropathology of transgenic APP/PS1 mice. *Behav. Brain Res.* **2015**, *281*, 32–42. [CrossRef] [PubMed]
59. Wang, D.M.; Liu, L.; Zhu, X.Y.; Wu, W.L.; Wang, Y. Hesperidin alleviates cognitive impairment, mitochondrial dysfunction and oxidative stress in a mouse model of Alzheimer's disease. *Cell. Mol. Neurobiol.* **2014**, *34*, 1209–1221. [CrossRef] [PubMed]

60. Javed, H.; Vaibhav, K.; Ahmed, M.E.; Khan, A.; Tabassum, R.; Islam, F.; Safhi, M.M.; Islam, F. Effect of hesperidin on neurobehavioral, neuroinflammation, oxidative stress and lipid alteration in intracerebroventricular streptozotocin induced cognitive impairment in mice. *J. Neurol. Sci.* **2015**, *348*, 51–59. [CrossRef] [PubMed]
61. Thenmozhi, A.J.; Raja, T.R.W.; Janakiraman, U.; Manivasagam, T. Neuroprotective effect of hesperidin on aluminium chloride induced Alzheimer's disease in wistar rats. *Neurochem. Res.* **2015**, *40*, 767–776. [CrossRef] [PubMed]
62. Justin Thenmozhi, A.; William Raja, T.R.; Manivasagam, T.; Janakiraman, U.; Mohamed Essa, M. Hesperidin ameliorates cognitive dysfunction, oxidative stress and apoptosis against aluminium chloride induced rat model of Alzheimer's disease. *Nutr. Neurosci.* **2016**. [CrossRef] [PubMed]
63. Chang, C.Y.; Lin, T.Y.; Lu, C.W.; Huang, S.K.; Wang, Y.C.; Chou, S.S.P.; Wang, S.J. Hesperidin inhibits glutamate release and exerts neuroprotection against excitotoxicity induced by kainic acid in the hippocampus of rats. *Neurotoxicology* **2015**, *50*, 157–169. [CrossRef] [PubMed]
64. Choi, E.J.; Ahn, W.S. Neuroprotective effects of chronic hesperetin administration in mice. *Arch. Pharm. Res.* **2008**, *31*, 1457–1462. [CrossRef] [PubMed]
65. Kiasalari, Z.; Khalili, M.; Baluchnejadmojarad, T.; Roghani, M. Protective effect of oral hesperetin against unilateral striatal 6-hydroxydopamine damage in the rat. *Neurochem. Res.* **2016**, *41*, 1065–1072. [CrossRef] [PubMed]
66. Rainey-Smith, S.; Schroetke, L.W.; Bahia, P.; Fahmi, A.; Skilton, R.; Spencer, J.P.; Rice-Evans, C.; Rattray, M.; Williams, R.J. Neuroprotective effects of hesperetin in mouse primary neurones are independent of creb activation. *Neurosci. Lett.* **2008**, *438*, 29–33. [CrossRef] [PubMed]
67. Vauzour, D.; Vafeiadou, K.; Rice-Evans, C.; Williams, R.J.; Spencer, J.P. Activation of pro-survival AKT and ERK1/2 signalling pathways underlie the anti-apoptotic effects of flavanones in cortical neurons. *J. Neurochem.* **2007**, *103*, 1355–1367. [CrossRef] [PubMed]
68. Hwang, S.L.; Yen, G.C. Neuroprotective effects of the Citrus flavanones against H_2O_2-induced cytotoxicity in PC12 cells. *J. Agric. Food Chem.* **2008**, *56*, 859–864. [CrossRef] [PubMed]
69. Khan, M.B.; Khan, M.M.; Khan, A.; Ahmed, M.E.; Ishrat, T.; Tabassum, R.; Vaibhav, K.; Ahmad, A.; Islam, F. Naringenin ameliorates Alzheimer's disease (AD)-type neurodegeneration with cognitive impairment (AD-TNDCI) caused by the intracerebroventricular-streptozotocin in rat model. *Neurochem. Int.* **2012**, *61*, 1081–1093. [CrossRef] [PubMed]
70. Baluchnejadmojarad, T.; Roghani, M. Effect of naringenin on intracerebroventricular streptozotocin-induced cognitive deficits in rat: A behavioral analysis. *Pharmacology* **2006**, *78*, 193–197. [CrossRef] [PubMed]
71. Heo, H.J.; Kim, D.O.; Shin, S.C.; Kim, M.J.; Kim, B.G.; Shin, D.H. Effect of antioxidant flavanone, naringenin, from *Citrus junos* on neuroprotection. *J. Agric. Food Chem.* **2004**, *52*, 1520–1525. [CrossRef] [PubMed]
72. Wu, L.H.; Lin, C.; Lin, H.Y.; Liu, Y.S.; Wu, C.Y.J.; Tsai, C.F.; Chang, P.C.; Yeh, W.L.; Lu, D.Y. Naringenin suppresses neuroinflammatory responses through inducing suppressor of cytokine signaling 3 expression. *Mol. Neurobiol.* **2016**, *53*, 1080–1091. [CrossRef] [PubMed]
73. Vafeiadou, K.; Vauzour, D.; Lee, H.Y.; Rodriguez-Mateos, A.; Williams, R.J.; Spencer, J.P. The *Citrus* flavanone naringenin inhibits inflammatory signalling in glial cells and protects against neuroinflammatory injury. *Arch. Biochem. Biophys.* **2009**, *484*, 100–109. [CrossRef] [PubMed]
74. Morelli, S.; Piscioneri, A.; Salerno, S.; Al-Fageeh, M.B.; Drioli, E.; de Bartolo, L. Neuroprotective effect of didymin on hydrogen peroxide-induced injury in the neuronal membrane system. *Cells Tissues Organs* **2014**, *199*, 184–200. [CrossRef] [PubMed]
75. Choi, B.S.; Sapkota, K.; Kim, S.; Lee, H.J.; Choi, H.S.; Kim, S.J. Antioxidant activity and protective effects of *Tripterygium regelii* extract on hydrogen peroxide-induced injury in human dopaminergic cells, SH-SY5Y. *Neurochem. Res.* **2010**, *35*, 1269–1280. [CrossRef] [PubMed]
76. Rong, W.; Wang, J.; Liu, X.; Jiang, L.; Wei, F.; Hu, X.; Han, X.; Liu, Z. Naringin treatment improves functional recovery by increasing bdnf and vegf expression, inhibiting neuronal apoptosis after spinal cord injury. *Neurochem. Res.* **2012**, *37*, 1615–1623. [CrossRef] [PubMed]
77. Golechha, M.; Chaudhry, U.; Bhatia, J.; Saluja, D.; Arya, D.S. Naringin protects against kainic acid-induced status epilepticus in rats: Evidence for an antioxidant, anti-inflammatory and neuroprotective intervention. *Biol. Pharm. Bull.* **2011**, *34*, 360–365. [CrossRef] [PubMed]

78. Brouillet, E.; Jacquard, C.; Bizat, N.; Blum, D. 3-Nitropropionic acid: A mitochondrial toxin to uncover physiopathological mechanisms underlying striatal degeneration in huntington's disease. *J. Neurochem.* **2005**, *95*, 1521–1540. [CrossRef] [PubMed]
79. Parhiz, H.; Roohbakhsh, A.; Soltani, F.; Rezaee, R.; Iranshahi, M. Antioxidant and anti-inflammatory properties of the *Citrus* flavonoids hesperidin and hesperetin: An updated review of their molecular mechanisms and experimental models. *Phytother. Res.* **2015**, *29*, 323–331. [CrossRef] [PubMed]
80. Youdim, K.A.; Dobbie, M.S.; Kuhnle, G.; Proteggente, A.R.; Abbott, N.J.; Rice-Evans, C. Interaction between flavonoids and the blood-brain barrier: In vitro studies. *J. Neurochem.* **2003**, *85*, 180–192. [CrossRef] [PubMed]
81. Herrmann, N.; Chau, S.A.; Kircanski, I.; Lanctot, K.L. Current and emerging drug treatment options for Alzheimer's disease a systematic review. *Drugs* **2011**, *71*, 2031–2065. [CrossRef] [PubMed]
82. Chin-Chan, M.; Navarro-Yepes, J.; Quintanilla-Vega, B. Environmental pollutants as risk factors for neurodegenerative disorders: Alzheimer and Parkinson diseases. *Front. Cell. Neurosci.* **2015**, *9*, 124. [CrossRef] [PubMed]
83. Mehta, A.; Prabhakar, M.; Kumar, P.; Deshmukh, R.; Sharma, P.L. Excitotoxicity: Bridge to various triggers in neurodegenerative disorders. *Eur. J. Pharmacol.* **2013**, *698*, 6–18. [CrossRef] [PubMed]
84. Lau, A.; Tymianski, M. Glutamate receptors, neurotoxicity and neurodegeneration. *Pflug. Arch. Eur. J. Phy.* **2010**, *460*, 525–542. [CrossRef] [PubMed]
85. De la Monte, S.M.; Tong, M. Mechanisms of nitrosamine-mediated neurodegeneration: Potential relevance to sporadic Alzheimer's disease. *J. Alzheimers Dis.* **2009**, *17*, 817–825. [PubMed]
86. Lester-Coll, N.; Rivera, E.J.; Soscia, S.J.; Doiron, K.; Wands, J.R.; de la Monte, S.M. Intracerebral streptozotocin model of type 3 diabetes: Relevance to sporadic Alzheimer's disease. *J. Alzheimers Dis.* **2006**, *9*, 13–33. [PubMed]
87. Choi, A.Y.; Choi, J.H.; Lee, J.Y.; Yoon, K.S.; Choe, W.; Ha, J.; Yeo, E.J.; Kang, I. Apigenin protects HT22 murine hippocampal neuronal cells against endoplasmic reticulum stress-induced apoptosis. *Neurochem. Int.* **2010**, *57*, 143–152. [CrossRef] [PubMed]
88. Braidy, N.; Grant, R.; Adams, S.; Guillemin, G.J. Neuroprotective effects of naturally occurring polyphenols on quinolinic acid-induced excitotoxicity in human neurons. *FEBS J.* **2010**, *277*, 368–382. [CrossRef] [PubMed]
89. Losi, G.; Puia, G.; Garzon, G.; de Vuono, M.C.; Baraldi, M. Apigenin modulates gabaergic and glutamatergic transmission in cultured cortical neurons. *Eur. J. Pharmacol.* **2004**, *502*, 41–46. [CrossRef] [PubMed]
90. Zhao, L.; Wang, J.L.; Liu, R.; Li, X.X.; Li, J.F.; Zhang, L. Neuroprotective, anti-amyloidogenic and neurotrophic effects of apigenin in an Alzheimer's disease mouse model. *Molecules* **2013**, *18*, 9949–9965. [CrossRef] [PubMed]
91. Liu, R.; Zhang, T.T.; Yang, H.G.; Lan, X.; Ying, J.A.; Du, G.H. The flavonoid apigenin protects brain neurovascular coupling against amyloid-β(25-35)-induced toxicity in mice. *J. Alzheimers Dis.* **2011**, *24*, 85–100. [PubMed]
92. Popovic, M.; Caballero-Bleda, M.; Benavente-Garcia, O.; Castillo, J. The flavonoid apigenin delays forgetting of passive avoidance conditioning in rats. *J. Psychopharmacol.* **2014**, *28*, 498–501. [CrossRef] [PubMed]
93. Taupin, P. Apigenin and related compounds stimulate adult neurogenesis. Mars, inc., the salk institute for biological studies: Wo2008147483. *Expert Opin Ther. Pat.* **2009**, *19*, 523–527. [CrossRef] [PubMed]
94. Patil, C.S.; Singh, V.P.; Satyanarayan, P.S.V.; Jain, N.K.; Singh, A.; Kulkarni, S.K. Protective effect of flavonoids against aging- and lipopolysaccharide-induced cognitive impairment in mice. *Pharmacology* **2003**, *69*, 59–67. [CrossRef] [PubMed]
95. Patil, S.P.; Jain, P.D.; Sancheti, J.S.; Ghumatkar, P.J.; Tambe, R.; Sathaye, S. Neuroprotective and neurotrophic effects of apigenin and luteolin in mptp induced Parkinsonism in mice. *Neuropharmacology* **2014**, *86*, 192–202. [CrossRef] [PubMed]
96. Liu, W.H.; Kong, S.Z.; Xie, Q.F.; Su, J.Y.; Li, W.J.; Guo, H.Z.; Li, S.S.; Feng, X.X.; Su, Z.R.; Xu, Y.; et al. Protective effects of apigenin against 1-methyl-4-phenylpyridinium ion-induced neurotoxicity in PC12 cells. *Int. J. Mol. Med.* **2015**, *35*, 739–746. [CrossRef] [PubMed]
97. Wu, P.S.; Yen, J.H.; Kou, M.C.; Wu, M.J. Luteolin and apigenin attenuate 4-hydroxy-2-nonenal-mediated cell death through modulation of UPR, Nrf2-ARE and MAPK pathways in PC12 cells. *PLoS ONE* **2015**, *10*, e0130599. [CrossRef] [PubMed]

98. Fu, X.B.; Zhang, J.Z.; Guo, L.; Xu, Y.G.; Sun, L.Y.; Wang, S.S.; Feng, Y.; Gou, L.S.; Zhang, L.; Liu, Y. Protective role of luteolin against cognitive dysfunction induced by chronic cerebral hypoperfusion in rats. *Pharmacol. Biochem. Behav.* **2014**, *126*, 122–130. [CrossRef] [PubMed]
99. Xu, B.; Li, X.X.; He, G.R.; Hu, J.J.; Mu, X.; Tian, S.; Du, G.H. Luteolin promotes long-term potentiation and improves cognitive functions in chronic cerebral hypoperfused rats. *Eur. J. Pharmacol.* **2010**, *627*, 99–105. [CrossRef] [PubMed]
100. Liu, Y.; Fu, X.B.; Lan, N.; Li, S.; Zhang, J.Z.; Wang, S.S.; Li, C.; Shang, Y.G.; Huang, T.H.; Zhang, L. Luteolin protects against high fat diet-induced cognitive deficits in obesity mice. *Behav. Brain Res.* **2014**, *267*, 178–188. [CrossRef] [PubMed]
101. Wang, H.M.; Wang, H.L.; Cheng, H.X.; Che, Z.Y. Ameliorating effect of luteolin on memory impairment in an Alzheimer's disease model. *Mol. Med. Rep.* **2016**, *13*, 4215–4220. [CrossRef] [PubMed]
102. Hu, L.W.; Yen, J.H.; Shen, Y.T.; Wu, K.Y.; Wu, M.J. Luteolin modulates 6-hydroxydopamine-induced transcriptional changes of stress response pathways in PC12 cells. *PLoS ONE* **2014**, *9*, e97880. [CrossRef] [PubMed]
103. Wruck, C.J.; Claussen, M.; Fuhrmann, G.; Romer, L.; Schulz, A.; Pufe, T.; Waetzig, V.; Peipp, M.; Herdegen, T.; Gotz, M.E. Luteolin protects rat PC12 and C6 cells against MPP^+ induced toxicity via an ERK dependent Keapl-Nrf2-ARE pathway. *J. Neural. Transm. Suppl.* **2007**, *72*, 57–67. [PubMed]
104. Rezai-Zadeh, K.; Ehrhart, J.; Bai, Y.; Sanberg, P.R.; Bickford, P.; Tan, J.; Shytle, R.D. Apigenin and luteolin modulate microglial activation via inhibition of STAT1-induced CD40 expression. *J. Neuroinflamm.* **2008**, *5*. [CrossRef] [PubMed]
105. Rezai-Zadeh, K.; Shytle, R.D.; Bai, Y.; Tian, J.; Hou, H.Y.; Mori, T.; Zeng, J.; Obregon, D.; Town, T.; Tan, J. Flavonoid-mediated presenilin-1 phosphorylation reduces Alzheimer's disease β-amyloid production. *J. Cell. Mol. Med.* **2009**, *13*, 574–588. [CrossRef] [PubMed]
106. Kao, T.K.; Ou, Y.C.; Lin, S.Y.; Pan, H.C.; Song, P.J.; Raung, S.L.; Lai, C.Y.; Liao, S.L.; Lu, H.C.; Chen, C.J. Luteolin inhibits cytokine expression in endotoxin/cytokine-stimulated microglia. *J. Nutr. Biochem.* **2011**, *22*, 612–624. [CrossRef] [PubMed]
107. Chen, H.Q.; Jin, Z.Y.; Wang, X.J.; Xua, X.M.; Deng, L.; Zhao, J.W. Luteolin protects dopaminergic neurons from inflammation-induced injury through inhibition of microglial activation. *Neurosci. Lett.* **2008**, *448*, 175–179. [CrossRef] [PubMed]
108. Zhu, L.H.; Bi, W.; Qi, R.B.; Wang, H.D.; Lu, D.X. Luteolin inhibits microglial inflammation and improves neuron survival against inflammation. *Int. J. Neurosci.* **2011**, *121*, 329–336. [CrossRef] [PubMed]
109. Zhu, L.H.; Bi, W.; Lu, D.; Zhang, C.J.; Shu, X.M.; Lu, D.X. Luteolin inhibits SH-SY5Y cell apoptosis through suppression of the nuclear transcription factor-κB, mitogen-activated protein kinase and protein kinase B pathways in lipopolysaccharide-stimulated cocultured BV2 cells. *Exp. Ther. Med.* **2014**, *7*, 1065–1070. [CrossRef] [PubMed]
110. Dirscherl, K.; Karlstetter, M.; Ebert, S.; Kraus, D.; Hlawatsch, J.; Walczak, Y.; Moehle, C.; Fuchshofer, R.; Langmann, T. Luteolin triggers global changes in the microglial transcriptome leading to a unique anti-inflammatory and neuroprotective phenotype. *J. Neuroinflamm.* **2010**, *7*. [CrossRef] [PubMed]
111. Nabavi, S.F.; Braidy, N.; Gortzi, O.; Sobarzo-Sanchez, E.; Daglia, M.; Skalicka-Wozniak, K.; Nabavi, S.M. Luteolin as an anti-inflammatory and neuroprotective agent: A brief review. *Brain Res. Bull.* **2015**, *119*, 1–11. [CrossRef] [PubMed]
112. Chao, C.C.; Hu, S.X. Tumor-necrosis-factor-alpha potentiates glutamate neurotoxicity in human fetal brain-cell cultures. *Dev. Neurosci.* **1994**, *16*, 172–179. [CrossRef] [PubMed]
113. Le, W.D.; Rowe, D.; Xie, W.J.; Ortiz, I.; He, Y.; Appel, S.H. Microglial activation and dopaminergic cell injury: An in vitro model relevant to Parkinson's disease. *J. Neurosci.* **2001**, *21*, 8447–8455. [PubMed]
114. Park, S.E.; Sapkota, K.; Kim, S.; Kim, H.; Kim, S.J. Kaempferol acts through mitogen-activated protein kinases and protein kinase B/AKT to elicit protection in a model of neuroinflammation in BV2 microglial cells. *Br. J. Pharmacol.* **2011**, *164*, 1008–1025. [CrossRef] [PubMed]
115. Yang, E.J.; Kim, G.S.; Jun, M.; Song, K.S. Kaempferol attenuates the glutamate-induced oxidative stress in mouse-derived hippocampal neuronal HT22 cells. *Food Funct.* **2014**, *5*, 1395–1402. [CrossRef] [PubMed]
116. Magalingam, K.B.; Radhakrishnan, A.; Haleagrahara, N. Rutin, a bioflavonoid antioxidant protects rat pheochromocytoma (PC-12) cells against 6-hydroxydopamine (6-OHDA)-induced neurotoxicity. *Int. J. Mol. Med.* **2013**, *32*, 235–240. [PubMed]

117. Song, K.; Kim, S.; Na, J.Y.; Park, J.H.; Kim, J.K.; Kim, J.H.; Kwon, J. Rutin attenuates ethanol-induced neurotoxicity in hippocampal neuronal cells by increasing aldehyde dehydrogenase 2. *Food Chem. Toxicol.* **2014**, *72*, 228–233. [CrossRef] [PubMed]
118. Yu, X.L.; Li, Y.N.; Zhang, H.; Su, Y.J.; Zhou, W.W.; Zhang, Z.P.; Wang, S.W.; Xu, P.X.; Wang, Y.J.; Liu, R.T. Rutin inhibits amylin-induced neurocytotoxicity and oxidative stress. *Food Funct.* **2015**, *6*, 3296–3306. [CrossRef] [PubMed]
119. Na, J.Y.; Kim, S.; Song, K.; Kwon, J. Rutin alleviates prion peptide-induced cell death through inhibiting apoptotic pathway activation in dopaminergic neuronal cells. *Cell. Mol. Neurobiol.* **2014**, *34*, 1071–1079. [CrossRef] [PubMed]
120. Nassiri-Asl, M.; Naserpour Farivar, T.; Abbasi, E.; Sadeghnia, H.R.; Sheikhi, M.; Lotfizadeh, M.; Bazahang, P. Effects of rutin on oxidative stress in mice with kainic acid-induced seizure. *J. Integr. Med.* **2013**, *11*, 337–342. [CrossRef] [PubMed]
121. Khan, M.M.; Raza, S.S.; Javed, H.; Ahmad, A.; Khan, A.; Islam, F.; Safhi, M.M.; Islam, F. Rutin protects dopaminergic neurons from oxidative stress in an animal model of Parkinson's disease. *Neurotox. Res.* **2012**, *22*, 1–15. [CrossRef] [PubMed]
122. Wang, S.W.; Wang, Y.J.; Su, Y.J.; Zhou, W.W.; Yang, S.G.; Zhang, R.; Zhao, M.; Li, Y.N.; Zhang, Z.P.; Zhan, D.W.; et al. Rutin inhibits β-amyloid aggregation and cytotoxicity, attenuates oxidative stress, and decreases the production of nitric oxide and proinflammatory cytokines. *Neurotoxicology* **2012**, *33*, 482–490. [CrossRef] [PubMed]
123. Xu, P.X.; Wang, S.W.; Yu, X.L.; Su, Y.J.; Wang, T.; Zhou, W.W.; Zhang, H.; Wang, Y.J.; Liu, R.T. Rutin improves spatial memory in Alzheimer's disease transgenic mice by reducing abeta oligomer level and attenuating oxidative stress and neuroinflammation. *Behav. Brain Res.* **2014**, *264*, 173–180. [CrossRef] [PubMed]
124. Machawal, L.; Kumar, A. Possible involvement of nitric oxide mechanism in the neuroprotective effect of rutin against immobilization stress induced anxiety like behaviour, oxidative damage in mice. *Pharmacol. Rep.* **2014**, *66*, 15–21. [CrossRef] [PubMed]
125. Moghbelinejad, S.; Nassiri-Asl, M.; Farivar, T.N.; Abbasi, E.; Sheikhi, M.; Taghiloo, M.; Farsad, F.; Samimi, A.; Hajiali, F. Rutin activates the MAPK pathway and BDNF gene expression on beta-amyloid induced neurotoxicity in rats. *Toxicol. Lett.* **2014**, *224*, 108–113. [CrossRef] [PubMed]
126. Habtemariam, S. Rutin as a natural therapy for Alzheimer's disease: Insights into its mechanisms of action. *Curr. Med. Chem.* **2016**, *23*, 860–873. [CrossRef] [PubMed]
127. Jesberger, J.A.; Richardson, J.S. Oxygen free-radicals and brain-dysfunction. *Int. J. Neurosci.* **1991**, *57*, 1–17. [CrossRef] [PubMed]
128. Shin, H.J.; Lee, J.Y.; Son, E.; Lee, D.H.; Kim, H.J.; Kang, S.S.; Cho, G.J.; Choi, W.S.; Roh, G.S. Curcumin attenuates the kainic acid-induced hippocampal cell death in the mice. *Neurosci. Lett.* **2007**, *416*, 49–54. [CrossRef] [PubMed]
129. Suematsu, N.; Hosoda, M.; Fujimori, K. Protective effects of quercetin against hydrogen peroxide-induced apoptosis in human neuronal SH-SY5Y cells. *Neurosci. Lett.* **2011**, *504*, 223–227. [CrossRef] [PubMed]
130. Roshanzamir, F.; Yazdanparast, R. Quercetin attenuates cell apoptosis of oxidant-stressed SK-N-MC cells while suppressing up-regulation of the defensive element, HIF-1α. *Neuroscience* **2014**, *277*, 780–793. [CrossRef] [PubMed]
131. Jembrek, M.J.; Vukovic, L.; Puhovic, J.; Erhardt, J.; Orsolic, N. Neuroprotective effect of quercetin against hydrogen peroxide-induced oxidative injury in P19 neurons. *J. Mol. Neurosci.* **2012**, *47*, 286–299. [CrossRef] [PubMed]
132. Sajad, M.; Zargan, J.; Zargar, M.A.; Sharma, J.; Umar, S.; Arora, R.; Khan, H.A. Quercetin prevents protein nitration and glycolytic block of proliferation in hydrogen peroxide insulted cultured neuronal precursor cells (NPCS): Implications on cns regeneration. *Neurotoxicology* **2013**, *36*, 24–33. [CrossRef] [PubMed]
133. Ansari, M.A.; Abdul, H.M.; Joshi, G.; Opii, W.O.; Butterfield, D.A. Protective effect of quercetin in primary neurons against Aβ(1-42): Relevance to Alzheimer's disease. *J. Nutr. Biochem.* **2009**, *20*, 269–275. [CrossRef] [PubMed]
134. Zhang, X.; Hu, J.; Zhong, L.; Wang, N.; Yang, L.; Liu, C.C.; Li, H.; Wang, X.; Zhou, Y.; Zhang, Y.; et al. Quercetin stabilizes apolipoprotein E and reduces brain Aβ levels in amyloid model mice. *Neuropharmacology* **2016**, *108*, 179–192. [CrossRef] [PubMed]

135. Lv, C.; Hong, T.; Yang, Z.; Zhang, Y.; Wang, L.; Dong, M.; Zhao, J.; Mu, J.; Meng, Y. Effect of quercetin in the 1-methyl-4-phenyl-1,2,3,6-tetrahydropyridine-induced mouse model of Parkinson's disease. *Evid. Based Complement. Altern. Med.* **2012**, *2012*, 928643. [CrossRef] [PubMed]
136. Chen, J.C.; Ho, F.M.; Pei-Dawn Lee, C.; Chen, C.P.; Jeng, K.C.; Hsu, H.B.; Lee, S.T.; Wen Tung, W.; Lin, W.W. Inhibition of iNOS gene expression by quercetin is mediated by the inhibition of IκB kinase, nuclear factor-kappa B and STAT1, and depends on heme oxygenase-1 induction in mouse Bv-2 microglia. *Eur. J. Pharmacol.* **2005**, *521*, 9–20. [CrossRef] [PubMed]
137. Kang, C.H.; Choi, Y.H.; Moon, S.K.; Kim, W.J.; Kim, G.Y. Quercetin inhibits lipopolysaccharide-induced nitric oxide production in BV2 microglial cells by suppressing the NF-κB pathway and activating the Nrf2-dependent HO-1 pathway. *Int. Immunopharmacol.* **2013**, *17*, 808–813. [CrossRef] [PubMed]
138. Bournival, J.; Francoeur, M.A.; Renaud, J.; Martinoli, M.G. Quercetin and sesamin protect neuronal PC12 cells from high-glucose-induced oxidation, nitrosative stress, and apoptosis. *Rejuvenation Res.* **2012**, *15*, 322–333. [CrossRef] [PubMed]
139. Xia, S.F.; Xie, Z.X.; Qiao, Y.; Li, L.R.; Cheng, X.R.; Tang, X.; Shi, Y.H.; Le, G.W. Differential effects of quercetin on hippocampus-dependent learning and memory in mice fed with different diets related with oxidative stress. *Physiol. Behav.* **2015**, *138*, 325–331. [CrossRef] [PubMed]
140. Lu, J.; Wu, D.M.; Zheng, Y.L.; Hu, B.; Zhang, Z.F.; Shan, Q.; Zheng, Z.H.; Liu, C.M.; Wang, Y.J. Quercetin activates AMP-activated protein kinase by reducing PP2C expression protecting old mouse brain against high cholesterol-induced neurotoxicity. *J. Pathol.* **2010**, *222*, 199–212. [CrossRef] [PubMed]
141. Zhang, Y.; Yi, B.; Ma, J.; Zhang, L.; Zhang, H.; Yang, Y.; Dai, Y. Quercetin promotes neuronal and behavioral recovery by suppressing inflammatory response and apoptosis in a rat model of intracerebral hemorrhage. *Neurochem. Res.* **2015**, *40*, 195–203. [CrossRef] [PubMed]
142. Arikan, S.; Ersan, I.; Karaca, T.; Kara, S.; Gencer, B.; Karaboga, I.; Hasan Ali, T. Quercetin protects the retina by reducing apoptosis due to ischemia-reperfusion injury in a rat model. *Arq. Bras. Oftalmol.* **2015**, *78*, 100–104. [CrossRef] [PubMed]
143. Tota, S.; Awasthi, H.; Kamat, P.K.; Nath, C.; Hanif, K. Protective effect of quercetin against intracerebral streptozotocin induced reduction in cerebral blood flow and impairment of memory in mice. *Behav. Brain Res.* **2010**, *209*, 73–79. [CrossRef] [PubMed]
144. Richetti, S.K.; Blank, M.; Capiotti, K.M.; Piato, A.L.; Bogo, M.R.; Vianna, M.R.; Bonan, C.D. Quercetin and rutin prevent scopolamine-induced memory impairment in zebrafish. *Behav. Brain Res.* **2011**, *217*, 10–15. [CrossRef] [PubMed]
145. Hu, P.; Wang, M.; Chen, W.H.; Liu, J.; Chen, L.; Yin, S.T.; Yong, W.; Chen, J.T.; Wang, H.L.; Ruan, D.Y. Quercetin relieves chronic lead exposure-induced impairment of synaptic plasticity in rat dentate gyrus in vivo. *Naunyn Schmiedebergs Arch. Pharmacol.* **2008**, *378*, 43–51. [CrossRef] [PubMed]
146. Barcelos, G.R.; Grotto, D.; Serpeloni, J.M.; Angeli, J.P.; Rocha, B.A.; de Oliveira Souza, V.C.; Vicentini, J.T.; Emanuelli, T.; Bastos, J.K.; Antunes, L.M.; et al. Protective properties of quercetin against DNA damage and oxidative stress induced by methylmercury in rats. *Arch. Toxicol.* **2011**, *85*, 1151–1157. [CrossRef] [PubMed]
147. Sachdeva, S.; Pant, S.C.; Kushwaha, P.; Bhargava, R.; Flora, S.J. Sodium tungstate induced neurological alterations in rat brain regions and their response to antioxidants. *Food Chem. Toxicol.* **2015**, *82*, 64–71. [CrossRef] [PubMed]
148. Sharma, D.R.; Wani, W.Y.; Sunkaria, A.; Kandimalla, R.J.; Verma, D.; Cameotra, S.S.; Gill, K.D. Quercetin protects against chronic aluminum-induced oxidative stress and ensuing biochemical, cholinergic, and neurobehavioral impairments in rats. *Neurotox. Res.* **2013**, *23*, 336–357. [CrossRef] [PubMed]
149. Sharma, D.R.; Sunkaria, A.; Wani, W.Y.; Sharma, R.K.; Verma, D.; Priyanka, K.; Bal, A.; Gill, K.D. Quercetin protects against aluminium induced oxidative stress and promotes mitochondrial biogenesis via activation of the PGC-1α signaling pathway. *Neurotoxicology* **2015**, *51*, 116–137. [CrossRef] [PubMed]
150. Sharma, D.R.; Wani, W.Y.; Sunkaria, A.; Kandimalla, R.J.; Sharma, R.K.; Verma, D.; Bal, A.; Gill, K.D. Quercetin attenuates neuronal death against aluminum-induced neurodegeneration in the rat hippocampus. *Neuroscience* **2016**, *324*, 163–176. [CrossRef] [PubMed]
151. Bavithra, S.; Selvakumar, K.; Pratheepa Kumari, R.; Krishnamoorthy, G.; Venkataraman, P.; Arunakaran, J. Polychlorinated biphenyl (PCBs)-induced oxidative stress plays a critical role on cerebellar dopaminergic receptor expression: Ameliorative role of quercetin. *Neurotox. Res.* **2012**, *21*, 149–159. [CrossRef] [PubMed]

152. Selvakumar, K.; Bavithra, S.; Ganesh, L.; Krishnamoorthy, G.; Venkataraman, P.; Arunakaran, J. Polychlorinated biphenyls induced oxidative stress mediated neurodegeneration in hippocampus and behavioral changes of adult rats: Anxiolytic-like effects of quercetin. *Toxicol. Lett.* **2013**, *222*, 45–54. [CrossRef] [PubMed]
153. Beckmann, D.V.; Carvalho, F.B.; Mazzanti, C.M.; Dos Santos, R.P.; Andrades, A.O.; Aiello, G.; Rippilinger, A.; Graca, D.L.; Abdalla, F.H.; Oliveira, L.S.; et al. Neuroprotective role of quercetin in locomotor activities and cholinergic neurotransmission in rats experimentally demyelinated with ethidium bromide. *Life Sci.* **2014**, *103*, 79–87. [CrossRef] [PubMed]
154. Nassiri-Asl, M.; Moghbelinejad, S.; Abbasi, E.; Yonesi, F.; Haghighi, M.R.; Lotfizadeh, M.; Bazahang, P. Effects of quercetin on oxidative stress and memory retrieval in kindled rats. *Epilepsy Behav.* **2013**, *28*, 151–155. [CrossRef] [PubMed]
155. Datla, K.P.; Christidou, M.; Widmer, W.W.; Rooprai, H.K.; Dexter, D.T. Tissue distribution and neuroprotective effects of *Citrus* flavonoid tangeretin in a rat model of Parkinson's disease. *Neuroreport* **2001**, *12*, 3871–3875. [CrossRef] [PubMed]
156. Shu, Z.P.; Yang, B.Y.; Zhao, H.; Xu, B.Q.; Jiao, W.J.; Wang, Q.H.; Wang, Z.B.; Kuang, H.X. Tangeretin exerts anti-neuroinflammatory effects via NF-κB modulation in lipopolysaccharide-stimulated microglial cells. *Int. Immunopharmacol.* **2014**, *19*, 275–282. [CrossRef] [PubMed]
157. Matsuzaki, K.; Yamakuni, T.; Hashimoto, M.; Haque, A.M.; Shido, O.; Mimaki, Y.; Sashida, Y.; Ohizumi, Y. Nobiletin restoring β-amyloid-impaired CREB phosphorylation rescues memory deterioration in Alzheimer's disease model rats. *Neurosci. Lett.* **2006**, *400*, 230–234. [CrossRef] [PubMed]
158. Onozuka, H.; Nakajima, A.; Matsuzaki, K.; Shin, R.W.; Ogino, K.; Saigusa, D.; Tetsu, N.; Yokosuka, A.; Sashida, Y.; Mimaki, Y.; et al. Nobiletin, a *Citrus* flavonoid, improves memory impairment and Aβ pathology in a transgenic mouse model of Alzheimer's disease. *J. Pharmacol. Exp. Ther.* **2008**, *326*, 739–744. [CrossRef] [PubMed]
159. Nakajima, A.; Aoyama, Y.; Nguyen, T.T.; Shin, E.J.; Kim, H.C.; Yamada, S.; Nakai, T.; Nagai, T.; Yokosuka, A.; Mimaki, Y.; et al. Nobiletin, a *Citrus* flavonoid, ameliorates cognitive impairment, oxidative burden, and hyperphosphorylation of tau in senescence-accelerated mouse. *Behav. Brain Res.* **2013**, *250*, 351–360. [CrossRef] [PubMed]
160. Nakajima, A.; Aoyama, Y.; Shin, E.J.; Nam, Y.; Kim, H.C.; Nagai, T.; Yokosuka, A.; Mimaki, Y.; Yokoi, T.; Ohizumi, Y.; et al. Nobiletin, a *Citrus* flavonoid, improves cognitive impairment and reduces soluble Aβ levels in a triple transgenic mouse model of Alzheimer's disease (3XTg-AD). *Behav. Brain Res.* **2015**, *289*, 69–77. [CrossRef] [PubMed]
161. Yamakuni, T.; Nakajima, A.; Ohizumi, Y. Preventive action of nobiletin, a constituent of AURANTII NOBILIS PERICARPIUM with anti-dementia activity, against amyloid-beta peptide-induced neurotoxicity expression and memory impairment. *Yakugaku Zasshi* **2010**, *130*, 517–520. [CrossRef] [PubMed]
162. Jeong, K.H.; Jeon, M.T.; Kim, H.D.; Jung, U.J.; Jang, M.C.; Chu, J.W.; Yang, S.J.; Choi, I.Y.; Choi, M.S.; Kim, S.R. Nobiletin protects dopaminergic neurons in the 1-methyl-4-phenylpyridinium-treated rat model of Parkinson's disease. *J. Med. Food* **2015**, *18*, 409–414. [CrossRef] [PubMed]
163. Cui, Y.; Wu, J.; Jung, S.C.; Park, D.B.; Maeng, Y.H.; Hong, J.Y.; Kim, S.J.; Lee, S.R.; Kim, S.J.; Kim, S.J.; et al. Anti-neuroinflammatory activity of nobiletin on suppression of microglial activation. *Biol. Pharm. Bull.* **2010**, *33*, 1814–1821. [CrossRef] [PubMed]
164. Yamamoto, Y.; Shioda, N.; Han, F.; Moriguchi, S.; Nakajima, A.; Yokosuka, A.; Mimaki, Y.; Sashida, Y.; Yamakuni, T.; Ohizumi, Y.; et al. Nobiletin improves brain ischemia-induced learning and memory deficits through stimulation of CaMKII and CREB phosphorylation. *Brain Res.* **2009**, *1295*, 218–229. [CrossRef] [PubMed]
165. Zhang, L.; Zhang, X.; Zhang, C.; Bai, X.; Zhang, J.; Zhao, X.; Chen, L.; Wang, L.; Zhu, C.; Cui, L.; et al. Nobiletin promotes antioxidant and anti-inflammatory responses and elicits protection against ischemic stroke in vivo. *Brain Res.* **2016**, *1636*, 130–141. [CrossRef] [PubMed]

8

3,5,6,7,8,3′,4′-Heptamethoxyflavone, a Citrus Flavonoid, Ameliorates Corticosterone-Induced Depression-Like Behavior and Restores Brain-Derived Neurotrophic Factor Expression, Neurogenesis and Neuroplasticity in the Hippocampus

Atsushi Sawamoto [1], Satoshi Okuyama [1,*], Kana Yamamoto [1], Yoshiaki Amakura [2], Morio Yoshimura [2], Mitsunari Nakajima [1] and Yoshiko Furukawa [1]

1 Department of Pharmaceutical Pharmacology, College of Pharmaceutical Sciences, Matsuyama University, 4-2 Bunkyo-cho, Matsuyama, Ehime 790-8578, Japan; 46140018@cc.matsuyama-u.ac.jp (A.S.); 66150087@cc.matsuyama-u.ac.jp (K.Y.) mnakajim@cc.matsuyama-u.ac.jp (M.N.); furukawa@cc.matsuyama-u.ac.jp (Y.F.)

2 Department of Pharmacognosy, College of Pharmaceutical Sciences, Matsuyama University, 4-2 Bunkyo-cho, Matsuyama, Ehime 790-8578, Japan; amakura@cc.matsuyama-u.ac.jp (Y.A.); myoshimu@cc.matsuyama-u.ac.jp (M.Y.)

* Correspondence: sokuyama@cc.matsuyama-u.ac.jp

Academic Editor: Luigia Trabace

Abstract: We previously reported that the citrus flavonoid 3,5,6,7,8,3′,4′-heptamethoxyflavone (HMF) increased the expression of brain-derived neurotrophic factor (BDNF) in the hippocampus of a transient global ischemia mouse model. Since the BDNF hypothesis of depression postulates that a reduction in BDNF is directly involved in the pathophysiology of depression, we evaluated the anti-depressive effects of HMF in mice with subcutaneously administered corticosterone at a dose of 20 mg/kg/day for 25 days. We demonstrated that the HMF treatment ameliorated (1) corticosterone-induced body weight loss, (2) corticosterone-induced depression-like behavior, and (3) corticosterone-induced reductions in BDNF production in the hippocampus. We also showed that the HMF treatment restored (4) corticosterone-induced reductions in neurogenesis in the dentate gyrus subgranular zone and (5) corticosterone-induced reductions in the expression levels of phosphorylated calcium-calmodulin-dependent protein kinase II and extracellular signal-regulated kinase1/2. These results suggest that HMF exerts its effects as an anti-depressant drug by inducing the expression of BDNF.

Keywords: heptamethoxyflavone; depression; corticosterone; hippocampus; brain-derived neurotrophic factor; neurogenesis

---

1. Introduction

The incidence of depression is increasing in every generation worldwide. A large number of studies have identified genetic factors, environmental factors, and stress as major risk factors for depression [1]. Stress induces the activation of the hypothalamic-pituitary-adrenal (HPA) axis [2], resulting in the over-secretion of glucocorticoids, which, in turn, leads to the depressive symptomatology [3]. Recent studies also showed that decreases in the levels of hippocampal brain-derived neurotrophic factor (BDNF), the most important neurotrophic factor in the brain, correlated with stress-induced depressive behavior; however, treatments with anti-depressants have been suggested to restore BDNF levels [4–6]. The BDNF hypothesis of depression was recently proposed based on these findings [7].

In addition to increasing evidence to show that BDNF is one of the representative molecules for depression, we previously demonstrated that 3,5,6,7,8,3′,4′-heptamethoxyflavone (HMF; Figure 1), a citrus polymethoxyflavone, has the potential to accelerate the synthesis of BDNF in the hippocampus following ischemia [8,9]. Therefore, we herein determined whether HMF ameliorates depressive-like behavior and depressive disorders in a depression mouse model. In the present study, a depression mice model was developed through the chronic administration of glucocorticoids, which was based on clinical observations that glucocorticoid levels are elevated in depressed patients [3]. Patients with elevated glucocorticoid levels (for example, by the administration of a high dose of corticosteroids) exhibit a depression-like state [10]. We previously reported that the repeated administration of corticosterone at a dose of 20 mg/kg for 3 weeks induced depressive conditions in mice [11]. These mice exhibited 1) depression-like behavior, 2) reduced body weight, and 3) decreases in the phosphorylated levels of extracellular signal-regulated kinase1/2 (ERK1/2), an important intracellular signal transduction molecule for neuronal function; cAMP response element-binding protein (CREB), a transcription factor that regulates neuronal function; and Akt, a critical factor in cell survival and apoptosis, in the hippocampus and cerebral cortex [11]. Moreover, the chronic administration of corticosterone at a dose of 32 mg/kg/day for 21 days [12] or the implantation of a corticosterone pellet (100 mg/kg/day for 21 days) [13] led to decreases in BDNF mRNA and protein levels in the hippocampus of the brain. These findings suggest that corticosterone-injected mice are a useful and reliable animal model for investigating the resilient effects of HMF on BDNF levels.

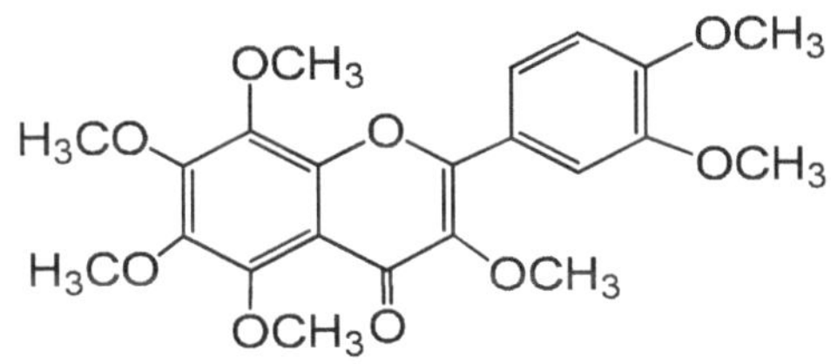

Figure 1. Structure of 3,5,6,7,8,3′,4′-heptamethoxyflavone (HMF).

We used fluoxetine (FLX), a selective serotonin reuptake inhibitor (SSRI), as a positive control of an anti-depressant drug in the present study. FLX was previously shown to increase not only serotonin concentrations in the synaptic cleft, but also BDNF concentrations [7,14,15].

2. Results

2.1. *Effects of Corticosterone and HMF on Body Weight Changes*

Figure 2 shows changes in the body weights of mice during the experimental period, indicating that the repeated administration of corticosterone significantly induced decreases in body weight before Day 7, as reported previously [11,16]. Body weight gain by Day 21 in the CORT group (1.1 ± 0.4 g) was approximately 50% that in the CON group (2.0 ± 0.2 g). Figure 2 also shows that this decrease was attenuated by the administration of HMF; body weight gain in the CORT + HMF group was 1.9 ± 0.3 g on Day 21, which was similar to that in the CON group. This result indicated that HMF significantly suppressed corticosterone-induced body weight loss. Body weight gain in the CORT + FLX group on Day 21 was 1.3 ± 0.4 g, indicating that the representative anti-depressant drug, FLX, did not suppress body weight loss during the experimental period.

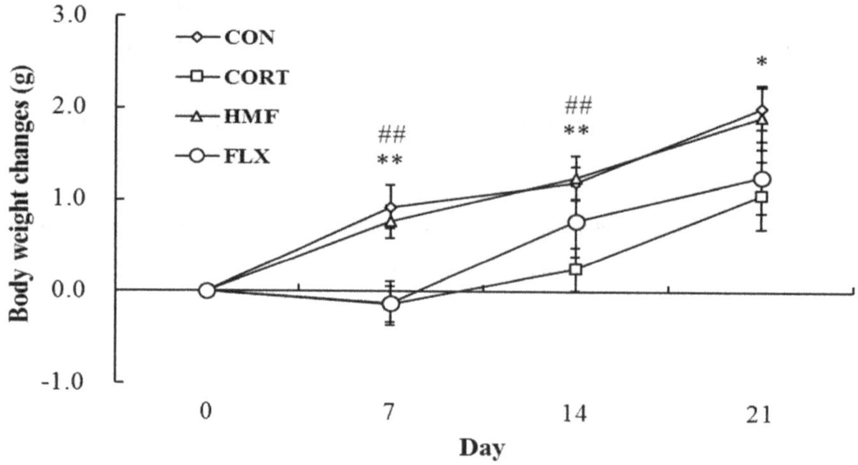

Figure 2. Body weight changes on Days 7, 14, and 21. Values are means ± SEM ($n = 8$). Symbols show significant differences between the following conditions: CON *vs.* CORT (* $p < 0.05$, ** $p < 0.01$) and CORT *vs.* CORT + HMF ($^{\#\#}$ $p < 0.01$).

2.2. Effects of Corticosterone and HMF on Depressive-Like Behavior

The depressive-like behavior of mice was evaluated in the forced swim and tail suspension tests. Immobility times in the forced swim test were examined on Day 22. Figure 3A shows that the immobility time in the CORT group (57.1 ± 9.8 s) was approximately two-fold that in the CON group (29.6 ± 5.7 s), and also that the corticosterone treatment significantly (* $p < 0.05$) prolonged immobility times in the forced swim test. The immobility time in the CORT + HMF group was 28.1 ± 5.3 s, indicating that HMF significantly ($^{\#}$ $p < 0.05$) suppressed corticosterone-induced depression-like behavior. In this test, the immobility time in the CORT + FLX group (70.1 ± 19.8 s) was markedly longer than that in the CORT group, which is consistent with previous findings [17].

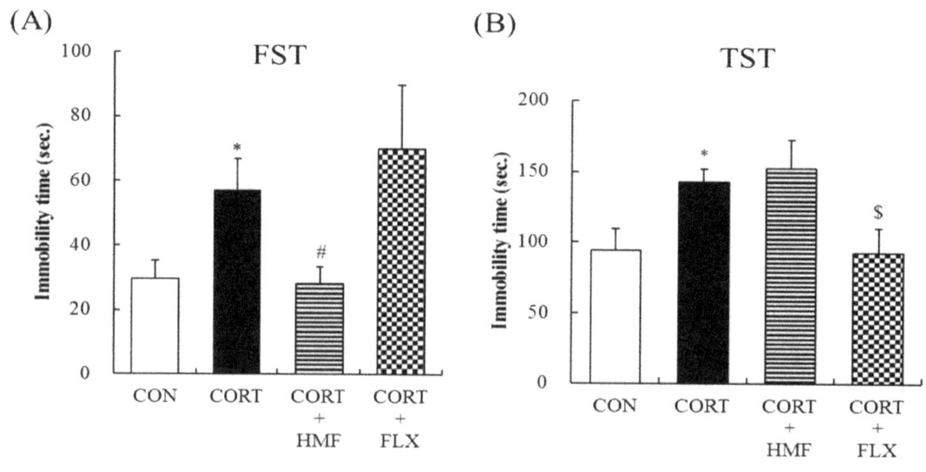

Figure 3. Effects of HMF on corticosterone-induced behavioral abnormalities in the forced swim test (**A**) and tail suspension test (**B**). Values are means ± SEM ($n = 7$–8). Symbols show significant differences between the following conditions: CON *vs.* CORT (* $p < 0.05$), CORT *vs.* CORT + HMF ($^{\#}$ $p < 0.05$), and CORT *vs.* CORT + FLX ($^{\$}$ $p < 0.05$).

As another method to assess depressive-like behavior, immobility times in the tail suspension test were examined on Day 23. Figure 3B shows that the immobility time in the CORT group (142.6 ± 9.6 s) was significantly (* $p < 0.05$) longer than that in the CON group (94.5 ± 14.7 s). Figure 3B also shows that the administration of FLX significantly ($^{\$}$ $p < 0.05$) attenuated corticosterone-induced increases in immobility times, whereas HMF did not.

2.3. Effects of Corticosterone and HMF on the Expression of BDNF in the Hippocampus

Previous studies indicated that modifications in the expression of BDNF in the hippocampus may correlate with depression [7,18], and our previous findings demonstrated that HMF enhanced the synthesis of BDNF in the hippocampus of the ischemic brain [8,9]. Therefore, we investigated the effects of HMF on the expression of BDNF in the hippocampus on Days 10, 17, and 26 using an immunofluorescence method. Figure 4A shows representative photographs of the hippocampal region on Day 26. The BDNF signal on Day 26 was markedly weaker in the CORT group (b) than in the CON group (a), while those in the CORT + HMF group (c) and CORT + FLX group (d) were stronger than that in the CORT group. A quantitative analysis of BDNF-positive signal density (Figure 4B) showed that although BDNF signals in the CORT group were not weaker on Day 10, their densities gradually became weaker on Day 17; corticosterone significantly (*** $p < 0.001$) reduced the expression of BDNF at Day 26, while HMF and FLX significantly ($^{\#\#}$ $p < 0.01$ and $^{\$\$}$ $p < 0.01$, respectively) attenuated this decrease. These results indicated that HMF attenuated the corticosterone-induced suppression of BDNF expression in the hippocampus, similar to FLX.

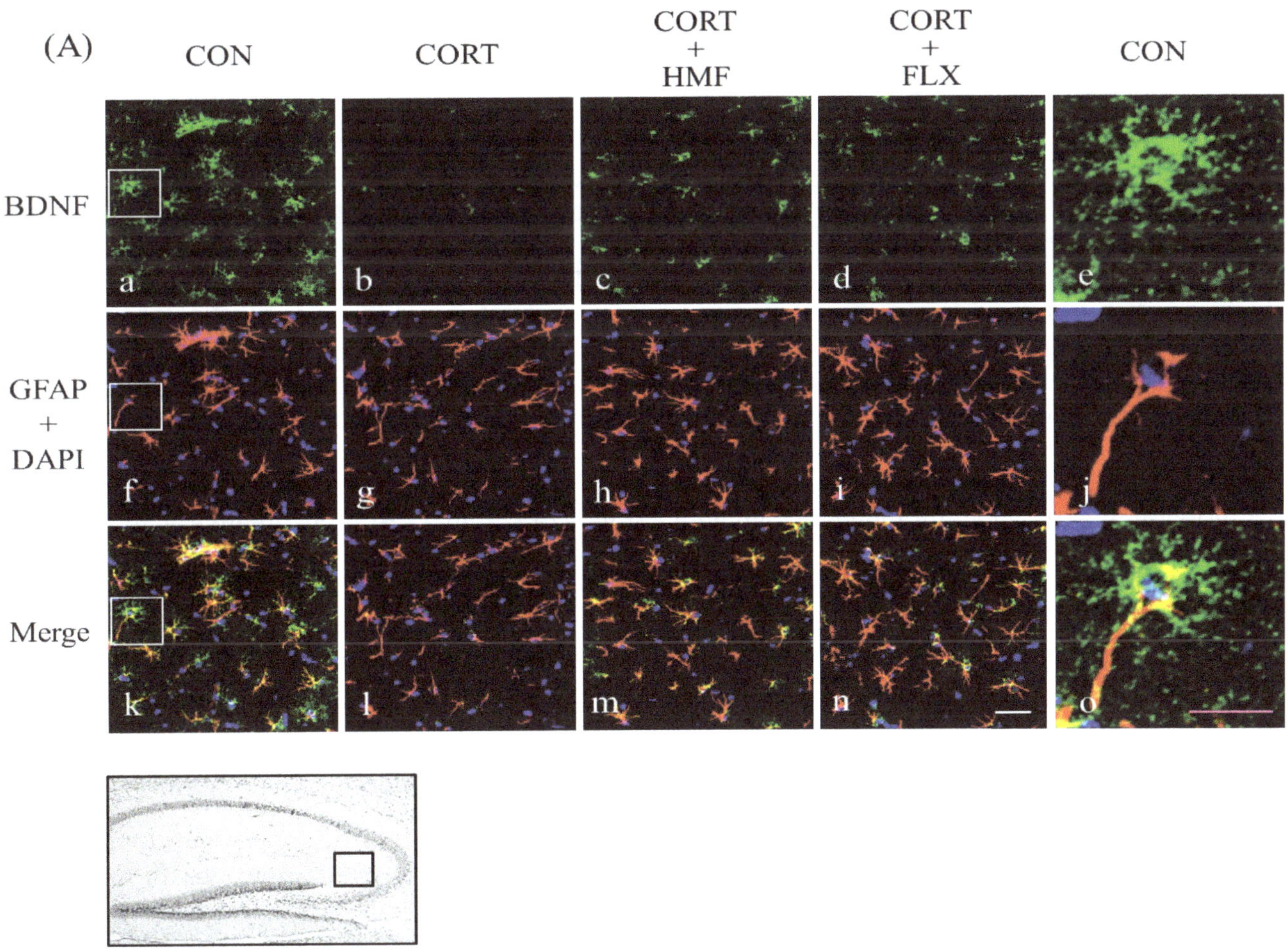

Figure 4. *Cont.*

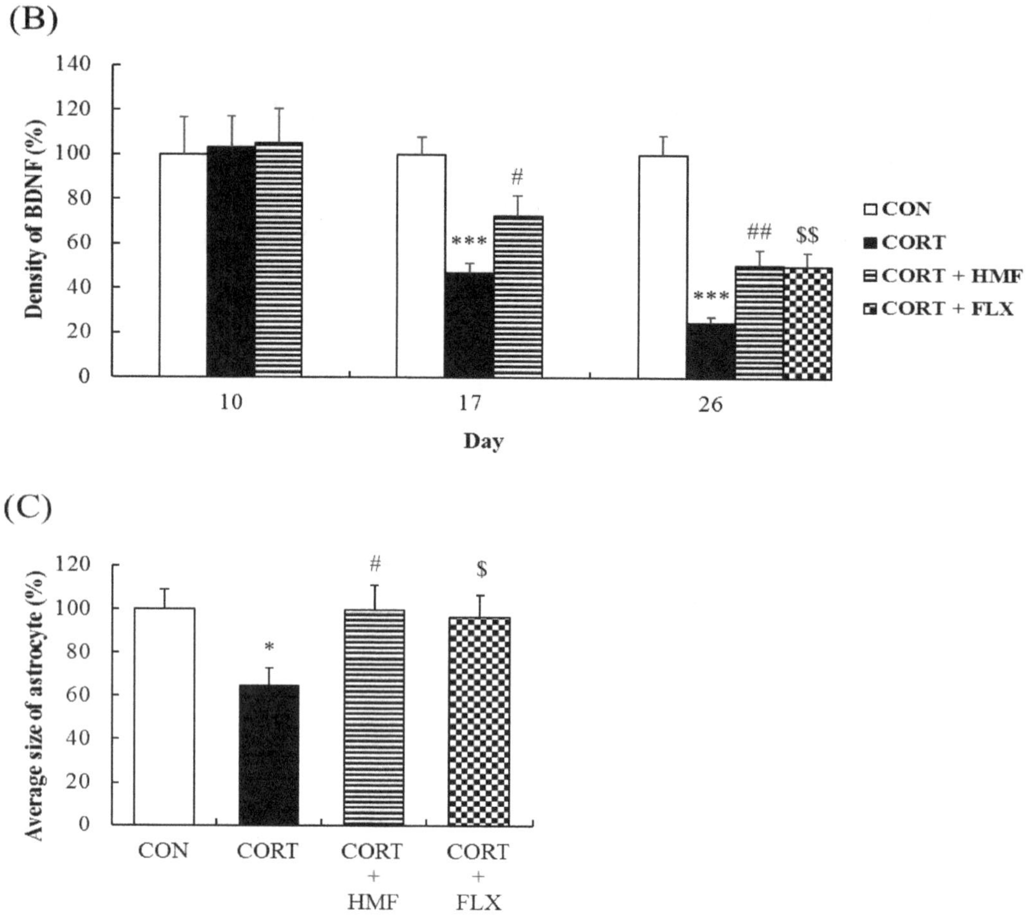

Figure 4. Effects of HMF on the expression of BDNF and GFAP immunoreactivity in the corticosterone-induced depressive mouse hippocampus. (A) Sagittal sections on Day 26 after continuous corticosterone injections were stained with specific antibodies, either anti-BDNF (green; a, b, c, d, e) or anti-GFAP with DAPI staining (red and blue, respectively; f, g, h, i, j). Each signal was merged in k, l, m, n and o, respectively. White squares in the CON group showed a typical astrocyte expressing BDNF, and each high-power magnification picture was shown as e, j, and o. The white and the pink scale bar show 50 μm and 25 μm, respectively. The location of the captured images in the hippocampus and quantification is shown with a square (0.22 mm^2). (**B**) A quantitative analysis of BDNF-positive signal densities using ImageJ software. Values are means ± SEM (Day 10; $n = 4$, Day 17; $n = 8$, Day 26; $n = 8$–10). Symbols show significant differences between the following conditions: CON *vs.* CORT (*** $p < 0.001$), CORT *vs.* CORT + HMF ($^{\#}$ $p < 0.05$, $^{\#\#}$ $p < 0.01$), and CORT *vs.* CORT + FLX ($^{\$\$}$ $p < 0.01$). A quantitative analysis of the average size (**C**) of GFAP-positive signals on Day 26 using ImageJ software. Values are means ± SEM ($n = 8$–10). Symbols show significant differences between the following conditions: CON *vs.* CORT (* $p < 0.05$), CORT *vs.* CORT + HMF ($^{\#}$ $p < 0.05$), and CORT *vs.* CORT + FLX ($^{\$}$ $p < 0.05$).

Figure 4A also shows that BDNF-positive cells (a, b, c, d) and glial fibrillary acidic protein (GFAP; a marker of activated astrocytes)-positive cells with DAPI staining (f, g, h, i) had nearly merged (k, l, m, n), and also that the size of GFAP-positive cells was markedly smaller in the CORT group (g) than in the CON group (f), CORT + HMF group (h), and CORP + FLX group (i). Figure 4C shows that corticosterone significantly (* $p < 0.05$) reduced the size of GFAP-positive cells and that HMF and FLX significantly ($^{\#}$ $p < 0.05$ and $^{\$}$ $p < 0.05$, respectively) attenuated this decrease. These results indicated that corticosterone inactivated astrocytes, resulting in a decrease in the expression of BDNF.

2.4. Effects of Corticosterone and HMF on Neurogenesis in the Hippocampus

Decreases in hippocampal neurogenesis have been reported in corticosterone-treated rats [19] and chronic stress-loaded rats [20]. Therefore, we herein investigated the effects of HMF on neurogenesis in the subgranular zone of the dentate gyrus in the hippocampus using an anti-doublecortin (DCX) antibody, which recognizes a microtubule-associated protein expressed by neuronal precursor cells, on Days 10, 17, and 26. We defined and manually counted DCX-positive cells, which had more than 10μm diameter, in the hippocampal dentate gyrus. Figure 5A shows representative photographs of the hippocampal dentate gyrus region on Day 26, indicating that the DCX signal was markedly weaker in the CORT group (b) than in the CON group (a), CORT + HMF group (c), and CORT + FLX group (d). Figure 5B shows that the DCX signal was not significantly different among the three groups on Day 10, but was significantly (** $p < 0.01$) weaker in the CORT group on Day 17. It was also significantly (** $p < 0.01$) weaker than that in the CON group on Day 26, while the HMF and FLX treatments significantly attenuated these changes (### $p < 0.001$ and $$ $p < 0.01$, respectively). These results indicated that HMF and FLX attenuated corticosterone-induced reductions in neurogenesis.

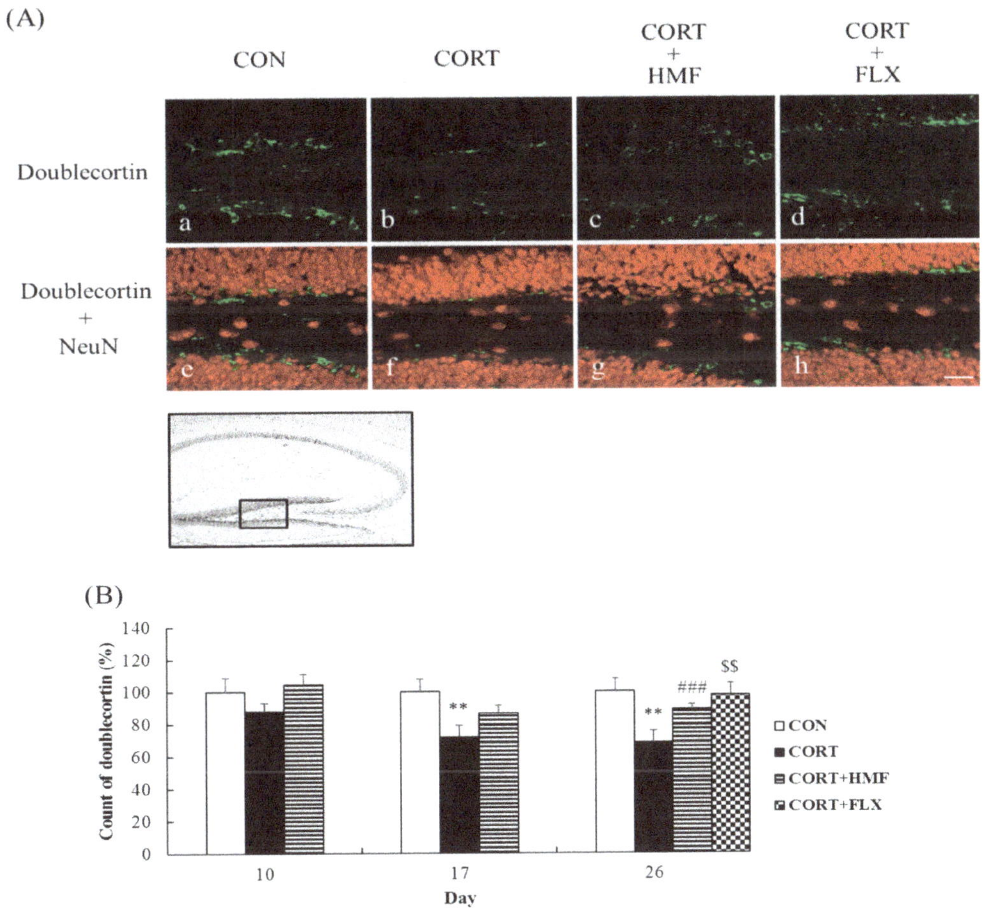

Figure 5. Effects of HMF on the expression of doublecortin immunoreactivity in the corticosterone-induced depressive mouse hippocampal dentate gyrus. (**A**) Sagittal sections on Day 26 after continuous corticosterone injections were stained with specific antibodies, either anti-doublecortin (green; a, b, c, d) or anti-NeuN (red; e, f, g, h). The scale bar shows 50 μm. The location of the captured images in the hippocampus is shown with a square (0.09 mm^2). (**B**) A quantitative analysis of doublecortin-positive cell counts was performed manually. Values are means ± SEM (Day 10; $n = 4$, Day 17; $n = 8$, Day 26; $n = 8$–10). Symbols show significant differences between the following conditions: CON *vs.* CORT (** $p < 0.01$), CORT *vs.* CORT + HMF (### $p < 0.001$), and CORT *vs.* CORT + FLX ($$ $p < 0.01$).

2.5. *Effects of Corticosterone and HMF on the Neuronal Network in the Hippocampus*

We evaluated the effects of corticosterone and HMF on the neuronal network in the hippocampus using experiments with an anti-phosphorylated calcium-calmodulin-dependent protein kinase II (p-CaMK II) antibody. CaMK II is one of the serine/threonine protein kinases, the autophosphorylation of which is known to be important for neuroplasticity [21]. Figure 6A shows representative photographs of the hippocampus on Day 26, indicating that the p-CaMK II signal was markedly weaker in the CORT group (b) than in the CON group (a). Figure 6A also shows that corticosterone-induced reductions in the intensity of the p-CaMK II signal were attenuated in the CORT + HMF group (c) and CORT + FLX group (d). The signal of NeuN, a neuronal marker, was similar among the four groups (e, f, g, h) on Day 26, suggesting that corticosterone did not injure neuronal cells.

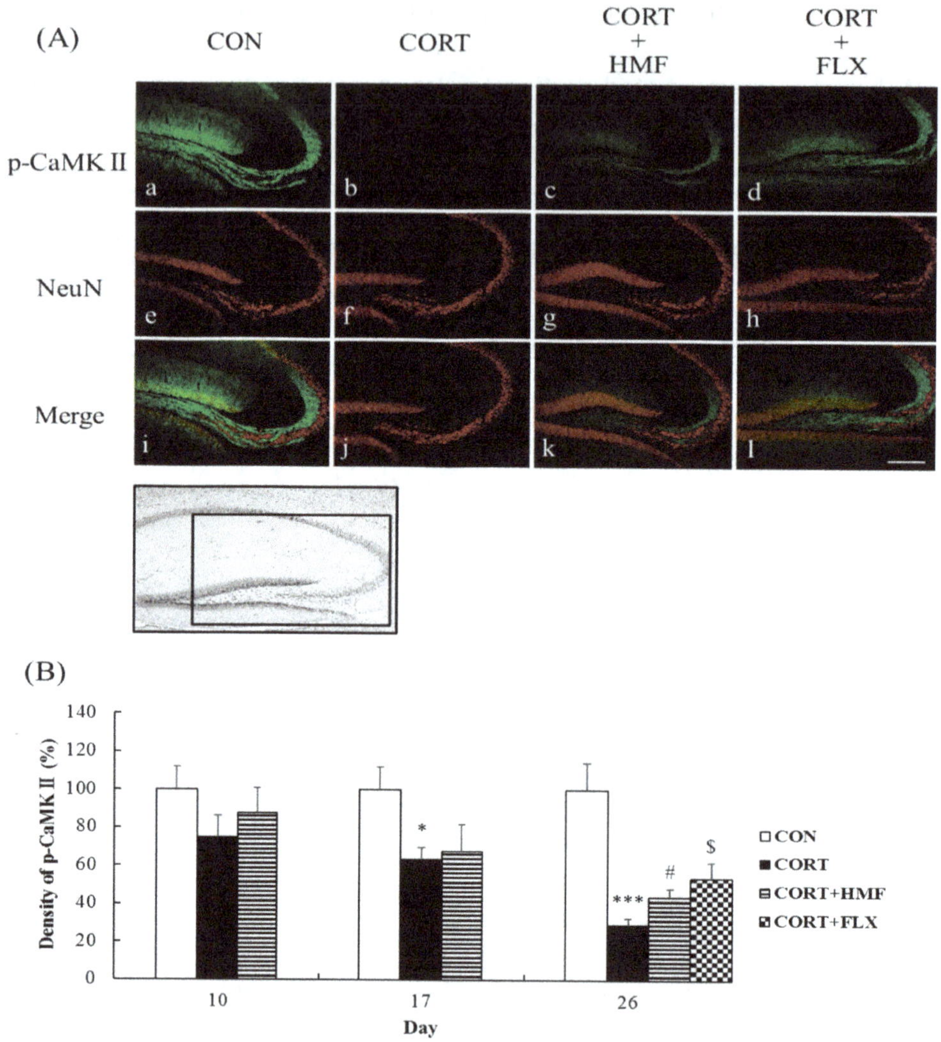

Figure 6. Effects of HMF on the expression of phosphorylated CaMK II and NeuN immunoreactivity in the corticosterone-induced depressive mouse hippocampus. (**A**) Sagittal sections on Day 26 after continuous corticosterone injections were stained with specific antibodies, either anti-phospho-CaMK II (green; a, b, c, d) or anti-NeuN (red; e, f, g, h). Each signal was merged in i, j, k and l, respectively. The scale bar shows 200 μm. The location of the captured images in the hippocampus and quantification is shown with a square (1.0 mm^2). (**B**) A quantitative analysis of phospho-CaMK II-positive signal density using ImageJ software. Values are means ± SEM (Day 10; $n = 4$, Day 17; $n = 8$, Day 26; $n = 8$–10). Symbols show significant differences between the following conditions: CON *vs.* CORT (* $p < 0.05$, *** $p < 0.001$), CORT *vs.* CORT + HMF ($^{\#}$ $p < 0.05$), and CORT *vs.* CORT + FLX ($^{\$}$ $p < 0.05$).

Figure 6B shows that the p-CaMK II signal was not significantly different among the three groups on Day 10, but was significantly (* $p < 0.05$) weaker in the CORT group on Day 17 (63.2% ± 6.2% of CON group). On Day 26, the p-CaMK II signal was significantly (*** $p < 0.001$) weaker in the CORT group than in the CON group, and this change was attenuated by the HMF and FLX treatments ($^{\#}$ $p < 0.05$ and $^{\$}$ $p < 0.05$, respectively).

2.6. Effects of Corticosterone and HMF on ERK1/2-Phosphorylation in the Hippocampus

ERK1/2 has been implicated in the depression-like symptoms elicited by stress-related insults [22,23]. We previously reported that HMF activates (phosphorylates) ERK1/2 in cortical neurons *in vitro* [24] and in the hippocampus *in vivo* [9], while corticosterone decreases the level of phosphorylated ERK1/2 (p-ERK1/2) [11]. Therefore, we herein investigated the effects of HMF on the activation of ERK1/2 in corticosterone-treated brains using a western blot analysis. The band intensity of p-ERK1/2 was not influenced by corticosterone or HMF on Day 10 (Figure 7A), whereas that in the CORT group significantly (** $p < 0.01$) reduced on Day 17 and the HMF treatment slightly restored phosphorylation levels (Figure 7B). These results suggested that HMF attenuated corticosterone-induced decreases in the activation of ERK1/2.

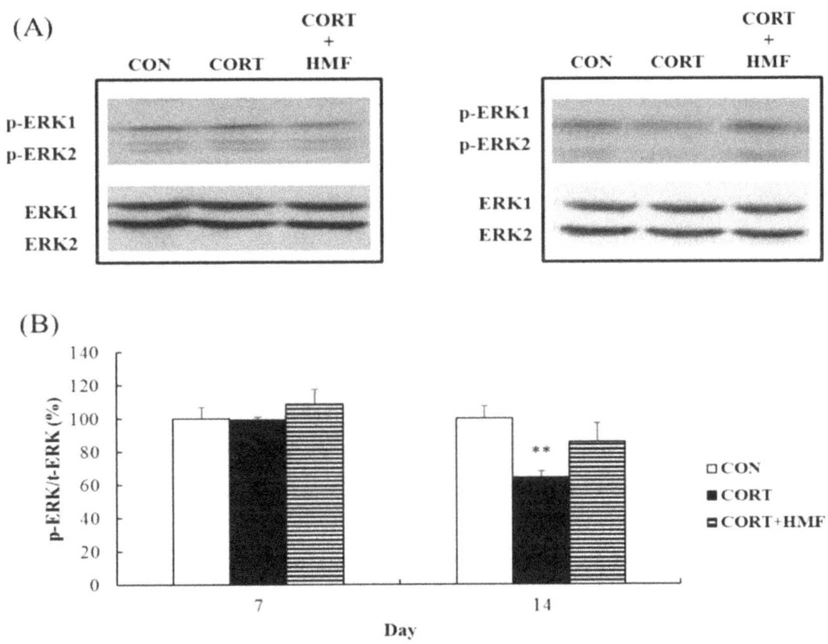

Figure 7. A Western blot analysis of the influence of HMF on the expression of phosphorylated ERK in the corticosterone-induced depressive mouse hippocampus. (**A**) Representative band patterns of p-ERK1/2 and ERK1/2. (**B**) A quantitative analysis of the p-ERK/ERK ratio using ImageJ software. Values are means ± SEM (Day 10; $n = 4$, Day 17; $n = 5$). Symbols show significant differences between the following conditions: CON *vs.* CORT (** $p < 0.01$).

3. Discussion

Several theories exist for the basis of depression. The monoamine hypothesis of depression suggests that mood disorders including depression are caused by an imbalance in monoamines, particularly serotonin, in the brain, and this imbalance may be corrected by the administration of anti-depressant drugs [25]. On the other hand, the neurotrophin hypothesis of depression suggests that a decrease in neurotrophins, particularly BDNF, is an important cause of depression, and that anti-depressant drugs exert their effects by increasing BDNF levels [7]. The neuroplastic hypothesis of depression suggests that alterations in the plasticity of neural networks are a relevant factor in mood disorders including depression [26], and FLX restores structural plasticity [27]. The cytokine hypothesis of depression implicates the immune system in the development of depression, and suggests that anti-depressant drugs prevent microembolism-induced changes in inflammation and behavior [28,29].

By focusing on the neurotrophin (BDNF) hypothesis of depression, we herein demonstrated that the HMF treatment attenuated corticosterone-induced reductions in BDNF levels in the hippocampus (Figure 4) as well as corticosterone-induced depression-like symptoms (Figures 2 and 3), suggesting that HMF has potential as an anti-depressant agent. BDNF is the most abundant neurotrophic factor in the brain and plays an important role not only in neural development, survival, and function, but also in neurogenesis and neuroplasticity, both of which are important targets for depressive disorder treatments [30]. Neurogenesis in the hippocampus was previously reported to be suppressed during depression [19,20], and chronic treatments with SSRIs increased the expression of BDNF, proliferation/differentiation of neuronal progenitor cells, and maturation of newborn neurons [31]. We showed that the HMF treatment attenuated corticosterone-induced reductions in the expression of DCX in the hippocampus (Figure 5). Neuroplasticity in the hippocampus is also known to be suppressed during depression [32,33], and anti-depressant drugs induce plastic changes in neuronal connectivity, which gradually lead to improvements in neuronal information processing and mood recovery. In the present study, we demonstrated that the HMF treatment attenuated corticosterone-induced reductions in the expression of p-CaMK II in the hippocampus (Figure 6).

Consistent with previous findings showing that SSRIs activate glial cells, particularly astrocytes [34], we found that the HMF treatment attenuated the corticosterone-induced inactivation of astrocytes in the hippocampus (Figure 4A and C). The results of the immunohistochemical study (Figure 4A) revealed that BDNF-positive cells merged with GFAP-positive cells. Collectively, our results and previous findings showed that HMF and SSRIs enhance neurogenesis and neuroplasticity in the depressive hippocampus via BDNF synthesized by astrocytes, and we are now investigating the mechanisms responsible for the effects of HMF on astrocytes *in vitro*.

Commonly used depressive-like behavioral tests are the forced swim test and tail suspension test, with increases in immobility times reflecting a depressive state. The results of the present study showed that the HMF treatment decreased corticosterone-induced increases in immobility times in the forced swim test, but not in the tail suspension test. In contrast, the FLX treatment decreased immobility times in the tail suspension test, but not in the forced swim test (Figure 3). This inconsistency suggests that HMF attenuates depressive-like behavior through different mechanism(s) to those of FLX.

A previous study that examined postmortem tissues demonstrated that hippocampal volumes were significantly smaller in patients with major depressive disorders [35]. The findings of a neuroimaging study also revealed smaller hippocampal volumes in depressed patients that were attenuated by an anti-depressant treatment [36]. We herein found that the average size of GFAP-positive cells were significantly reduced in the hippocampus in the CORT group, but were attenuated by the HMF treatment (Figure 4). Since 1) the total number, somal volume, and protrusion length of GFAP-positive astrocytes correlate with hippocampal volume [37], and 2) astrocytes contribute to enhancements in neurotrophic support and associated augmentations in synaptic plasticity [38], the HMF treatment may effectively maintain astrocyte function, and this may be followed by the production of BDNF.

On the other hand, ERK1/2, a signal transduction factor for several receptors, was previously reported to contribute to depression. The treatment of mice with corticosterone was previously shown to selectively decrease p-ERK1/2 levels in the dentate gyrus, but not in the CA1/CA3 regions; therefore, decreases in the levels of p-ERK1/2 temporally coincided with depressive-like behavioral responses [22]. The phosphorylation level of ERK1/2 may mediate the efficacy of anti-depressant drugs in depressed humans and animal models of depression [23]. We herein showed that the HMF treatment attenuated corticosterone-induced reductions in p-ERK1/2 levels in the hippocampus (Figure 7).

The results of the present study suggest the potential of HMF as a novel anti-depressant drug based on the "BDNF hypothesis of depression".

4. Materials and Methods

4.1. Animals

Male C57BL/6 strain mice (seven weeks old) were purchased from Japan SLC, Inc. (Hamamatsu, Shizuoka, Japan). Stock diets and tap water were freely available during the experimental period. Mice were kept at 23 ± 1 °C on a 12-h light/dark cycle (lights on 8:00–20:00). All animal experiments were carried out in accordance with the Guidelines for Animal Experimentation and approved by the Animal Care and Use Committee of Matsuyama University. Mice were divided into 10 experimental groups, and each group contained 5–8 mice.

4.2. Administration of Corticosterone and Test Drugs

Mice in the seven groups were subcutaneously (s.c.) administered corticosterone (Wako Pure Chemical Industries, Ltd., Osaka, Japan) at a dose of 20 mg/kg/day in a volume of 5 mL/kg once a day. The administration periods used were 9 days for two groups, 16 days for another two groups, and 25 days for the last three groups. The remaining three groups were administered vehicle (DMSO/polyethylene glycol (PEG)-300 (3:7) solution). The administration periods used were 9 days, 16 days, and 25 days for each group.

HMF was prepared from orange oil (Wako Pure Chemical Industries, Ltd., Osaka, Japan) as described previously [24]. FLX was purchased from LKT Laboratories, Inc. (St. Paul, MN, USA). Both chemicals were dissolved in DMSO/PEG-300 (3:7) solution. In the corticosterone plus HMF-treated group (CORT + HMF group) or corticosterone plus FLX-treated group (CORT + FLX group), HMF (50 mg/kg/day) or FLX (10 mg/kg/day) was s.c. administered simultaneously with corticosterone for 9, 16, or 25 days. The control group (CON group) and corticosterone-treated group (CORT group) were s.c. administered the same volume of vehicle (DMSO/PEG-300 solution).

4.3. Forced Swim Test

On Day 22, 30 min after the administration of corticosterone/test drugs, mice were subjected to the forced swim test with a minor modification to the methods described by Porsolt [39]. Mice were individually placed in the center of a plastic cylinder (10 (Φ) × 25 (H) cm) filled with water (up to 15 cm in height) at an ambient temperature, and allowed to swim freely for 6 min. Immobility times were manually counted during the last 4 min. Mice were judged to be immobile when only making small movements necessary, namely, moving their limbs subtly, in order to keep their heads above the water and also when floating.

4.4. Tail Suspension Test

On Day 23, mice were subjected to the tail suspension test according to previously described methods [40] 30 min after the administration of corticosterone/test drugs. Mice were individually suspended 10 cm above a tabletop with a peg positioned 2 cm from the tip of the tail for 6 min, and immobility times were manually counted in the last 4 min. Mice were judged to be immobile when they hung passively and completely motionless.

4.5. Immunofluorescence for Confocal Microscopy

Mice were transcardially perfused with ice-cold phosphate buffered-saline (PBS) 1 day after the final administration of samples (Day 10, 17, or 26), and their brains were used in immunohistochemical and biochemical analyses. In the immunohistochemical analysis, brains were postfixed as previously described [41], and sagittal sections at 30 μm were incubated with the following primary antibodies; mouse anti-GFAP (1:200; Sigma-Aldrich, St. Louis, MO, USA), rabbit anti-BDNF (dilution 1:150; Epitomics, Burlingame, CA, USA), mouse anti-NeuN (1:300; Millipore, Billerica, MA, USA), rabbit anti-phospho CaMK II (p-Thr286, 1:500; Sigma-Aldrich), and goat anti-DCX (1:50; Santa Cruz

Biotechnology, Santa Cruz, CA, USA). As secondary antibodies, Alexa Fluor 488 goat anti-rabbit IgG (H + L) (1:300; Invitrogen, Carlsbad, CA, USA), Alexa Fluor 488 donkey anti-goat IgG (H + L) (1:300), Alexa Fluor 568 goat anti-rabbit IgG (H + L) (1:300), and Alexa Fluor 568 goat anti-mouse IgG (H + L) (1:300) were used. A mounting medium with DAPI was employed (Vectashield; Vector Laboratories, Burlingame, CA, USA), and images were captured with a confocal fluorescence microscopy system (LSM510; Zeiss, Oberkochen, Germany). ImageJ software (NIH, Bethesda, Rockville, MD, USA) was used for the quantification of fluorescence signals for BDNF and phospho-CaMK II in images as described previously [8]. The fluorescence signals of doublecortin-positive cells were manually counted with a confocal fluorescence microscopy system. The location of the captured images and quantification is shown with a square in each figure.

4.6. Western Blot Analysis

Hippocampal regions after perfusion were weighed and homogenized in 10 volumes of RIPA buffer (20 mM Tris-HCl, pH 7.5, 0.1% SDS, 150 mM NaCl, 1% NP-40, 1% sodium deoxycholate, 2 mM EDTA, and a protease inhibitor cocktail (Roche, Mannheim, Germany)). Lysates were then centrifuged at 20,000× g at 4 °C for 30 min, and supernatant solutions were collected as the protein extract. SDS-polyacrylamide gel electrophoresis was used to separate equal amounts of protein (20 µg), which were then electroblotted onto an Immuno-Blot^{TM} PVDF Membrane (Bio-Rad, Hercules, CA, USA) as previously described [9]. The primary antibodies used were rabbit antibodies against 44/42 ERK1/2 (Millipore), which recognize 44-kDa ERK1 and 42-kDa ERK2, and phospho-44/42 MAPK (Thr202/Tyr204; Cell Signaling, Woburn, MA, USA), which recognize phosphorylated ERK1 and ERK2. The secondary antibody was horseradish peroxidase-linked anti-rabbit IgG (Cell Signaling). Immunoreactive bands were visualized by ECL-prime (GE Healthcare, Chalfont St. Giles, UK), and band intensities were measured using a LAS-3000 imaging system (Fujifilm, Tokyo, Japan).

4.7. Statistical Analysis

Data for individual groups were expressed as means ± SEM. Data were analyzed using an unpaired t-test, and a value of $p < 0.05$ was considered significant.

5. Conclusions

HMF attenuated corticosterone-induced body weight loss, corticosterone-induced depressive-like behavior, the corticosterone-induced down-regulation of BDNF and GFAP, and corticosterone-induced reductions in the expression of DCX, p-CaMK II, and ERK1/2 in the hippocampus. These results suggest that HMF enhances the production of BDNF in the hippocampus, resulting in the attenuation of corticosterone-induced depression through enhancements in the production of BDNF.

Acknowledgments: The Research Promotion Fund of Ehime Industrial Promotion Foundation supported this work.

Author Contributions: A.S., S.O. and Y.F. conceived and designed the experiments; A.S., S.O., K.Y., Y.A., M.Y., and M.N. performed the experiments; A.S., S.O. and Y.F. wrote the paper.

References

1. Charney, D.S.; Manji, H.K. Life stress, genes, and depression: Multiple pathways lead to increased risk and new opportunities for intervention. *Sci. STKE* **2004**, *225*, re5. [CrossRef] [PubMed]
2. Pariante, C.M.; Lightman, S.L. The HPA axis in major depression: Classical theories and new developments. *Trends Neurosci.* **2008**, *31*, 464–468. [CrossRef] [PubMed]
3. Dinan, T.G. Glucocorticoids and the genesis of depressive illness. A psychobiological model. *Br. J. Psychiatry* **1994**, *164*, 365–371. [CrossRef] [PubMed]

4. Duman, R.; Monteggia, I. A neurotrophic model for stress-related mood disorders. *Biol. Psychiatry* **2006**, *59*, 1116–1127. [CrossRef] [PubMed]
5. Ye, Y.; Wang, G.; Wang, H.; Wang, X. Brain-derived neurotrophic factor (BDNF) infusion restored astrocytic plasticity in the hippocampus of a rat model of depression. *Neurosci. Lett.* **2011**, *503*, 15–19. [CrossRef] [PubMed]
6. Paizanis, E.; Hamon, M.; Lanfumey, L. Hippocampal neurogenesis, depressive disorders, and antidepressant therapy. *Neural Plast.* **2007**, *2007*. [CrossRef] [PubMed]
7. Martinowich, K.; Manji, H.; Lu, B. New insights into BDNF function in depression and anxiety. *Nat. Neurosci.* **2007**, *10*, 1089–1093. [CrossRef] [PubMed]
8. Okuyama, S.; Morita, M.; Miyoshi, K.; Nishigawa, Y.; Kaji, M.; Sawamoto, A.; Terugo, T.; Toyoda, N.; Makihata, N.; Amakura, Y.; *et al.* 3,5,6,7,8,3′,4′-Heptamethoxyflavone, a citrus flavonoid, on protection against memory impairment and neuronal cell death in a global cerebral ischemia mouse model. *Neurochem. Int.* **2014**, *70*, 30–38. [CrossRef] [PubMed]
9. Okuyama, S.; Shimada, N.; Kaji, M.; Morita, M.; Miyoshi, K.; Minami, S.; Amakura, Y.; Yoshimura, M.; Yoshida, T.; Watanabe, S.; *et al.* Heptamethoxyflavone, a citrus flavonoid, enhances brain-derived neurotrophic factor production and neurogenesis in the hippocampus following cerebral global ischemia in mice. *Neurosci. Lett.* **2012**, *528*, 190–195. [CrossRef] [PubMed]
10. Antonijevic, I.A.; Steiger, A. Depression-like change of the sleep-EEG during high dose corticosteroid treatment in patients with multiple sclerosis. *Psychoneuroendocrinology* **2003**, *28*, 780–795. [CrossRef]
11. Shibata, S.; Iinuma, M.; Soumiya, H.; Fukumitsu, H.; Furukawa, Y.; Furukawa, S. A novel 2-decenoic acid thioester ameliorates corticosterone-induced depression- and anxiety-like behaviors and normalizes reduced hippocampal signal transduction in treated mice. *Pharmacol. Res. Perspect.* **2015**, *3*, e00132. [CrossRef] [PubMed]
12. Jacobsen, J.P.; Mørk, A. Chronic corticosterone decreases brain-derived neurotrophic factor (BDNF) mRNA and protein in the hippocampus, but not in the frontal cortex, of the rat. *Brain Res.* **2006**, *1110*, 221–225. [CrossRef] [PubMed]
13. Dwivedi, Y.; Rizavi, H.S.; Pandey, G.N. Antidepressants reverse corticosterone-mediated decrease in brain-derived neurotrophic factor expression: Differential regulation of specific exons by antidepressants and corticosterone. *Neuroscience* **2006**, *139*, 1017–1029. [CrossRef] [PubMed]
14. Mostert, J.P.; Koch, M.W.; Heerings, M.; Heersema, D.J.; de Keyser, J. Therapeutic potential of fluoxetine in neurological disorders. *CNS Neurosci. Ther.* **2008**, *14*, 153–164. [CrossRef] [PubMed]
15. Shen, J.D.; Ma, L.G.; Hu, C.Y.; Pei, Y.Y.; Jin, S.L.; Fang, X.Y.; Li, Y.C. Berberine up-regulates the BDNF expression in hippocampus and attenuates corticosterone-induced depressive-like behavior in mice. *Neurosci. Lett.* **2016**, *614*, 77–82. [CrossRef] [PubMed]
16. Zhao, Y.; Ma, R.; Shen, J.; Su, H.; Xing, D.; Du, L. A mouse model of depression induced by repeated corticosterone injections. *Eur. J. Pharmacol.* **2008**, *581*, 113–120. [CrossRef] [PubMed]
17. Cryan, J.F.; Valentino, R.J.; Lucki, I. Assessing substrates underlying the behavioral effects of antidepressants using the modified rat forced swimming test. *Neurosci. Biobehav. Rev.* **2005**, *29*, 547–569. [CrossRef] [PubMed]
18. Kimpton, J. The brain derived neurotrophic factor and influences of stress in depression. *Psychiatr. Danub.* **2012**, *24*, 169–171.
19. Mayer, J.L.; Klumpers, L.; Maslam, S.; de Kloet, E.R.; Joëls, M.; Lucassen, P.J. Brief treatment with the glucocorticoid receptor antagonist mifepristone normalises the corticosterone-induced reduction of adult hippocampal neurogenesis. *J. Neuroendocrinol.* **2006**, *18*, 629–631. [CrossRef] [PubMed]
20. Oomen, C.A.; Mayer, J.L.; de Kloet, E.R.; Joëls, M.; Lucassen, P.J. Brief treatment with the glucocorticoid receptor antagonist mifepristone normalizes the reduction in neurogenesis after chronic stress. *Eur. J. Neurosci.* **2007**, *26*, 3395–3401. [CrossRef] [PubMed]
21. Lučić, V.; Greif, G.J.; Kennedy, M.B. Detailed State Model of CaMKII Activation and Autophosphorylation. *Eur. Biophys. J.* **2008**, *38*, 83–98. [CrossRef] [PubMed]
22. Gourley, S.L.; Wu, F.J.; Taylor, J.R. Corticosterone regulates pERK1/2 map kinase in a choronic depression model. *Ann. N. Y. Acad. Sci.* **2008**, *1148*, 509–514. [CrossRef] [PubMed]
23. Gourley, S.L.; Wu, F.J.; Kiraly, D.D.; Ploski, J.E.; Kedves, A.T.; Duman, R.S.; Taylor, J.R. Regionally specific regulation of ERK MAP kinase in a model of antidepressant-sensitive chronic depression. *Biol. Psychiatry* **2008**, *63*, 353–359. [CrossRef] [PubMed]

24. Furukawa, Y.; Okuyama, S.; Amakura, Y.; Watanabe, S.; Fukata, T.; Nakajima, M.; Yoshimura, M.; Yoshida, T. Isolation and characterization of activators of ERK/MAPK from citrus plants. *Int. J. Mol. Sci.* **2012**, *13*, 1832–1845. [CrossRef] [PubMed]
25. Cryan, J.F.; Mombereau, C. In search of a depressed mouse: Utility of models for studying depression-related behavior in genetically modified mice. *Mol. Psychiatry* **2004**, *9*, 326–357. [CrossRef] [PubMed]
26. Castrén, E. Is mood chemistry? *Nat. Rev. Neurosci.* **2005**, *6*, 241–246. [CrossRef] [PubMed]
27. Maya Vetencourt, J.F.; Sale, A.; Viegi, A.; Baroncelli, L.; De Pasquale, R.; O'Leary, O.F.; Castrén, E.; Maffei, L. The antidepressant fluoxetine restores plasticity in the adult visual cortex. *Science* **2008**, *320*, 385–388. [CrossRef] [PubMed]
28. Haase, J.; Brown, E. Integrating the monoamine, neurotrophin and cytokine hypotheses of depression–a central role for the serotonin transporter? *Pharmacol. Ther.* **2015**, *147*. [CrossRef] [PubMed]
29. Nemeth, C.L.; Miller, A.H.; Tansey, M.G.; Neigh, G.N. Inflammatory mechanisms contribute to microembolism-induced anxiety-like and depressive-like behaviors. *Behav. Brain Res.* **2016**, *303*, 160–167. [CrossRef] [PubMed]
30. Pittenger, C.; Duman, R.S. Stress, depression, and neuroplasticity: A convergence of mechanisms. *Neuropsychopharmacology* **2008**, *33*, 88–109. [CrossRef] [PubMed]
31. Sairanen, M.; Lucas, G.; Ernfors, P.; Castrén, M.; Castrén, E. Brain-derived neurotrophic factor and antidepressant drugs have different but coordinated effects on neuronal turnover, proliferation, and survival in the adult dentate gyrus. *J. Neurosci.* **2005**, *25*, 1089–1094. [CrossRef] [PubMed]
32. Djordjevic, A.; Djordjevic, J.; Elaković, I.; Adzic, M.; Matić, G.; Radojcic, M.B. Effects of fluoxetine on plasticity and apoptosis evoked by chronic stress in rat prefrontal cortex. *Eur. J. Pharmacol.* **2012**, *693*, 37–44. [CrossRef] [PubMed]
33. Freitas, A.E.; Machado, D.G.; Budni, J.; Neis, V.B.; Balen, G.O.; Lopes, M.W.; de Souza, L.F.; Dafre, A.L.; Leal, R.B.; Rodrigues, A.L. Fluoxetine modulates hippocampal cell signaling pathways implicated in neuroplasticity in olfactory bulbectomized mice. *Behav. Brain Res.* **2013**, *237*, 176–184. [CrossRef] [PubMed]
34. Czéh, B; di Benedetto, B. Antidepressants act directly on astrocytes: Evidences and functional consequences. *Eur. Neuropsychopharmacol.* **2013**, *23*, 171–185.
35. Cobb, J.A.; Simpson, J.; Mahajan, G.J.; Overholser, J.C.; Jurjus, G.J.; Dieter, L.; Herbst, N.; May, W.; Rajkowska, G.; Stockmeier, C.A. Hippocampal volume and total cell numbers in major depressive disorder. *J. Psychiatr. Res.* **2013**, *47*, 299–306. [CrossRef] [PubMed]
36. Sheline, Y.I.; Gado, M.H.; Kraemer, H.C. Untreated depression and hippocampal volume loss. *Am. J. Psychiatry* **2003**, *160*, 1516–1518. [CrossRef] [PubMed]
37. Zhang, H.; Zhao, Y.; Wang, Z. Chronic corticosterone exposure reduces hippocampal astrocyte structural plasticity and induces hippocampal atrophy in mice. *Neurosci. Lett.* **2015**, *592*, 76–81. [CrossRef] [PubMed]
38. Rial, D.; Lemos, C.; Pinheiro, H.; Duarte, J.M.; Gonçalves, F.Q.; Real, J.I.; Prediger, R.D.; Gonçalves, N.; Gomes, C.A.; Canas, P.M.; *et al.* Depression as a Glial-Based Synaptic Dysfunction. *Front. Cell. Neurosci.* **2016**, *9*. [CrossRef] [PubMed]
39. Porsolt, R.D.; Bertin, A.; Jalfre, M. Behavioral despair in mice: A primary screening test for antidepressants. *Arch. Int. Pharmacodyn.* **1997**, *229*, 327–336.
40. Steru, L.; Chermat, R.; Thierry, B.; Simon, P. The tail suspension test: A new method for screening antidepressants in mice. *Psychopharmacology* **1985**, *85*, 367–370. [CrossRef] [PubMed]
41. Sato, S.; Xu, J.; Okuyama, S.; Martinez, L.B.; Walsh, S.M.; Jacobsen, M.T.; Swan, R.J.; Schlautman, J.D.; Ciborowski, P.; Ikezu, T. Spatial learning impairment, enhanced CDK5/p35 activity, and downregulation of NMDA receptor expression in transgenic mice expressing tau-tubulin kinase 1. *J. Neurosci.* **2008**, *28*, 14511–14521. [CrossRef] [PubMed]

9

The Anticonvulsant Activity of a Flavonoid-Rich Extract from Orange Juice Involves both NMDA and GABA-Benzodiazepine Receptor Complexes

Rita Citraro [1], Michele Navarra [2,*], Antonio Leo [1], Eugenio Donato Di Paola [1], Ermenegildo Santangelo [1], Pellegrino Lippiello [3], Rossana Aiello [1], Emilio Russo [1] and Giovambattista De Sarro [1]

1 Department of Science of Health, School of Medicine and Surgery, University of Catanzaro, Catanzaro I-88100, Italy; citraro@unicz.it (R.C.); aleo@unicz.it (A.L.); donatodipaola@unicz.it (E.D.D.P.); santangelo@unicz.it (E.S.); aiellorossana@gmail.com (R.A.); erusso@unicz.it (E.R.); desarro@unicz.it (G.D.S.)
2 Department of Chemical, Biological, Pharmaceutical and Environmental Sciences, University of Messina, Messina I-98168, Italy
3 Department of Pharmacy, University of Naples Federico II, Naples I-80131, Italy; plippiello@gmail.com
* Correspondence: mnavarra@unime.it

Academic Editor: Derek J. McPhee

Abstract: The usage of dietary supplements and other natural products to treat neurological diseases has been growing over time, and accumulating evidence suggests that flavonoids possess anticonvulsant properties. The aim of this study was to examine the effects of a flavonoid-rich extract from orange juice (OJe) in some rodent models of epilepsy and to explore its possible mechanism of action. The genetically audiogenic seizures (AGS)-susceptible DBA/2 mouse, the pentylenetetrazole (PTZ)-induced seizures in ICR-CD1 mice and the WAG/Rij rat as a genetic model of absence epilepsy with comorbidity of depression were used. Our results demonstrate that OJe was able to exert anticonvulsant effects on AGS-sensible DBA/2 mice and to inhibit PTZ-induced tonic seizures, increasing their latency. Conversely, it did not have anti-absence effects on WAG/Rij rats. Our experimental findings suggest that the anti-convulsant effects of OJe are likely mediated by both an inhibition of NMDA receptors at the glycine-binding site and an agonistic activity on benzodiazepine-binding site at $GABA_A$ receptors. This study provides evidences for the antiepileptic activity of OJe, and its results could be used as scientific basis for further researches aimed to develop novel complementary therapy for the treatment of epilepsy in a context of a multitarget pharmacological strategy.

Keywords: orange; *Citrus sinensis*; flavonoids; audiogenic seizures; absence epilepsy; spike-wave discharges; natural products; complementary and alternative medicines; orange juice

---

1. Introduction

Epilepsy is one of the most common serious neurological disorders encountered in clinical practice. It is known that both GABA and glutamate receptors may play an important role in seizure initiation, maintenance and arrest [1]. Moreover, excessive activation of excitatory amino-acid receptors determines the generation of reactive oxygen (ROS) and reactive nitrogen (RNS) species that in turn can provoke seizure genesis and related cell death [2,3]. Thus, intervention with antioxidants could be a potential beneficial approach in the treatment of epilepsy [4]. Previous studies have suggested a protective role of antioxidants, such as ascorbic acid, vitamin E, α-tocopherol, curcumin, *trans*-resveratrol, melatonin and α-lipoic acid against seizures induced by different convulsive agents [5–7].

It is well known that flavonoids, plant secondary metabolites commonly found in the fruits and vegetables regularly consumed by humans, exert a broad spectrum of biological activities by both interaction with specific molecular targets and their antioxidant properties. Moreover, it is known that flavonoids are biologically active molecules in the central nervous system (CNS) [8] and that may act as ligands for benzodiazepine receptors [9]. Tea, as well as *Citrus* fruits and their juices, are the main food sources of flavonoids [10]. The health properties of *Citrus* flavonoids have been extensively studied, especially as regards their anticancer, cardiovascular and anti-inflammatory activity [11], however, to the best of our knowledge, the anticonvulsant potential of *Citrus* juices has not been investigated.

Citrus sinensis var. Tarocco, commonly known as "half-blood" orange is native to Italy and mainly cultivated in eastern Sicily. Its health properties have long been studied and were recently reviewed by Grosso et al. [12]. Very recently we studied the antioxidant activity of a flavonoid-rich extract from half-blood orange juice (OJe), demonstrating its capability to: (i) reduce the levels of both reactive oxygen species and membrane lipid peroxidation; (ii) improve mitochondrial functionality and (iii) prevent DNA-oxidative damage in A549 cells incubated with H_2O_2 [13]. We have also shown the chelating property of OJe and its ability to induce the antioxidant catalase, thus blocking iron oxidative-induced injury [14].

Based on this background, we have evaluated the potential anticonvulsant effects of an OJe on some animal models of seizures and epilepsy, investigating on its possible mechanism of action. Since hesperidin (HES) and narirutin (NRTN) were the flavonoids present in highest amounts in our extract, some anticonvulsant effects were also evaluated after their administration.

2. Results

2.1. OJe HES Mitigates Pentylenetetrazole (PTZ)-Induced Seizures

Following PTZ administration, all animals in the control group underwent both clonic and tonic seizures, and 75% died within 30 min (Table 1).

Administering OJe (40 mg/kg i.p.) 30 min before PTZ significantly ($p < 0.01$) induced an increase of latency (Table 2) and significantly suppressed tonic but not clonic seizures (Table 1A). Eighty mg/kg OJe significantly rise latency of tonus ($p < 0.05$), but not reduces the incidence of seizure phase (Table 1). On the contrary, both the dosage of 100 and 120 mg/kg significantly decrease the incidence of both clonus and tonus seizures ($p < 0.01$; Table 1A). Similarly, latency to both tonus and death episodes were significantly enhanced by OJe at the doses of 40, 80, 100 and 120 mg/kg (Table 2). Conversely, nor OJe at the dosage of 20 mg/kg neither HES or NRTN (40 and 80 mg/kg) significantly affected the incidence of seizures (Table 1A,B). Also OJe, HES or NRTN (all at 40 mg/kg concentration) administered 60 or 120 min before PTZ were ineffective. However, 80 mg/kg HES significantly enhanced the latency of tonus seizures and death ($p < 0.05$; Table 2A). Interestingly, oral treatment with both 20 and 40 mg/kg/day OJe for 5 consecutive days significantly ($p < 0.05$) inhibited both tonic seizures and death ($p < 0.05$ and $p < 0.01$, respectively; Table 1B) as well as the higher dose significantly increase their latency ($p < 0.05$; Table 2B). Similarly, oral administration of HES at 80 mg/kg/day concentration for 5 consecutive days significantly reduced the incidence of tonic seizures ($p < 0.01$; Table 1B) and increased their latency ($p < 0.05$; Table 2B), while the dose of 40 mg/kg/day appeared to reduce the incidence of tonic seizures and increase latency without reaching a significant level. On the contrary, NRTN (40 and 80 mg/kg/day) did not exert significant protection against PTZ-induced seizures (Tables 1 and 2).

Table 1. Effects of OJe, HES or NRTN administered by i.p. (**A**) or per os (**B**) on the PTZ-induced seizures in CD1 mice. * $p < 0.05$; ** $p < 0.01$.

A

Treatment (mg/kg; i.p.)		Time(min)	Seizure Phase (%)			Number of Mice
			Clonus	Tonus	Death	
Vehicle	Saline	30	100	100	75	8
OJe	20	30	100	87.5	75	8
	40	30	75	37.5 **	37.5 **	8
	80	30	75	50 *	75	8
	100	30	50 *	25 **	25 **	8
	120	30	25 **	0 **	0 **	8
	40	60	100	75	75	8
	40	120	100	100	100	8
HES	40	30	100	87.5	75	8
	80	30	100	50 *	50 *	8
	100	30	62.5	25 **	25 **	8
	120	30	25 **	12.5 **	0 **	8
	40	60	100	100	87.5	8
	40	120	100	100	87.5	8
NRTN	40	30	100	100	75	8
	80	30	100	75	75	8
	100	30	87.5	50 *	50 *	8
	120	30	62.5	25 **	37.5 **	8
	40	60	100	100	100	8
	40	120	100	100	100	8
HES + NRTN	120 + 120	30	37.5 **	12.5 **	12.5 **	8

B

Treatment (mg/kg; os)		Time (Days)	Seizure Phase (%)			Number of Mice
			Clonus	Tonus	Death	
Vehicle	Saline	5	100	100	100	10
OJe	20	5	100	60 *	40 **	10
	40	5	80	20 **	20 **	10
HES	40	5	100	75	50 *	8
	80	5	90	40 **	30 **	10
NRTN	40	5	100	100	80	10
	80	5	100	100	75	8

Table 2. Effects of OJe, HES or NRTN administered i.p. (**A**) or os (**B**) 30 min before PTZ on latency of clonus, tonus and death (n = 8–10 mice for each group) The latency of clonic, tonic and death episodes were statistically evaluated according to Kruskal-Wallis. * $p < 0.05$.

A

Treatment (mg/kg; i.p.)		Latency (s)		
		Clonus	Tonus	Death
Vehicle	Saline	164 (152–177)	681 (618–750)	706 (586–851)
OJe	20	174 (158–192)	712 (584–868)	776 (645–934)
	40	194 (176–214)	852 (695–1044) *	918 (746–1130) *
	80	211 (192–230)	868 (684–1102) *	909 (684–1208) *
HES	40	176 (156–198)	734 (592–910)	804 (672–962)
	80	184 (160–211.6)	845 (683–1110) *	878 (724–1064.8) *
NRTN	40	168 (150–201)	756 (564–900)	801 (644–966)
	80	179 (155–206.7)	784 (598–1027.8)	834 (696–999.4)

Table 2. *Cont.*

B

Treatment (mg/kg; 5 Days; os)		Latency (s)		
		Clonus	Tonus	Death
Vehicle	Saline	158 (140–178)	664 (598–737)	712 (604–839)
OJe	20	160 (140–180)	670 (494–697)	788 (602–946)
	40	224 (198–253)	928 (715–1204) *	998 (776–1284) *
HES	40	168 (150–201)	756 (564–900)	801 (644–966)
	80	218 (200–248)	899 (709–1198) *	995 (788–1226) *
NRTN	40	155 (146–198)	744 (526–897)	798 (625–978)
	80	196 (150–201)	767 (602–916)	802 (627–974)

2.2. Effects of OJe, HES or NRTN in Audiogenic Seizure Prone DBA/2 Mice

OJe administration at dosage of 20 mg/kg (i.p.) 30 and 60 min before auditory stimulation did not influence the incidence of wild running and clonus of audiogenic seizures in DBA/2 mice. Instead, the administration of OJe at concentration of 40 mg/kg or higher 30 min before auditory stimulation significantly protected against tonus and clonus ($p < 0.01$; Figure 1), that were further reduced by the dosage of 100 and 120 mg/kg ($p < 0.01$).

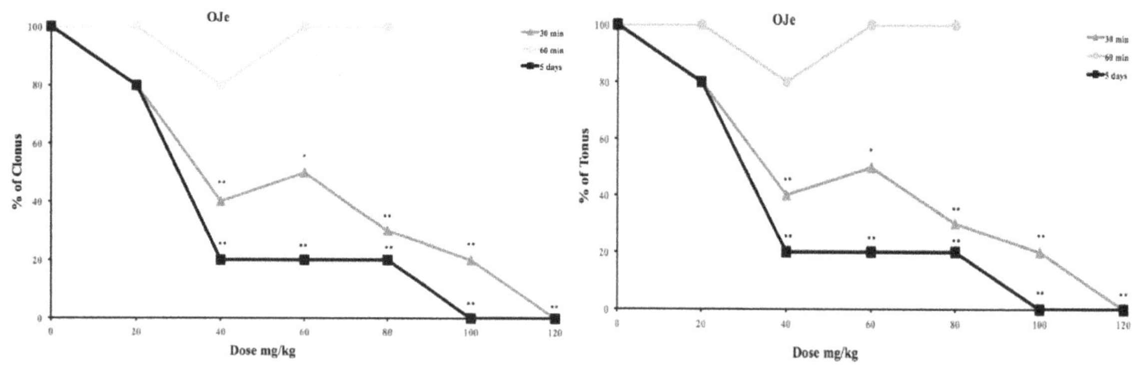

Figure 1. Effects of OJe against clonus and tonus in audiogenic seizure of DBA/2 mice.

Conversely, using the same experimental protocol, the administration of HES (up to 40 mg/kg) or NRTN (up to 60 mg/kg) with did not produce significant anticonvulsant effects against tonus and clonus (data not shown). Only a dose of HES of 120 mg/kg was able to significant protect against the clonic phase of audiogenic seizures, whereas NRTN was unable to protect against clonus at doses up to 120 mg/kg. The ED_{50} values of OJe, HES and NRTN against the tonus and clonus of audiogenic seizures were reported in Table 3.

Table 3. ED_{50} values (±95% confidence limits) of the OJe, HES and NRTN on audiogenic seizures in DBA/2 mice. All data are expressed in mg/kg and were calculated according to the method of Litchfield and Wilcoxon (1949). The significant changes were statistically evaluated according to Lichtfield and Wilcoxon. ** $p < 0.01$.

Treatment	Time (min)	ED_{50} Values	
		Clonus	Tonus
OJe	30	71.89 (56.75–91.08) **	36.34 (25.49–51.82) **
HES	30	112.05 (81.85–153.40)	57.54 (47.33–69.95)
NRTN	30	>120	66.65 (48.49–91.22)

Oral treatment for 5 consecutive days with OJe (20 mg/kg/day) before auditory stimulation did not exert marked anticonvulsant effects against the tonic and clonic phases of audiogenic seizures in DBA/2 mice. Of note, OJe administration at the doses of 40–120 mg/kg/day significantly reduced the incidence of both tonic and clonic seizures ($p < 0.01$; Figure 1 and Table 3). The same treatment with HES produced similar effects, but higher doses were necessary to produce similar antiseizure activity (Table 3), whereas NRTR was the weakest effective.

2.2.1. Interactions between NMDA Antagonists (CPPene, D-Cycloserine, Felbamate) and OJe against Audiogenic Seizures in DBA/2 Mice

CPPene (0.6–4.2 mg/kg; i.p.) produced a dose-dependent protection against tonic and clonic phases of audiogenic seizures in DBA/2 mice when administered 45 min before auditory stimulation (Figure 2A,B) with an ED_{50} of 1.76 mg/kg for clonus and 0.79 mg/kg for tonus (Table 4).

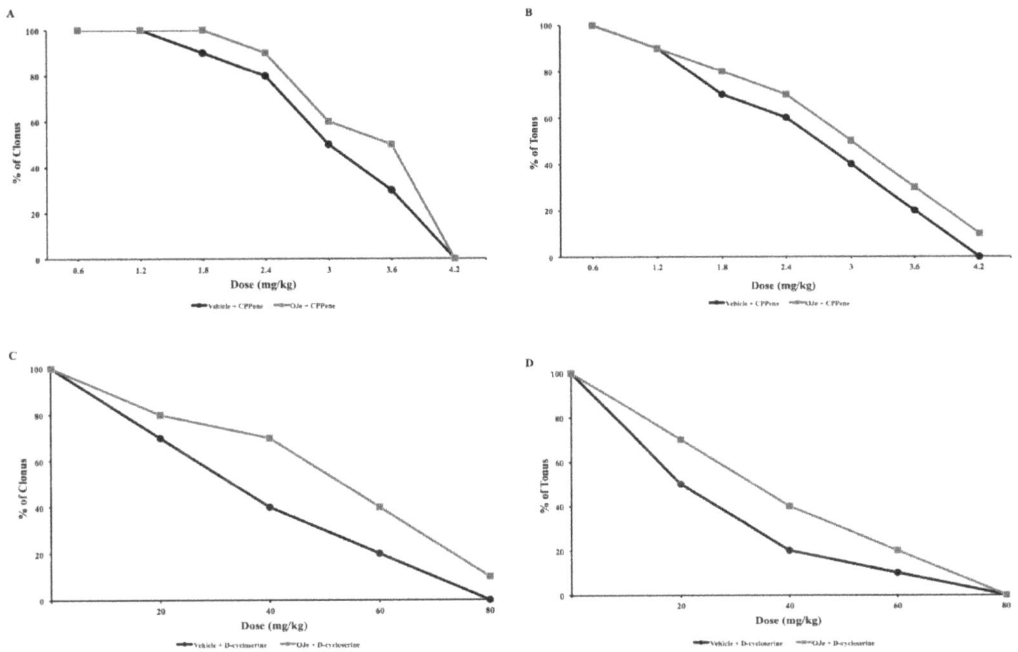

Figure 2. Influence of CPPene or D-cycloserine and their co-administration with OJe on the clonic (**A** and **C**) and the tonic (**B** and **D**) seizures in DBA/2 mice.

Table 4. ED_{50} values (±95% confidence limits) of the OJe co-administrated with NMDA antagonists on audiogenic seizures in DBA/2 mice. All data are expressed in mg/kg and were calculated according to the method of Litchfield and Wilcoxon (1949). The significant changes were statistically evaluated according to Lichtfield and Wilcoxon. * $p < 0.05$; ** $p < 0.01$.

Treatment			ED_{50} Values	
			Clonus	Tonus
CPPene	plus	Saline	1.76 (1.21–2.26)	0.79 (0.44–1.43)
	plus	OJe	2.69 (2.30–3.15) **	2.61 (2.04–3.33) **
D-cycloserine	plus	Saline	27.6 (17.7–43.2)	14.4 (7.8–26.5)
	plus	OJe	58.7 (37.4–92.3) **	28.3 (20.1–39.8) **
Felbamate	plus	Saline	48.8 (35.4–67.2)	23.1 (12.1–44.0)
	plus	OJe	105.6 (64.9–171.7) **	65.9 (38.5–112.8) **
NBQX	plus	Saline	4.9 (3.2–7.5)	2.2 (1.4–3.6)
	plus	OJe	4.1 (2.6–6.49)	2.8 (2.05–3.73)
CFM-2	plus	Saline	10.04 (11.3–13.1)	9.42 (7.34–12.09)
	plus	OJe	15.9 (11.3–22.46) *	10.78 (7.59–15.30)

In another group of experiments, we evaluated anticonvulsant effects of D-cycloserine (DCS), exposing the animals to auditory test. DCS (20–80 mg/kg; i.p.) administered 60 min before auditory testing induced a dose-dependent protection against the clonic and tonic phases of audiogenic seizure response in DBA/2 mice, with an ED_{50} of 27.6 mg/kg for clonus and 14.4 for tonus (Figure 2C,D and Table 4). Felbamate (30–300 mg/kg; i.p.) administered 45 min before auditory stimulation, dose-dependently reduced the severity of the audiogenic seizures in DBA/2 mice (Figure 3A,B). Felbamate antagonized audiogenic seizures with an ED_{50} value of 23.1 mg/kg for tonus and 48.8 mg/kg for clonus (Table 4).

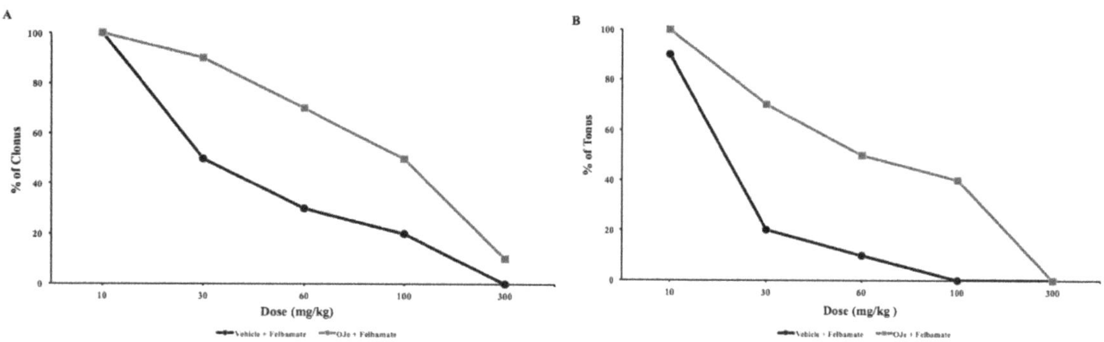

Figure 3. Influence of felbamate in presence or absence of OJe on both clonic (**A**) and tonic (**B**) seizures in DBA/2 mice.

In order to study the possible mechanism of action of OJe, the extract was administered at the not effective dose of 20 mg/kg in combination with DCS, felbamate or CPPene, 30 min before auditory stimulation. As shown in Figures 1 and 2, OJe was able to produce a consistent shift to the right of the dose-response curves of CPPene, DCS and felbamate. Evidence that the maximum shift was observed when OJe was co-administered with felbamate and DCS, suggests that the decrease in anticonvulsant activity by OJe was prevalently mediated at the glycine site of NMDA receptor complex (Figures 2 and 3). Accordingly, ED_{50} values were increased in co-administration protocols (Table 4).

2.2.2. Interaction between NBQX and CFM-2, Two AMPA Receptor Antagonists and OJe

NBQX (5–20 mg/kg; i.p.) administered 30 min before auditory stimulation, was able to suppress the severity of the audiogenic seizures in a dose-dependent manner (Figure 4A,B). Similarly, a pre-treatment of 30 min with CFM-2 (3–50 mg/kg; i.p.) produced a significant dose-dependent protection against tonic and clonic phases of the audiogenic seizures in DBA/2 mice ($p < 0.05$; Figure 4C,D). The ED_{50} values for NBQX and CFM-2 against clonic and tonic seizures are reported in Table 4. Co-administration of OJe (20 mg/kg; i.p.) with the two competitive AMPA receptor antagonist 30 min before auditory stimulation was unable to produce a consistent shift of the dose-response curves for both drugs (Figure 4 and Table 4) The only case of significant increase ($p < 0.05$) of ED_{50} value for clonus was observed when OJe was co-administered with CFM-2.

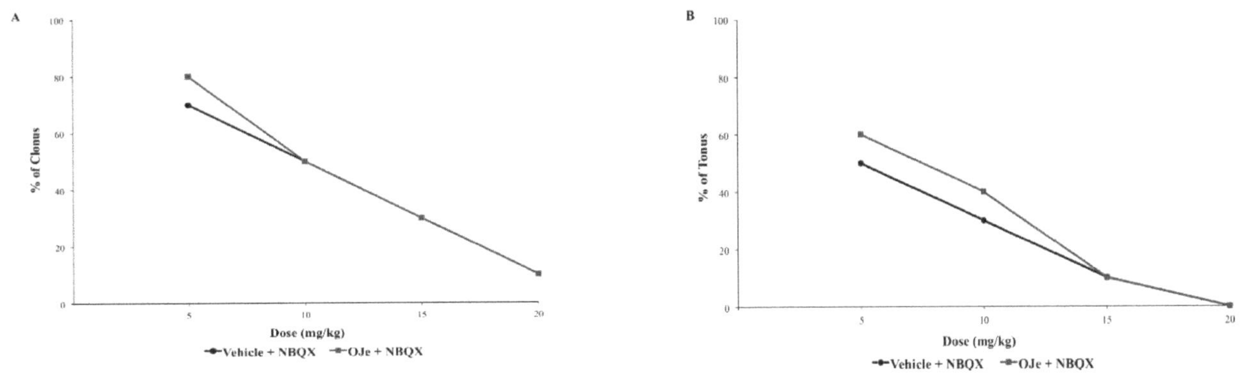

Figure 4. *Cont.*

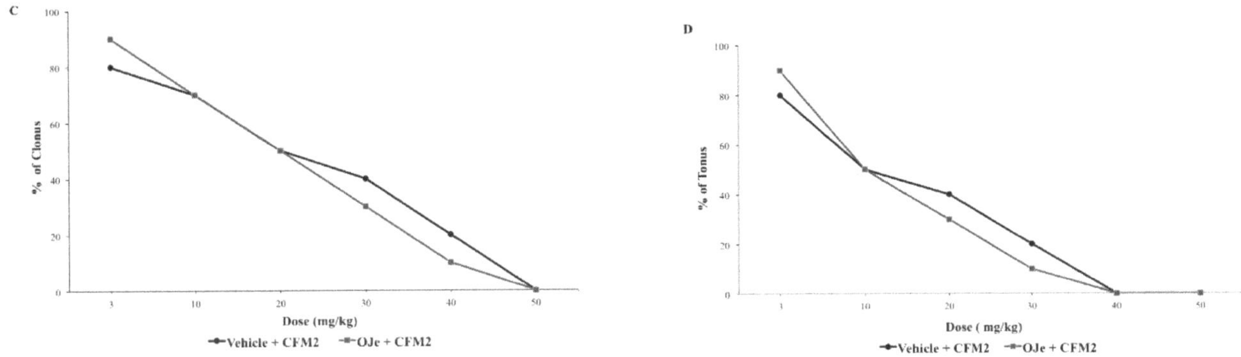

Figure 4. Influence of NBQX or CFM2 and co-administration with OJe on the clonic (**A** and **C**) and the tonic (**B** and **D**) seizures in DBA/2 mice.

2.2.3. Treatment with Flumazenil

To ascertain the possible involvement of GABA-benzodiazepine receptor complex in the antiseizure activity of OJe, the latter was administered 15 min before flumazenil. As shown in Figure 5, the anticonvulsant effect of OJe (40 mg/kg; i.p.) was reduced by a treatment with 2.5 mg/kg flumazenil. Flumazenil administered i.p. 15 min before HES or NRTN antagonized the modest pharmacological effects of these flavonoids (data not shown).

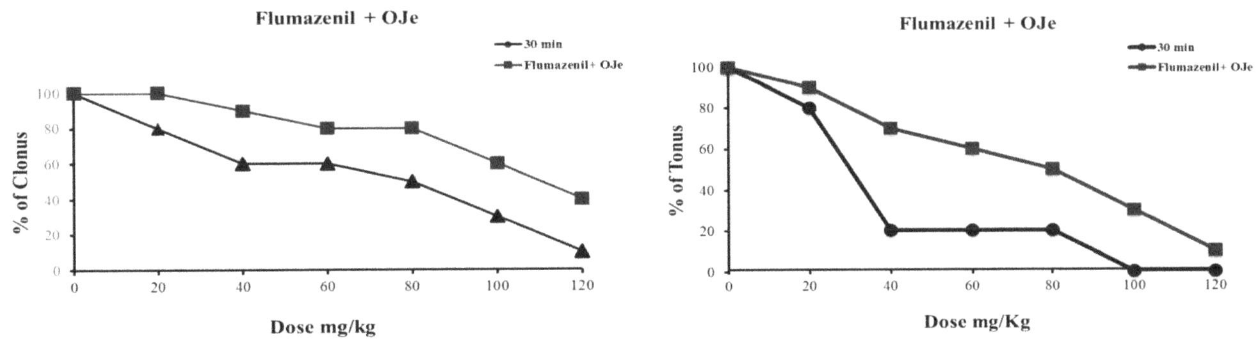

Figure 5. Influence of flumazenil together or not with OJe on both clonic and tonic seizures in DBA/2 mice.

2.3. *Effects of OJe on Absence Seizures in WAG/Rij Rats*

At 6 months of age, all WAG/Rij rats exhibited spontaneously occurring SWDs on EEGs; the mean number of SWDs (nSWDs) for a 30 min epoch was 5.82 $\pm$ 0.84 min seizures with a mean total duration (dSWDs) of 12.23 ± 5.34 s. The i.p. administration of OJe (20 and 40 mg/kg), HSE or NRTN (40 and 80 mg/kg) did not modify the number and duration of SWDs in comparison to control group (data not shown).

3. Discussion

In this study, for the first time, we report the anticonvulsant effects of a flavonoid-rich extract from *Citrus sinensis* juice in some experimental models of epilepsy. Our results support the effects of OJe in the CNS, showing that more than a single mechanism of action might contribute to its anti-seizure properties. The main mechanisms involved in the anticonvulsant activity exerted by OJe seems to be linked to its effects on both $GABA_A$ and NMDA receptors.

It is well known that several natural products widely used in traditional, folk and alternative medicine exert a broad spectrum of biological activities, so many plant extracts are currently used for the prevention or treatment of certain diseases. Very often their pharmacological activity is due to the presence of flavonoids, plant secondary metabolites commonly found in the fruits and vegetables regularly consumed by humans. In this line, we have recently shown the anti-tumor effects of the flavonoid fraction of *Citrus reticulata* (mandarin) juice [15], as well as we demonstrated that the anti-cancer activity of the *Citrus bergamia* (bergamot) juice (BJ) exerted both in vitro [16,17] and in vivo [18] is related to its flavonoids [19]. Interestingly, evidence that a flavonoid-rich extract from bergamot juice (BJe) is able to exert antioxidant and anti-inflammatory activity both in vitro [20,21] and in animal models [22,23] increases the potential of the *Citrus* juice as a tool for pharmacological intervention in some pathologies [24,25]. *Citrus sinensis* var. Tarocco, commonly known as "half-blood" orange is native to Italy and mainly cultivated in eastern Sicily. Its health properties were studied and are recently reviewed by Grosso et al. [12]. The OJe employed in this experimental research has demonstrated antioxidant properties, realized by different complementary routes via scavenging free radicals, chelating metal ions and boosting the cellular antioxidant defense [13,14].

Data from the present study demonstrate the anticonvulsant activity of OJe in PTZ-induced seizures in CD-1 mice and in audiogenic seizures in DBA/2 mice, but not against absence seizures in WAG/Rij rats. However, OJe not always induced a dose-dependent response, and we can't exclude that other effects might appear at higher dosages. Since OJe is a pool of flavonoids, it is likely that more than a single bioactive molecules present in the extract could contribute to the observed effects. Accordingly, hesperidin, the major component of our extract, was found to be effective against PTZ-kindling at dosages (100–200 mg/kg) much higher than the one used in our experiments (about 10 mg/kg) [26]. In addition, OJe appeared more potent and effective than HES and NRTN, suggesting that other components are involved in the antiseizure effects. This was supported by the evidence that a much higher dose of HES or NRTN given alone or in combination is needed to obtain comparable pharmacological results to those observed using the OJe. These findings strengthen the hypothesis that the complex mixtures of phytochemicals present in an extract could be more effective than their individual constituents, enhancing each other's pharmacological activity. Moreover, a phytocomplex has the advantage that the individual active substances are present in a much lower concentration than that would be required to achieve the same effectiveness with a single active principle, with possible impact on the safety of the natural drug. Finally, the presence of numerous molecules that simultaneously can act on different targets and by diverse mechanisms of action may enhance the potential of phytocomplexes in a context of a multitarget pharmacological strategy.

GABA and glutamate are the major neurotransmitters in the brain, and are involved in the pathophysiology of epilepsy [27]. In order to explore the mechanism through which OJe exerts its antiseizure activity, first we used the flumazenil, a benzodiazepine receptor antagonist [28]. Evidence that this drug was able to antagonize most of OJe effects indicate that the *Citrus* extract act as agonist of the GABA-benzodiazepine receptor complex. Also HES and NRTN appears to act in this manner.

The excitatory neurotransmitter glutamate has been implicated in early changes that lead to the initiation of hyperactivity, but also to the amplification and spread of the excitatory hyperactivity acting through two main families of receptors, the ionotropic and metabotropic glutamate receptors [29]. Both types of receptors have been implicated in the etiology of different seizures types [30,31]. In this light, in the DBA/2 mice, a genetic animal model of audiogenic seizures, we have studied OJe activity on glutamate ionotropic receptors by combination of our extract with various antagonists of these receptors. OJe at a concentration of 40 mg/kg administrated 30 min before auditory stimulation possesses anticonvulsant properties in DBA/2 mice with significant protection only against tonus. At least 80 mg/kg were necessary to protect against clonus. Moreover, oral treatment for 5 consecutive days protected DBA/2 mice from sound-induced tonic extension. Then, we have used the not effective dose of 20 mg/kg in combination with glutamate receptor antagonists. It is known that CPPene, felbamate, DCS, NBQX and CFM-2 are effective anticonvulsants in DBA/2 mice [32–34]. Among these drugs, OJe interacted with both DCS and felbamate, which are known to bind at the glycine modulatory site on the NMDA receptor complex [35]. At odds, OJe interacts very slightly with CPPene, acting on the glutamate binding site on the NMDA receptors, and not at all with NBQX or CFM-2, two competitively and non-competitively blockers of AMPA receptors, respectively. These data suggest that the anticonvulsant activity of OJe was also mediated by the interaction with the glycine site of NMDA receptor complex.

Taken together, our results demonstrate that the flavonoid-rich extract from orange juice employed in this study possesses antiepileptic effects in PTZ-induced seizures and in AGS-sensible DBA/2 mice, which are very likely mediated by both the inhibition of NMDA receptors at the glycine-binding site and the agonistic activity on benzodiazepine-binding site at $GABA_A$ receptors. However, other mechanisms of action contributing to the effects exerted by OJe cannot be excluded, and further studies will be necessary to explore the detailed mechanism of OJe action at the CNS.

This study provides evidences for the antiepileptic activity of OJe, and its results could be used as scientific basis for further researches aimed to develop novel complementary therapy for the treatment of epilepsy in a context of a multitarget pharmacological strategy.

4. Materials and Methods

4.1. Animals

Male DBA/2 mice (3 weeks of age), CD-1 mice (6 weeks of age) and WAG/Rij rats (6–7 months old, 250–300 g) were purchased from Harlan Italy Srl (Correzzana, Milan, Italy). Animals were housed in groups under stable conditions of humidity (60% ± 5%) and temperature (21 ± 2 °C), with a reversed light/dark (12/12 h) cycle (light on at 19.00) with free access to standard laboratory chow and tap water until the time of experiments. Procedures involving animals and their care were conducted in conformity with the international and national laws and policies (EU Directive 2010/63/EU for animal experiments, ARRIVE guidelines and the Basel Declaration including the 3R concept). All efforts were made to minimize animal suffering and to use only the number of animals necessary to produce reliable scientific data.

4.2. Drugs

The OJe was provided by the company "Agrumaria Corleone" (Palermo, Italy) that used fruits of *Citrus sinensis* (L.) Osbeck (sweet orange) var. Tarocco coming from crops grown in the south-eastern part of Sicily (Italy). The extract was produced in its liquid form by passing the fresh orange juice through columns equipped with adsorbent resins that retain flavonoids. The latter were then eluted with NaOH and immediately passed through cationic resins, thus obtaining the biomolecules in their acid form. Finally, the extract was collected, filtered, centrifuged, transformed into a powder by spray drying and then stored at −20 °C. Immediately prior to use, it was defrosted, diluted in saline solution until the desired concentration and administered orally by gavage or intraperitoneally, depending on the test. Qualitative and quantitative composition of OJe was previous reported [13]. The flavanones hesperidin and narirutin were the flavonoids present in highest amounts (232 and 90 mg/g, respectively), followed by the flavone *C*-glucosides vicenin-2 and lucenin-2 methyl ether (43 and 22 mg/g of dried extract, respectively). Didymin and nobiletin were the flavanone *O*-glycosides and the polymetoxyflavone present in quite large quantities, respectively (15 mg/g of dried extract for both). Their chemical structures are shown in Figure 6.

CPPene (3-((F)-2-carboxypiperazin-4-yl)-1-phosphonic acid) was supplied by Novartis Pharmaceutical Development (Basel, Switzerland) and D-Cycloserine (D-4-amino-3-isoxazolidone, DCS) was purchased from Sigma (Milan, Italy). Felbamate was supplied by Schering-Plough (Milan, Italy), 2,3-dihydroxy-6-nitro-7-sulphamoyl-benzo(F)quinoxoline (NBQX) by Novo Nordisk (Malov, Denmark), CFM-2, (1-(4-aminophenyl)-3,5-dihydro-7,8-dimethoxy-4*H*-2,3-benzodiazepin-4-one) was synthesized in the A. Chimirri laboratories (University of Messina, Italy). Flumazenil (ethyl-8-fluoro-5,6-dihydro-5-methyl-6-oxo-4*H*-imidazo[1,5-a][1,4]benzodiazepine-3-carboxylate) was obtained from Hoffmann-LaRoche (Basel, Switzerland). Hesperidin (HES) and narirutin (NRTN) were purchased from Sigma (Milan, Italy). HES was suspended in 0.5% *w*/*v* sodium carboxymethylcellulose (CMC), while NRTN was dissolved in sterile saline; both flavonoids were administered orally (p.o.) by gavage or intraperitoneally (i.p.), depending on the test. HES and NAR were administered at the same times of OJe before some convulsant tests. All the other compounds were given i.p. (0.1 mL/10 g of mouse's body weight). CPPene and DCS were dissolved in sterile saline and given i.p. as freshly prepared solution. Felbamate and CFM-2 were administered as a freshly prepared solution in 50% dimethylsulphoxide (DMSO) and 50% sterile saline (0.9% NaCl). NBQX was dissolved in a minimum quantity of NaOH 1 N. The final volume was made up with sodium phosphate buffer (67 mM). When necessary, the pH was adjusted to 7.3–7.4 by adding HC1 0.2 N.

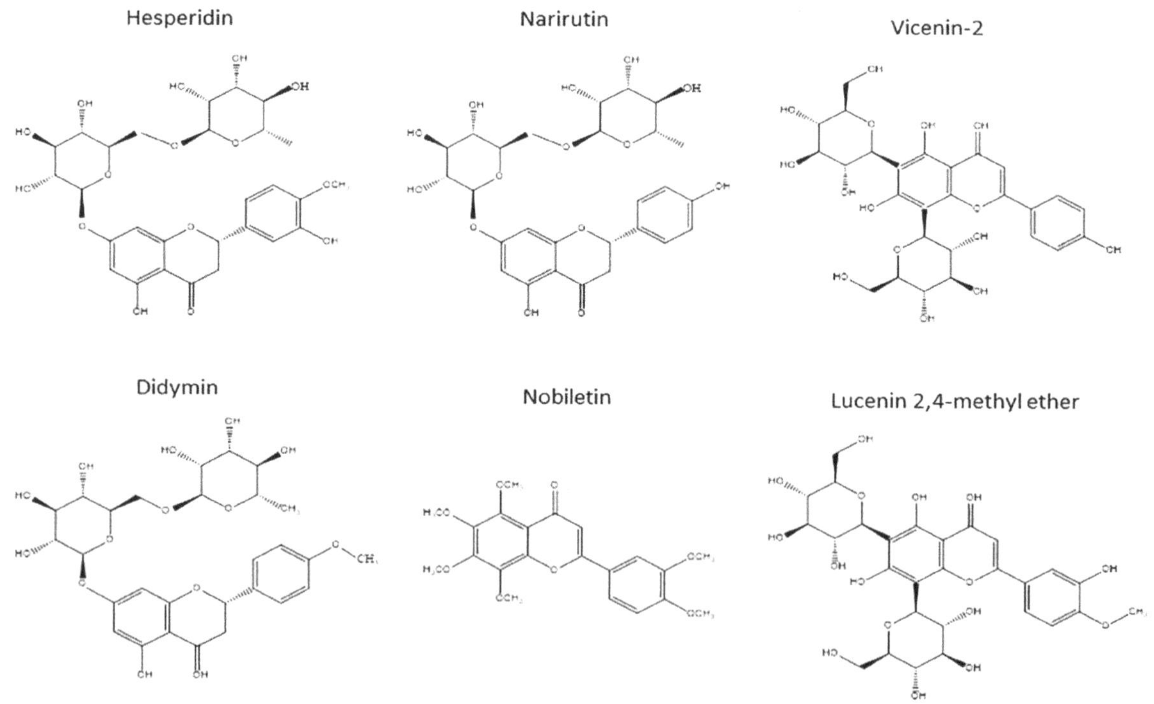

Figure 6. Chemical structures of the main flavonoids in OJe.

4.3. *Pentylenetetrazole (PTZ)-Induced Seizures in CD-1 Mice*

In order to investigate the effects of OJe treatment on PTZ-induced seizures, we used two different administration protocols.

4.3.1. Experiment 1 (Acute Treatment)

The effect of acute systemic OJe, HES or NRTN administration on PTZ-induced seizures was investigated in CD-1 mice, that received OJe, HES or NRTN (20, 40, 80, 100 or 120 mg/kg i.p. $n = 8$ mice per dose) or its vehicle (sterile saline solution 0.9% NaCl i.p.), 30, 60 or 120 min before the injection of PTZ (65 mg/kg; i.p.) [36]. Animals were placed in a 30 × 30 × 30 cm Plexiglas box and observed for 30 min to evaluate the occurrence of clonic and tonic seizure and their latency; a threshold convulsion has been considered as an episode of clonic spasms lasting for at least 5 s [28]. Absence of this threshold convulsion over 30 min indicated that the animal was protected from the convulsant-induced seizures [37].

4.3.2. Experiment 2 (Subchronic Treatment)

OJe, HES, NRTN or vehicle were orally administered for 5 consecutive days (20 or 40 mg/kg/day; $n = 10$ mice per dose) and the last administration was 30 min before PTZ (dose of 60 mg/kg) injection as previously described [36,37]. The animals were evaluated for the appearance of behavioral seizures, as described above.

4.4. Audiogenic Seizures in DBA/2 Mice

Experimental groups, consisting of 10 animals, were assigned according to a randomized schedule, and each mouse was used only once. Control animals were always tested on the same day with respective experimental groups, as previously described [37].

For acute treatment (Experiment 1), DBA/2 mice were exposed to auditory stimulation 30, 45, 60 and 120 min following intraperitoneal (i.p.) administration of OJe, HES or NRTN at the doses of 20, 40, 60, 80, 100 and 120 mg/kg ($n = 10$ mice per dose). Each mouse was placed under a hemispheric Perspex dome (diameter 58 cm) and 1 min was allowed for habituation and assessment of locomotor activity. Auditory stimulation (12–16 kHz, 109 dB) was applied for 1 min or until tonic extension occurred. The seizure response was assessed using the following scale: 0 = no response, 1 = wild running, 2 = clonus, 3 = tonus, 4 = respiratory arrest, as previously reported [38]. The maximum response was recorded for each animal.

For subchronic treatment (Experiment 2), DBA/2 mice were divided into four groups and orally pretreated, for 5 days, with OJe, HES or NRTN (20, 40, 60, 80, 100 and 120 mg/kg/day; $n = 10$ mice per dose) before auditory testing, as above described.

4.4.1. Administration of NMDA and AMPA Receptor Antagonists with OJe in DBA/2 Mice

For NMDA and AMPA antagonist receptors testing, DBA/2 mice were exposed to auditory stimulation 45 min following administration of vehicle, CPPene (at least $n = 60$ mice for each group) or felbamate ($n = 50$ mice for each group), 60 min following injection of DCS ($n = 50$ mice for each group) and 30 min following injection of NBQX ($n = 40$ mice for each group). or CFM-2 ($n = 60$ mice for each group). For co-administration, DBA/2 mice were pretreated with OJe (20 mg/kg, i.p.), 15 min before CPPene or felbamate administration, and 30 min before DCS, NBQX or CFM-2 administration. Auditory stimulation and seizure evaluation were performed as above described.

4.4.2. Co-Administration of Flumazenil with OJe in DBA/2 Mice

DBA/2 mice were administered i.p. with OJe, HES or NRTN (10–80 mg/kg $n = 10$ mice per dose) 15 min before flumazenil (2.5mg/kg i.p.), and auditory test was performed 30 min later. The dose of flumazenil, used in the present experiments was chosen according to our previous article because it does not worsen audiogenic seizures when administered alone. Total number of mice that developed seizures was tallied at each dose [28].

4.5. Experiments in WAG/Rij Rats

WAG/Rij rats of about 6 months of age and a body weight of approximately 280 g were chronically implanted, under anesthesia obtained by administration of a mixture of tiletamine/zolazepam (1:1; Zoletil 100®; 50 mg/kg i.p.; VIRBAC Srl, Milan, Italy), using a Kopf stereotaxic instrument, with five cortical electrodes for EEG recordings, as previously described [39]. All animals were allowed to at least 1 week of recovery and handled twice a day. In order to habituate the animals to the recording conditions, rats were connected to the recording cables, for at least 3 days before the experiments. The animals were connected to a multichannel amplifier (Stellate Harmonie Electroencephalograph; Montreal, QC, Canada) by a flexible recording cable and an electric swivel, fixed above the cages, permitting free movements for the animals [40]. WAG/Rij rats were intraperitoneally (i.p.) administered with different doses of OJe (20 and 40 mg/kg). Separate groups of rats ($n = 6$ for each dose) were used to determine the effects of vehicle (saline) and drug on the number and duration of SWDs. Every EEG recording session lasted 5 h:1 h baseline without injection, and 4 h after the i.p. administration of OJe, HES or NRTN or vehicle [39]. All EEG signals were amplified and conditioned by analog filters (filtering: below 1 Hz and above 30 Hz at 6 dB/octave) and subjected to an analog-to-digital conversion with a sampling rate of 300 Hz. The quantification of absence seizures was based on the number and the duration of electroencephalogram spike-wave discharges (SWDs), as previously described [41].

4.6. Statistical Analysis

All statistical procedures were performed using SPSS 15.0. software (Windows version 15.0, SPSS Inc., Chicago, IL, USA). In DBA/2 mice, statistical comparisons between control and drug-treated groups, were made using Fisher's exact probability test (incidence of the seizure phases). The percentage incidence of each phase of the audiogenic seizure was determined for each dose of compound administered, and dose-response curves were fitted using linear regression analysis of percentage response. ED_{50} values (±95% confidence limits) for each compound and each phase of seizure response were estimated using the method of Litchfield and Wilcoxon (1949) [42]. The relative anticonvulsant activities were determined by comparison of respective ED_{50} values [43]. Means ± SEM. were calculated for all relevant measures. Seizure severity scores and latencies were compared between groups using a Kruskall-Wallis nonparametric analysis of variance (ANOVA) followed by a Mann-Whitney U-test. For experiments in WAG/Rij rats, EEG recordings were subdivided into 30 min epochs, and the duration and number of SWDs were treated separately for every epoch. These values were averaged and data obtained were expressed as mean ± SEM for each dose group. Treated animals were compared by one-way ANOVA with treatment as the only variable, followed by a Bonferroni's post hoc test. All tests were two-sided, with $p < 0.05$ being considered significant.

Acknowledgments: This research was supported by grants from Sicily Region (PO FESR Sicilia 2007/2013, CUP G73F11000050004, project "MEPRA", N. 133 of Linea d'Intervento 4.1.1.1). The authors would like to thank Santa Cirmi for drawing the chemical structures in Figure 6.

Author Contributions: G.D.S. conceived and designed the experiments. R.C., A.L., E.S. P.L., R.A. and E.R. performed the experiments; G.D.S., M.N. and E.D.D.P. contributed reagents/materials/analysis tools. M.N. wrote the paper.

References

1. Sierra-Paredes, G.; Sierra-Marcuno, G. Extrasynaptic GABA and glutamate receptors in epilepsy. *CNS Neurol. Disorders Drug Targets* **2007**, *6*, 288–300. [CrossRef]
2. Costello, D.J.; Delanty, N. Oxidative injury in epilepsy: Potential for antioxidant therapy? *Exp. Rev. Neurother.* **2004**, *4*, 541–553. [CrossRef] [PubMed]

3. Obay, B.D.; Tasdemir, E.; Tumer, C.; Bilgin, H.; Atmaca, M. Dose dependent effects of ghrelin on pentylenetetrazole-induced oxidative stress in a rat seizure model. *Peptides* **2008**, *29*, 448–455. [CrossRef] [PubMed]
4. Wu, Z.; Xu, Q.; Zhang, L.; Kong, D.; Ma, R.; Wang, L. Protective effect of resveratrol against kainate-induced temporal lobe epilepsy in rats. *Neurochem. Res.* **2009**, *34*, 1393–1400. [CrossRef] [PubMed]
5. Aguiar, C.C.; Almeida, A.B.; Araujo, P.V.; de Abreu, R.N.; Chaves, E.M.; do Vale, O.C.; Macedo, D.S.; Woods, D.J.; Fonteles, M.M.; Vasconcelos, S.M. Oxidative stress and epilepsy: Literature review. *Oxid. Med. Cell. Longev.* **2012**, *2012*, 795259. [CrossRef] [PubMed]
6. Xu, K.; Stringer, J.L. Antioxidants and free radical scavengers do not consistently delay seizure onset in animal models of acute seizures. *Epilepsy Behav.* **2008**, *13*, 77–82. [CrossRef] [PubMed]
7. Tome, A.R.; Feng, D.; Freitas, R.M. The effects of alpha-tocopherol on hippocampal oxidative stress prior to in pilocarpine-induced seizures. *Neurochem. Res.* **2010**, *35*, 580–587. [CrossRef] [PubMed]
8. Hou, Y.; Aboukhatwa, M.A.; Lei, D.L.; Manaye, K.; Khan, I.; Luo, Y. Anti-depressant natural flavonols modulate bdnf and beta amyloid in neurons and hippocampus of double tgad mice. *Neuropharmacology* **2010**, *58*, 911–920. [CrossRef] [PubMed]
9. Hanrahan, J.R.; Chebib, M.; Johnston, G.A. Flavonoid modulation of GABA(A) receptors. *Br. J. Pharmacol.* **2011**, *163*, 234–245. [CrossRef] [PubMed]
10. Yao, L.H.; Jiang, Y.M.; Shi, J.; Tomas-Barberan, F.A.; Datta, N.; Singanusong, R.; Chen, S.S. Flavonoids in food and their health benefits. *Plant Foods Hum. Nutr.* **2004**, *59*, 113–122. [CrossRef] [PubMed]
11. Benavente-Garcia, O.; Castillo, J. Update on uses and properties of *Citrus* flavonoids: New findings in anticancer, cardiovascular, and anti-inflammatory activity. *J. Agric. Food Chem.* **2008**, *56*, 6185–6205. [CrossRef] [PubMed]
12. Grosso, G.; Galvano, F.; Mistretta, A.; Marventano, S.; Nolfo, F.; Calabrese, G.; Buscemi, S.; Drago, F.; Veronesi, U.; Scuderi, A. Red orange: Experimental models and epidemiological evidence of its benefits on human health. *Oxida. Med. Cell. Longev.* **2013**, *2013*, 157240. [CrossRef] [PubMed]
13. Ferlazzo, N.; Visalli, G.; Smeriglio, A.; Cirmi, S.; Lombardo, G.E.; Campiglia, P.; Di Pietro, A.; Navarra, M. Flavonoid fraction of orange and bergamot juices protect human lung epithelial cells from hydrogen peroxide-induced oxidative stress. *Evid. Based Compl. Alt.* **2015**, *2015*, 957031. [CrossRef] [PubMed]
14. Ferlazzo, N.; Visalli, G.; Cirmi, S.; Lombardo, G.E.; Lagana, P.; Di Pietro, A.; Navarra, M. Natural iron chelators: Protective role in a549 cells of flavonoids-rich extracts of citrus juices in Fe^{3+}-induced oxidative stress. *Environ. Toxicol. Pharmacol.* **2016**, *43*, 248–256. [CrossRef] [PubMed]
15. Celano, M.; Maggisano, V.; De Rose, R.F.; Bulotta, S.; Maiuolo, J.; Navarra, M.; Russo, D. Flavonoid fraction of *Citrus reticulata* juice reduces proliferation and migration of anaplastic thyroid carcinoma cells. *Nutr. Cancer* **2015**, *67*, 1183–1190. [CrossRef] [PubMed]
16. Delle Monache, S.; Sanità, P.; Trapasso, E.; Ursino, M.R.; Dugo, P.; Russo, M.; Ferlazzo, N.; Calapai, G.; Angelucci, A.; Navarra, M. Mechanisms underlying the anti-tumoral effects of *Citrus bergamia* juice. *PLoS ONE* **2013**, *8*, e61484. [CrossRef] [PubMed]
17. Ferlazzo, N.; Cirmi, S.; Russo, M.; Trapasso, E.; Ursino, M.R.; Lombardo, G.E.; Gangemi, S.; Calapai, G.; Navarra, M. NF-κB mediates the antiproliferative and proapoptotic effects of bergamot juice in HepG2 cells. *Life Sci.* **2016**, *146*, 81–91. [CrossRef] [PubMed]
18. Navarra, M.; Ursino, M.R.; Ferlazzo, N.; Russo, M.; Schumacher, U.; Valentiner, U. Effect of *Citrus bergamia* juice on human neuroblastoma cells *in vitro* and in metastatic xenograft models. *Fitoterapia* **2014**, *95*, 83–92. [CrossRef] [PubMed]
19. Visalli, G.; Ferlazzo, N.; Cirmi, S.; Campiglia, P.; Gangemi, S.; Di Pietro, A.; Calapai, G.; Navarra, M. Bergamot juice extract inhibits proliferation by inducing apoptosis in human colon cancer cells. *Anti-Cancer Agents Med. Chem.* **2014**, *14*, 1402–1413. [CrossRef]
20. Risitano, R.; Currò, M.; Cirmi, S.; Ferlazzo, N.; Campiglia, P.; Caccamo, D.; Ientile, R.; Navarra, M. Flavonoid fraction of bergamot juice reduces LPS-induced inflammatory response through SIRT1-mediated NF-κB inhibition in THP-1 monocytes. *PloS ONE* **2014**, *9*, e107431. [CrossRef]
21. Currò, M.; Risitano, R.; Ferlazzo, N.; Cirmi, S.; Gangemi, C.; Caccamo, D.; Ientile, R.; Navarra, M. *Citrus bergamia* juice extract attenuates β-amyloid-induced pro-inflammatory activation of THP-1 cells through MAPK and AP-1 pathways. *Sci. Rep.* **2016**, *6*, 20809. [CrossRef] [PubMed]

22. Impellizzeri, D.; Bruschetta, G.; Di Paola, R.; Ahmad, A.; Campolo, M.; Cuzzocrea, S.; Esposito, E.; Navarra, M. The anti-inflammatory and antioxidant effects of bergamot juice extract (BJe) in an experimental model of inflammatory bowel disease. *Clin. Nutr.* **2015**, *34*, 1146–1154. [CrossRef] [PubMed]
23. Impellizzeri, D.; Cordaro, M.; Campolo, M.; Gugliandolo, E.; Esposito, E.; Benedetto, F.; Cuzzocrea, S.; Navarra, M. Anti-inflammatory and antioxidant effects of flavonoid-rich fraction of bergamot juice (BJe) in a mouse model of intestinal ischemia/reperfusion injury. *Front. Pharmacol.* **2016**, *7*, 203. [CrossRef] [PubMed]
24. Cirmi, S.; Bisignano, C.; Mandalari, G.; Navarra, M. Anti-infective potential of citrus bergamia risso et poiteau (bergamot) derivatives: A systematic review. *Phytother. Res.* **2016**, *30*, 1404–1411. [CrossRef] [PubMed]
25. Marino, A.; Paterniti, I.; Cordaro, M.; Morabito, R.; Campolo, M.; Navarra, M.; Esposito, E.; Cuzzocrea, S. Role of natural antioxidants and potential use of bergamot in treating rheumatoid arthritis. *Pharma. Nutr.* **2015**, *3*, 53–59. [CrossRef]
26. Kumar, A.; Lalitha, S.; Mishra, J. Possible nitric oxide mechanism in the protective effect of hesperidin against pentylenetetrazole (PTZ)-induced kindling and associated cognitive dysfunction in mice. *Epilepsy Behav.* **2013**, *29*, 103–111. [CrossRef] [PubMed]
27. Meldrum, B.S.; Rogawski, M.A. Molecular targets for antiepileptic drug development. *Neurotherapeutics* **2007**, *4*, 18–61. [CrossRef] [PubMed]
28. De Sarro, G.; Carotti, A.; Campagna, F.; McKernan, R.; Rizzo, M.; Falconi, U.; Palluotto, F.; Giusti, P.; Rettore, C.; De Sarro, A. Benzodiazepine receptor affinities, behavioral, and anticonvulsant activity of 2-aryl-2,5-dihydropyridazino[4,3-b]indol-3(3*H*)-ones in mice. *Pharmacol. Biochem. Behav.* **2000**, *65*, 475–487. [CrossRef]
29. Dingledine, R. Glutamatergic Mechanisms Related to Epilepsy: Ionotropic Receptors. In *Jasper's Basic Mechanisms of the Epilepsies*, 4th ed.; Noebels, J.L., Avoli, M., Rogawski, M.A., Olsen, R.W., Delgado-Escueta, A.V., Eds.; National Center for Biotechnology Information: Bethesda, MD, USA, 2012.
30. Citraro, R.; Russo, E.; Gratteri, S.; Di Paola, E.D.; Ibbadu, G.F.; Curinga, C.; Gitto, R.; Chimirri, A.; Donato, G.; De Sarro, G. Effects of non-competitive AMPA receptor antagonists injected into some brain areas of WAG/Rij rats, an animal model of generalized absence epilepsy. *Neuropharmacology* **2006**, *51*, 1058–1067. [CrossRef] [PubMed]
31. Russo, E.; Gitto, R.; Citraro, R.; Chimirri, A.; De Sarro, G. New AMPA antagonists in epilepsy. *Exp. Opin. Investig. Drugs* **2012**, *21*, 1371–1389. [CrossRef] [PubMed]
32. De Sarro, G.; Chimirri, A.; Meldrum, B.S. Group III mGlu receptor agonists potentiate the anticonvulsant effect of AMPA and NMDA receptor block. *Eur. J. Pharmacol.* **2002**, *451*, 55–61. [CrossRef]
33. De Sarro, G.; Gratteri, S.; Naccari, F.; Pasculli, M.P.; De Sarro, A. Influence of D-cycloserine on the anticonvulsant activity of some antiepileptic drugs against audiogenic seizures in DBA/2 mice. *Epilepsy Res.* **2000**, *40*, 109–121. [CrossRef]
34. Ferreri, G.; Chimirri, A.; Russo, E.; Gitto, R.; Gareri, P.; De Sarro, A.; De Sarro, G. Comparative anticonvulsant activity of *N*-acetyl-1-aryl-6,7-dimethoxy-1,2,3,4-tetrahydroisoquinoline derivatives in rodents. *Pharmacol. Biochem. Behav.* **2004**, *77*, 85–94. [CrossRef] [PubMed]
35. Watson, G.B.; Bolanowski, M.A.; Baganoff, M.P.; Deppeler, C.L.; Lanthorn, T.H. D-cycloserine acts as a partial agonist at the glycine modulatory site of the NMDA receptor expressed in xenopus oocytes. *Brain Res.* **1990**, *510*, 158–160. [CrossRef]
36. Russo, E.; Scicchitano, F.; Citraro, R.; Aiello, R.; Camastra, C.; Mainardi, P.; Chimirri, S.; Perucca, E.; Donato, G.; De Sarro, G. Protective activity of α-lactoalbumin (ALAC), a whey protein rich in tryptophan, in rodent models of epileptogenesis. *Neuroscience* **2012**, *226*, 282–288. [CrossRef] [PubMed]
37. De Sarro, G.; Ibbadu, G.F.; Marra, R.; Rotiroti, D.; Loiacono, A.; Donato Di Paola, E.; Russo, E. Seizure susceptibility to various convulsant stimuli in dystrophin-deficient mdx mice. *Neurosci. Res.* **2004**, *50*, 37–44. [CrossRef] [PubMed]
38. Russo, E.; Donato di Paola, E.; Gareri, P.; Siniscalchi, A.; Labate, A.; Gallelli, L.; Citraro, R.; De Sarro, G. Pharmacodynamic potentiation of antiepileptic drugs' effects by some hmg-coa reductase inhibitors against audiogenic seizures in DBA/2 mice. *Pharmacol. Res.* **2013**, *70*, 1–12. [CrossRef] [PubMed]
39. Citraro, R.; Russo, E.; Ngomba, R.T.; Nicoletti, F.; Scicchitano, F.; Whalley, B.J.; Calignano, A.; De Sarro, G. CB1 agonists, locally applied to the cortico-thalamic circuit of rats with genetic absence epilepsy, reduce epileptic manifestations. *Epilepsy Res.* **2013**, *106*, 74–82. [CrossRef] [PubMed]

40. Citraro, R.; Chimirri, S.; Aiello, R.; Gallelli, L.; Trimboli, F.; Britti, D.; De Sarro, G.; Russo, E. Protective effects of some statins on epileptogenesis and depressive-like behavior in WAG/Rij rats, a genetic animal model of absence epilepsy. *Epilepsia* **2014**, *55*, 1284–1291. [CrossRef] [PubMed]
41. Citraro, R.; Leo, A.; de Fazio, P.; De Sarro, G.; Russo, E. Antidepressants but not antipsychotics have antiepileptogenic effects with limited effects on comorbid depressive-like behavior in the wag/rij rat model of absence epilepsy. *Br. J. Pharmacol.* **2015**, *172*, 3177–3188. [CrossRef] [PubMed]
42. Litchfield, J.T., Jr.; Wilcoxon, F. A simplified method of evaluating dose-effect experiments. *J. Pharmacol. Exp. Ther.* **1949**, *96*, 99–113. [PubMed]
43. De Sarro, G.; Paola, E.D.; Gratteri, S.; Gareri, P.; Rispoli, V.; Siniscalchi, A.; Tripepi, G.; Gallelli, L.; Citraro, R.; Russo, E. Fosinopril and zofenopril, two angiotensin-converting enzyme (ACE) inhibitors, potentiate the anticonvulsant activity of antiepileptic drugs against audiogenic seizures in dba/2 mice. *Pharmacol. Res.* **2012**, *65*, 285–296. [CrossRef] [PubMed]

10

Natural Phytochemicals in the Treatment and Prevention of Dementia

Rosaliana Libro, Sabrina Giacoppo, Thangavelu Soundara Rajan, Placido Bramanti and Emanuela Mazzon *

IRCCS Centro Neurolesi "Bonino-Pulejo", Via Provinciale Palermo, Contrada Casazza, 98124 Messina, Italy; rosalianalibro@hotmail.it (R.L.); giacoppo.sabrina@hotmail.it (S.G.); tsrajanpillai@gmail.com (T.S.R.); bramanti.dino@gmail.com (P.B.)

* Correspondence: emazzon.irccs@gmail.com

Academic Editor: Derek J. McPhee

Abstract: The word dementia describes a class of heterogeneous diseases which etiopathogenetic mechanisms are not well understood. There are different types of dementia, among which, Alzheimer's disease (AD), vascular dementia (VaD), dementia with Lewy bodies (DLB) and frontotemporal dementia (FTD) are the more common. Currently approved pharmacological treatments for most forms of dementia seem to act only on symptoms without having profound disease-modifying effects. Thus, alternative strategies capable of preventing the progressive loss of specific neuronal populations are urgently required. In particular, the attention of researchers has been focused on phytochemical compounds that have shown antioxidative, anti-amyloidogenic, anti-inflammatory and anti-apoptotic properties and that could represent important resources in the discovery of drug candidates against dementia. In this review, we summarize the neuroprotective effects of the main phytochemicals belonging to the polyphenol, isothiocyanate, alkaloid and cannabinoid families in the prevention and treatment of the most common kinds of dementia. We believe that natural phytochemicals may represent a promising sources of alternative medicine, at least in association with therapies approved to date for dementia.

Keywords: dementia; phytochemicals; polyphenols; isothiocyanates; alkaloids; cannabinoids

---

1. Introduction

The Etiopathogenesis of Dementia

Dementia is an age-related irreversible condition resulting in a progressive cognitive decline that reduces a person's ability to perform daily activities. Despite the progress made in the field of dementia in the last decades, the precise pathogenetic mechanisms of dementia are still not well understood. Dementia affects nearly 47.5 million patients worldwide and its incidence is predicted to increase significantly in the next decades since the average age of the population is increasing [1]. There are many different forms of dementia classified by the National Institute of Health: Alzheimer's disease (AD), vascular dementia (VaD), dementia with Lewy bodies (DLB), frontotemporal dementia (FTD), and mixed dementias [2].

AD is the most common form of dementia worldwide, accounting for approximately 60% of all dementia cases, followed by VaD (20%), DLB (10%) and FTD (2%) [3]. AD is characterized by a gradual degeneration of the cholinergic neurons, in particular in the hippocampus and cortex areas that imply a loss of cognitive function causing symptoms such as memory loss, impaired judgement, depression and mental deterioration. The main pathological hallmarks of AD, including senile plaques, resulted from the extracellular accumulation of the amyloid beta (Aβ) protein, and the neurofibrillary tangles (NFTs), formed by hyperphosphorylated and aggregated Tau protein [4]. Aβ accumulation generates a cascade of events including oxidative stress and inflammation [5]. Furthermore, microglia activated by Aβ release pro-inflammatory cytokines, reactive oxygen species (ROS) and reactive nitrogen species (RNS), which cause mitochondrial dysfunction, leading to glutamate release and excitotoxic neuronal death. Additionally, NFTs form insoluble filaments that limit the transportation of neurotransmitters like acetylcholine (ACh) and interfere with communication between neurons contributing with Aβ oligomers to affect synaptic transmission, leading to cognitive impairment. Conventional therapies for AD are mainly symptomatic and consist of acetylcholinesterase inhibitors (AChEIs), among which donepezil (Aricept®), rivastigmine (RIV, Exelon®) and galantamine (GAL, Reminyl®) are widely used in AD patients. AChEIs enhance cholinergic transmission and show modest but statistically significant improvements on cognition and global functioning in mild to moderate AD [6]. To date another treatment recognized for moderate to severe AD is memantine (Namenda®), an antagonist of the *N*-methyl-D-aspartate (NMDA) receptor that has proven beneficial effects on the cognition, behavior and activities of daily living of AD patients [7].

VaD refers to a whole spectrum of cognitive dysfunctions, ranging from mild cognitive impairment to more severe cases that are characterized by a cerebrovascular etiology (cerebral ischemia, stroke). Reduced blood flow in the brain generates hypoxia and oxidative stress that trigger inflammatory responses and damage endothelial vessels, glial and neuronal cells [8]. In addition, cholinergic deficits have been reported in VaD patients. Although cholinergic therapies have shown promising effects on cognitive improvement [9], until now these treatments have not been validated for VaD. Current treatment approaches for VaD are aimed at preventing future vascular insults by controlling the major risk factors such as hypertension, hypercholesterolemia and diabetes mellitus [10].

DLB is a neurodegenerative dementia that generally occurs during the course of Parkinson's disease, characterized by the abnormal aggregation of the α-synuclein (α-Syn) protein in neuronal cells, known as Lewy bodies [11]. The pathogenetic mechanisms involved in DLB are multifactorial, although genetic mutations in the α-Syn family genes have been implicated in the formation of Lewy bodies [12]. Clinically, DLB is characterized by cognitive decline, fluctuations in alertness and cognition, recurrent visual hallucinations, sleep disturbances, slowed movements, stiff limbs, and tremors (Parkinsonism). Neurodegeneration associated with DLB involves multiple brain areas including both dopaminergic and cholinergic neurons and for these reasons, it is often misdiagnosed as AD or other forms of dementia. Moreover, oxidative stress is significantly involved in the pathology of DLB [13]. In particular, α-Syn accumulation causes mitochondrial degeneration, which leads to the induction of oxidative stress followed by neurodegeneration. Current DLB therapies are directed at alleviating the symptoms and consist of drugs that restore dopamine signaling, such as levodopa, dopamine agonists and dopamine reuptake inhibitors [14].

FTD is a dementia characterized by early onset, and thus considered a dementia of the presenile age (<65 years of age). FTD is genetically and pathologically heterogeneous, characterized by progressive atrophy in the frontal or temporal lobes resulting in a gradual and progressive decline in behavior or language. In addition, neurovascular dysfunction contributes to FTD [1]. However, therapies for FTD are still missing and antipsychotics or antidepressants are typically administered to manage the symptoms [15].

The exact etiopathogenetic mechanisms leading to dementia have not yet been completely identified and the ongoing therapeutic strategies are generally based on the different aspects of dementia: to reduce protein aggregation, including β-amyloidosis and abnormal Tau phosphorylation in AD, and α-Syn deposition in DLB; to prevent further cerebrovascular and ischemic events in VaD and FTD; to restore specific neurotransmitter impairment, including cholinergic abnormalities in AD, and dysfunction of glutamatergic and dopaminergic system in DLB.

As already cited, conventional drugs used for most forms of dementia seem to act solely on symptoms, without having any profound disease-modifying effects. Although such treatments are effective in the early stages of the disease, long-term therapy has been associated with serious adverse effects [16,17]. Moreover, given the involvement of Aβ-induced oxidative stress in the etiology and pathology of dementia, one of the promising approaches of preventive interventions for dementia may be represented by antioxidant therapy which inhibits the detrimental effects of excess ROS through induction of endogenous antioxidant enzymes. Over the last decade, in an attempt to discover new alternative therapies for the most common form of dementia, basic science has focused on the discovery of natural compounds as potential candidates that can protect neurons against various insults and exert beneficial effects on neuronal cells. It is very likely that a dietary intake of foods or plant-based extracts with antioxidant as well as anti-inflammatory properties might have beneficial effects on human health and improve brain functions.

This review summarizes and discusses major *in vitro/in vivo* studies and clinical data demonstrating the neuroprotective effects of the most common natural phytochemicals belonging to the polyphenol, isothiocyanate, alkaloid and cannabinoid families in the prevention and/or in the treatment of the most common forms of dementia.

2. Polyphenols

Polyphenols are a class of natural compounds found mainly in fruits, vegetables, cereals and beverages, and considered the most abundant dietary antioxidants with an average consumption of around 1 g/day per person [18]. Polyphenol compounds can be classified into two main groups: non-flavonoids and flavonoids. More than 8000 phenolic structures are currently known and among them, more than 4000 flavonoids have been identified [19]. Non-flavonoid compounds include phenolic acids, stilbenes, lignans and other polyphenols (Table 1) [20]. Flavonoids are classified into six subgroups: flavones, flavonols, flavanols, flavanones, isoflavones, and anthocyanins [21].

Table 1. Polyphenols are classified into two main groups: non-flavonoids and flavonoids. Non-flavonoids include phenolic acids, stilbenes, and lignans. Flavonoids are distinct in six subgroups: flavones, flavonols, flavanols, flavanones, isoflavones, and anthocyanins.

Subclass	Polyphenols *Non-Flavonoids* Phytochemical	Source
Stilbenes	resveratrol	grapeskin, red wine, blueberries and blackberries
Lignans	secoisolariciresinol	linseed, cereals and grain
	Flavonoids	
Flavones	apigenin, luteolin	parsley and celery
Flavonols	kaempferol, quercetin	onions, leeks and broccoli
Flavanols	catechin, epicatechin, epigallocatechin and epigallocatechin gallate	green tea, red wine and chocolate
Flavanones	hesperetin, naringenin	citrus fruits and tomatoes
Isoflavones	daidzein, genistein, glycetin	soy and soy products
Anthocyanins	pelargonidin, cyanidin, malvidin	red wine and berry fruits

The first evidence of the beneficial role of polyphenols in human health came from investigations in the 1960s and 1970s [22,23]. Further epidemiological studies have indicated that polyphenol consumption can be associated with a decreased risk to develop cancer [24], cardiovascular diseases [25] and neurodegenerative disorders [26]. Over the last decade, polyphenols have been suggested in the prevention and treatment of cognitive diseases, due to their antioxidative and anti-amyloidogenic features [27,28].

We performed a literature search using PubMed to identify articles about polyphenols and dementia, and found three most investigated polyphenols. By using the keywords "curcumin and dementia" 225 publications were found; by "resveratrol and dementia" 109 publications were found; and by searching for "epigallocatechin 3-gallate and dementia" 61 publications were found.

2.1. Curcumin: A Non-Flavonoid

Curcumin (CUR) or diferuloylmethane is extracted from *Curcuma longa*, a member of the ginger family, used for centuries in traditional Indian and Chinese medicine as a herbal remedy to cure inflammation of the skin and muscles [29]. The observation that Indian people aged 70–79 years consuming a diet rich in CUR had an incidence about 4.4-fold lower to develop AD than American people of the same age [30], led us to suppose that CUR could exert a neuroprotective role [31]. Indeed, numerous studies suggest CUR as a promising candidate for dementia therapy due to its neuroprotective activities including antioxidative, anti-inflammatory and anti-amyloidogenic effects [32,33]. The antioxidant properties of CUR are ascribed mainly to the presence of a phenolic group attached to two methoxy groups (Figure 1), which confers CUR the ability to transfer hydrogen atoms or sequentially transfer an electron and a proton [34]. CUR can scavenge hydroxyl and superoxide radicals *in vitro* and its antioxidant activity is considered to be around fourfold higher than α-tocopherol, a form of vitamin E [35]. CUR can act also as metal-chelator *in vivo* by binding with the redox-active metals iron and copper, and prevents neuroinflammation via metal induction inhibition of the Nuclear Factor Kappa B (NFκB) pathway in the brain of AD animal models [36].

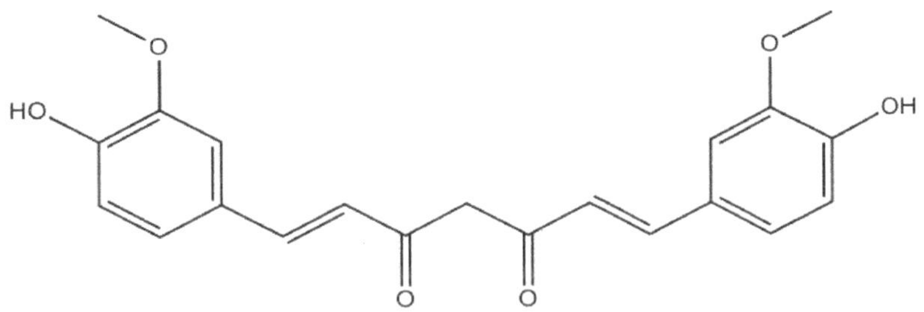

Figure 1. Molecular structure of curcumin.

Jin *et al.* [37] investigated the effect of CUR pre-treatment in lipopolysaccharide (LPS)-stimulated BV2 microglia cells. They found that CUR prevented the increased expression of inducible nitric oxide synthase (iNOS) and cyclooxygenase 2 (COX-2) which inhibited the consequent production of nitric oxide (NO) and prostaglandin E2 (PGE2), respectively. Moreover, CUR reduced the transcription levels of the pro-inflammatory cytokines interleukin-1beta (IL-1β), interleukin-6 (IL-6), and Tumor Necrosis Factor-alpha (TNF-α) by NFκB signaling inhibition. Similar results by Shi *et al.* [38] demonstrated that CUR protected mouse primary microglia cells from Aβ-toxicity in a dose-dependent manner by attenuating the release of IL-β, IL-6 and TNF-α via p38 mitogen-activated protein kinase (MAPK) and extracellular-signal-regulated kinases (ERK) inhibition. Parallel to these *in vitro* studies, CUR-mediated anti-inflammatory effects have been reported in *in vivo* models. The effect of CUR supplementation in diet at low (160 ppm) or at high doses (5000 ppm) for 6 months was investigated in Tg2576, an AD transgenic mouse model by Lim *et al.* [39]. The authors found that both doses of CUR decreased the expression of the pro-inflammatory cytokines, such as IL-1β, that was elevated in Tg2576 brains, as well as reduced the levels of oxidized proteins. Furthermore, they observed that animal treated with CUR at low doses showed a reduction of both insoluble amyloid and plaque burden as well as reduced levels of the glial fibrillary acidic protein (GFAP), a well-known marker of activated astrocytes. Rinwa *et al.* [40] investigated the effect of daily administration of CUR (20 mg/kg for 14 days) in another AD mouse model obtained by intracerebroventricular (icv) administration of streptozocin (STZ) (icv-STZ mouse). They found that CUR supplementation in this model reduced memory deficits by decreasing oxidative stress and AChE activity. In addition, they investigated the role of peroxisome proliferator-activated receptor gamma (PPAR-γ), an important negative regulator of inflammation [41], in CUR-stimulated anti-inflammatory effects. They found that icv-STZ AD mice pretreated with PPARγ antagonist failed to show the protective effect of CUR, suggesting a crucial role of PPARγ receptor in CUR-triggered anti-inflammatory effects [40].

Furthermore, several *in vitro* and *in vivo* studies highlighted the anti-amyloidogenic properties of CUR. Park and coauthors [42] reported that CUR pre-treatment (10 μg/mL for 1 h) reduced oxidative stress, intracellular calcium influx, and Tau hyperphosphorylation induced by Aβ exposure in rat pheocromocytoma PC12 cells. In human neuroblastoma cells SH-SY5Y expressing the Swedish mutant of the Amyloid Precursor Protein (APP_{swe}), CUR treatment significantly reduced Aβ production in a dose- and time-dependent manner and this Aβ reduction was mediated by serine 9 residue phosphorylation of Glycogen Synthase Kinase 3 (GSK3β), a key enzyme involved in the phosphorylation of the Amyloid Precursor Protein (APP) and Tau proteins [43]. In murine neuroblastoma cells Neuro2a overexpressing the mutant APP_{swe} (N2a/APP_{swe}), CUR treatment decreased the expression of presenilin-1 (PS1; γ-secretase) and beta-site amyloid precursor protein cleaving enzyme 1 (BACE-1; β-secretase), proteases involved in the synthesis of Aβ plaques [44].

Indeed, similar anti-amyloidogenic feature of CUR has been also demonstrated in *in vivo* models. 1,7-Bis(4′-hydroxy-3′-trifluoromethoxyphenyl)4-methoxycarbonylethyl-1,6-heptadiene-3,5-dione) (FMeC1), a novel curcumin derivative, significantly decreased the insoluble Aβ deposits, glial activation, and ameliorated the cognitive deficits in APP/PS1 double transgenic AD mice [45]. Another interesting study performed by Wang *et al.* [46] demonstrated that CUR may exert anti-amyloidogenic effects by inhibiting Phosphatidylinositol 3-Kinase (PI3K), phosphorylated protein kinase B (Akt) and mammalian target of rapamycin (mTOR) pathway (PI3K/Akt/mTOR pathway)-mediated formation of Aβ deposits in APP/PS1 AD mice [46]. Moreover, enzymes required for Aβ degradation, such as insulin-degrading enzymes and neprilysin, were found to be increased in these mice administered with CUR, which eventually improved the spatial learning and memory abilities [47]. Data reported by Garcia-Alloza *et al.* [48] provided further evidences for the anti-amyloidogenic effect of CUR. They showed that CUR crossed the blood brain barrier (BBB) and label Aβ, which eventually causes Aβ degradation in APP/PS1 AD mice. Furthermore, *in vivo* administration of CUR was shown to reduce high-cholesterol, a well-known risk factor for VaD and AD [49]. Tian *et al.* [50] showed that CUR administration lowered the cholesterol levels and ameliorated the vascular cognitive impairment in rat with chronic cerebral hypoperfusion (CCH), a VaD model [51,52]. They found that CUR decreased cholesterol levels by inducing the expression of the ATP-binding cassette transporter and apolipoprotein A1, which mediate cholesterol transmembrane transportation. The summary of molecular mechanisms underlying CUR-induced antioxidative, anti-inflammatory and anti-amyloidogenic effects discussed above is listed in Table 2.

Significant preclinical data obtained from *in vitro* and *in vivo* studies made clinicians to explore the therapeutic efficacy of CUR in dementia patients [53–57]. However, these clinical trials have failed to produce any convincing protection in AD patients. Possible reasons behind the unsuccessful results of these clinical trials are: (1) the molecular pathology underlying animal models with dementia is not same as that of humans; (2) the metabolism of CUR in rodents and in humans may differ.

Besides, the role of CUR in VaD, DLB and FTD patients is yet to be investigated. In summary, we propose the urgent need of compelling animal models of dementia, which reflect the similar pathology in dementia patients in order to successfully evaluate the therapeutic efficacy of CUR.

Table 2. Preclinical studies of curcumin-mediated neuroprotective effects.

Model	CUR-Mediated Protective Effects	Proposed Mechanisms Involved	Up/Down	References
		In vitro		
LPS-stimulated rat BV2 microglia	antioxidative, anti-inflammatory	iNOS, NO, COX-2, PGE2, IL-1β, IL-6, TNF-α	↓	[37]
Aβ-induced murine primary microglia	anti-inflammatory, anti-amyloidogenic	IL-1β, IL-6, TNF-α, MAPK, ERK1/2	↓	[38]
Aβ-induced rat PC12 cells	anti-amyloidogenic	intracellular calcium, Tau hyperphosphorylation	↓	[42]
Mutant APP_{swe} over expression in SH-SY5Y	anti-amyloidogenic	GSK3β activity, APP and Tau hyperphosphorylation	↓	[43]
Mutant APP_{swe} over expression in Neuro2A	anti-amyloidogenic	PS1, BACE-1, Aβ plaques	↓	[37]
		In vivo		
Tg2576 mice expressing mutant APP	anti-inflammatory, anti-amyloidogenic	IL-1β, GFAP, amyloid plaques	↓	[39]
Icv-STZ mice model for AD	anti-inflammatory, antioxidative	AChE, oxidative stress, memory deficits PPARγ receptor activation	↓ ↑	[40]
APP/PS1 double transgenic AD mice	anti-amyloidogenic	Aβ deposits, cognitive deficit	↓	[38]
APP/PS1 double transgenic AD mice	anti-amyloidogenic	PI3K/Akt/mTOR pathway	↓	[46]
APP/PS1 double transgenic AD mice	anti-amyloidogenic	insulin-degrading enzymes and neprilysin	↑	[47]
CCH rats	anti-cholesterol	ATP-binding cassette transporter and Apolipoprotein A1	↑	[50]

2.2. *Resveratrol: A Non-Flavonoid*

Resveratrol (RESV) belongs to a non-flavonoids class of polyphenolic compounds, called stilbenes, found in more than 70 different plants [58], including gnetum, butterfly orchid tree, white hellebore, Scots pine, corn lily, eucalyptus, spruce, and also in a lot of fruits and beverages, including grapes, cranberry, and wine. RESV is a phytoalexin synthesized from plants after exposure to stress, such as injury, fungal infections and UV radiation [58]. RESV can cross the BBB and produce neuroprotective effects against cerebral injury [59]. Structural studies demonstrated that the antioxidant properties of RESV depend on the presence of three hydroxyl groups in positions 3, 4 and 5 attached to the aromatic rings that offer RESV the ability to remove free radical species [60] (Figure 2). The antioxidant properties of RESV have been associated also with its ability to stimulate the expression of endogenous antioxidant enzymes. In healthy rats, RESV administration increased the activity of some detoxifying enzymes, such as superoxide dismutase (SOD) and catalase (CAT), while decreasing the activity of the pro-oxidant enzyme malondialdehyde (MDA) in mouse brain [61].

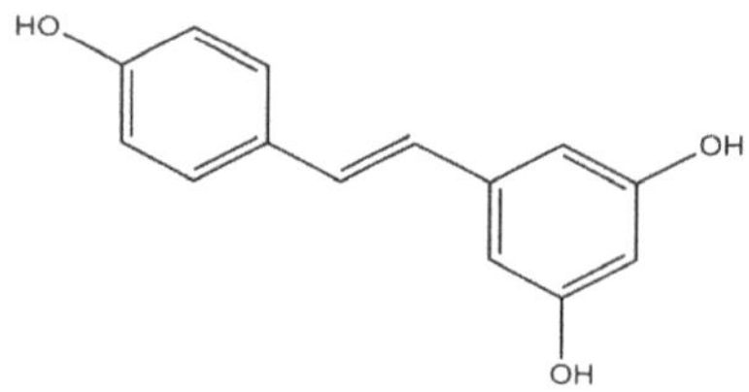

Figure 2. Molecular structure of resveratrol.

Many *in vitro* and *in vivo* studies have demonstrated the therapeutic efficacy of RESV in dementia models associated with AD. Kim *et al.* [62] found that pre-incubation with RESV (20 μM) in rat C6 glioma cells protected them against Aβ toxicity, by inhibiting iNOS and COX-2 expression and consequently reducing the production of PGE2 and NO. In PC12 cells exposed to Aβ toxicity, RESV pre-treatment (25 μM) protected cells against Aβ-induced oxidative cell death, by decreasing ROS accumulation, by attenuating the increased expression of pro-apoptotic proteins such as the Bcl-2-associated X protein (Bax), and by blocking the activation of the c-Jun N-terminal kinases (JNK) and NFκB [63]. Han *et al.* [64] showed that RESV treatment in rat hippocampal cells attenuated Aβ-induced cell-death in a concentration-dependent manner. Furthermore, they demonstrated that cells pre-treated with the protein kinase C (PKC) inhibitor significantly reduced the neuroprotective effect of RESV, suggesting the role of PKC in RESV-mediated neuroprotection [65]. RESV treatment in HEK293 and Neuro2a cells transfected with APP_{swe} variant attenuated Aβ accumulation by activating 5′ adenosine monophosphate-activated protein kinase (AMPK), a crucial regulator of cellular energy metabolism [66]. AMPK activation inhibits mTOR signaling and promotes autophagy and lysosomal degradation of Aβ [67]. Similar AMPK pathway activation by RESV has been reported in *in vivo* AD models. In senescence accelerated mouse (SAMP8) model of AD, dietary administration (1 g/kg) of RESV reduced the Aβ burden and Tau hyperphosphorylation via AMPK activation. These results were paralleled with the reduction in cognitive impairment. Moreover, activation of Sirtuin 1 (SIRT1), a class III histone deacetylase enzyme implicated in ROS control [68], was observed in RESV treatment [69]. In APP/PS1 mice model of AD, oral chronic administration of RESV reduced Aβ deposits and increased the protein levels of the mitochondrial complex IV, by activating both SIRT-1 and AMPK pathways [70]. These results suggested that RESV-induced reduction in cognitive impairment in AD models may have resulted via activation of AMPK pathway-mediated Aβ clearance and SIRT1 pathway-mediated prevention of oxidative stress and forkhead transcription factors-induced apoptosis.

Antioxidative and anti-apoptotic effects of RESV have also been investigated in *in vivo* VaD models. Ma *et al.* [71] showed that daily intragastric administration of RESV (25 mg/kg) improved learning and memory ability in a CCH rat model of VaD, by decreasing oxidative stress through MDA reduction, and SOD and glutathione (GSH) upregulation in the hippocampus and cerebral cortex [71]. A recent study reported similar data that in CCH rats, RESV treatment (10 mg/kg) prevented oxidative stress by decreasing lipid peroxidation and restoring the reduced glutathione-S-transferase (GST) level [72]. Sun *et al.* [73] reported that oral doses of RESV (25 mg/kg) attenuated memory impairment in the CCH rat model. This protective effect was supported by the reduction of expression of pro-apoptotic proteins, such as Bax, cleaved caspase-3 and cleaved poly(ADP-ribose) polymerase (PARP). RESV pre-treatment (40 mg/kg) in CCH rats ameliorated spatial learning and memory abilities by restoring the synaptic plasticity, by increasing the activity of protein kinase A (PKA) and by inducing the phosphorylation of the cAMP-responsive element-binding protein (CREB), a critical transcriptional factor involved in the memory process [74]. The summary of molecular mechanisms underlying RESV-induced antioxidative, anti-apoptotic, and anti-amyloidogenic effects discussed above is listed in Table 3. Although all these evidences suggest that RESV possesses a lot of neuroprotective features against dementia, the efficacy of RESV in dementia patients has not yet been demonstrated.

Accordingly, we recommend that clinical trials with dementia patients to evaluate the therapeutic features of RESV may provide more information in the context of the therapeutic implications of RESV in dementia.

Table 3. Preclinical studies of resveratrol-mediated neuroprotective effects.

Model	RESV-Mediated Protective Effects	Proposed Mechanisms Involved	Up/Down	References
	In vitro			
Aβ-induced rat C6 glioma cells	anti-inflammatory	iNOS, NO, COX-2, PGE2	↓	[62]
Aβ-induced rat PC12 cells	anti-apoptotic anti-inflammatory	ROS, Bax, JNK, NFκB	↓	[63]
Aβ-induced rat hippocampal cells	anti-apoptotic	PKCphosphorylation	↑	[64]
Mutant APP_{swe} over expression in Neuro 2A and in HEK293 cells	anti-amyloidogenic	AMPK	↑	[66]
	In vivo			
Healthy rats	antioxidative	SOD, CAT MDA	↑ ↓	[61]
SAMP8 mice	anti-amyloidogenic antioxidative	AMPK, SIRT-1	↑	[68]
APP/PS1 double transgenic AD mice	anti-amyloidogenic antioxidative	AMPK, SIRT-1	↑	[69]
CCH rats	antioxidative	MDA GSH, SOD, GST	↓ ↑	[71] [72]
CCH rats	anti-apoptotic	Bax, PARP	↓	[73]
CCH rats	spatial learning and memory improvement	PKA, CREB phosphorylation	↑	[74]

2.3. *Epigallocatechin-3-Gallate: A Flavonoid*

The flavanol epigallocatechin-3-gallate (EGCG) is the most abundant catechin found in tea, extracted from *Camellia sinensis*, a member of the Theaceae family. EGCG is considered a powerful antioxidant for its direct scavenging properties due to the presence of the trihydroxyl group in the B ring and the gallate moiety esterified at the 3rd position in the C ring [75] (Figure 3). In addition, EGCG possesses the indirect antioxidant ability by activating the nuclear erythroid-2 related factor (Nrf2) and its downstream antioxidant phase II enzymes, including glutathione peroxidase (GPx), glutamate cysteine ligase (GCLC), GST, SOD, NAD(P)H:quinone oxidoreductase 1 (NQO1), and heme oxygenase-1 (HO-1) [76].

Antioxidative and anti-inflammatory effects of EGCG have been investigated in *in vitro* and *in vivo* models associated with AD and dementia. Cheng-Chung *et al.* [77] demonstrated that EGCG treatment of mouse microglia cells (EOC 13.31) suppressed Aβ-induced inflammatory response of microglia by inhibiting the expression of TNF-α, IL-1β, IL-6, and iNOS. Additionally, EGCG protected Neuro2a cells against microglia-mediated neurotoxicity by restoring the levels of Nrf2 and HO-1. In IL-1β/Aβ exposed human astrocytoma cells (U373MG), pre-incubation of EGCG (20 μM) reduced the level of IL-6, IL-8, Vascular Endothelial Growth Factor (VEGF), PGE, and COX2. Activation of NFκB, MAPK and JNK signaling pathways were also inhibited by EGCG [78]. EGCG administration in APP/PS1 mice reduced Aβ level and restored the mitochondrial respiratory rates by decreasing ROS production and by increasing ATP levels in mitochondria derived from the hippocampus, cortex and striatum [79]. Improvement in cognitive impairment and reduction in ROS and AChE activity was observed in icv-STZ rats treated with EGCG (10 mg/kg/day for 4 weeks) [80]. Lee *et al.* [81] showed that EGCG pre-treatment (1.5 mg/kg for three weeks) prevented cognitive impairment in Aβ-treated-mice. In addition, they noticed that EGCG treatment (3 mg/kg for one week) ameliorated the cognitive deficits in AD (PS2-mutant) transgenic mice. *A*β plaques were decreased in both experimental AD mouse models. Interestingly, they found that EGCG inhibited the activation of ERK/NFκB pathway, which resulted in the reduction of Aβ-synthesizing β- and γ-secretases, and increased the activity of non-amyloidogenic α-secretase. Another important study in APP/PS1 mice demonstrated that EGCG may reduce Aβ levels and ameliorate cognitive impairment via two putative mechanisms: (1) neurogenesis induction via nerve growth factor (NGF)-Tropomyosin receptor kinase A (TrkA) pathway activation, which regulates c-Raf/ERK1-2/CREB cascade; (2) apoptosis inhibition, via suppression of pro-apoptotic full length neurotrophin receptor ($p75^{NTR}$)/intracellular domain fragment neurotrophin receptor ($p75^{ICD}$) and reduction of JNK2/cleaved-caspase 3 activity [82]. The summary of molecular mechanisms underlying EGCG-induced antioxidative, anti-inflammatory, and anti-amyloidogenic effects discussed above is listed in Table 4.

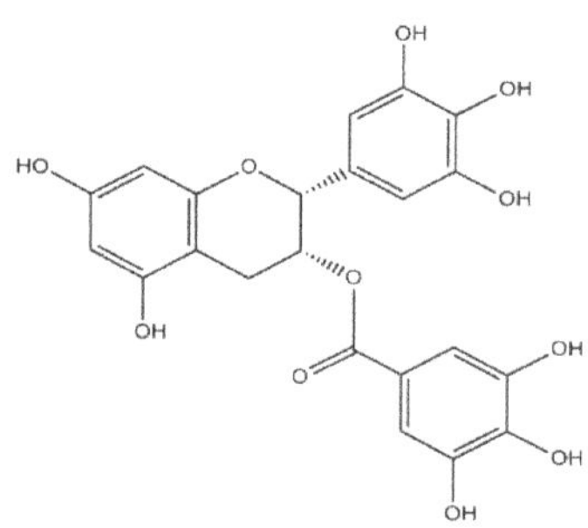

Figure 3. Molecular structure of epigallocatechin-3-gallate.

Table 4. Preclinical studies of the epigallocatechin 3-Gallate-mediated neuroprotective effects.

Model	EGCG-Mediated Protective Effects	Proposed Mechanisms Involved	Up/Down	References
		In vitro		
EOC 13.31	anti-inflammatory	TNF-α, IL-1β, IL-6, iNOS.	↓	[77]
Neuro2a	antioxidative	Nrf2, HO-1	↑	[77]
IL-1β/Aβ exposed U373MG cells	anti-inflammatory	IL-6, IL-8, VEGF, PGE, COX2. NFκB, MAPK, JNK	↓	[78]
		In vivo		
APP/PS1 double transgenic AD mice	antioxidative anti-amyloidogenic	ROS ATP	↓ ↑	[79]
icv-STZ rats	anti-amyloidogenic anti-oxidative	ROS, AChE	↓	[80]
AD (PS2-mutant) transgenic mice; Aβ-treated mice	anti-amyloidogenic	ERK/NFκB, γ-secretases, β-secretases	↓	[81]
APP/PS1 double transgenic AD mice	neurogenesis anti-amyloidogenic anti-apoptotic	NGF, TrKa $p75^{NTR}$, JNK/cleaved-caspase 3	↑ ↓	[82]

Although significant preclinical data from *in vitro* and *in vivo* studies have shown the neuroprotective effects of EGCG, it is important to mention that EGCG, at concentrations of 500 mg/kg body weight and above, has been recognized to be hepatotoxic in mice [83], and sporadic incidents of hepatotoxicity in humans have also been reported [84]. However, clinical trials with EGCG, at daily doses of 800 mg, in AD patients have shown no adverse effects (ClinicalTrials.gov identifier: NCT00951834), and the results of these clinical trials have not been reported yet.

3. Isothiocyanates

Isothiocyanates (ITCs), belonging mainly to the family of the Brassicacae (Brussels sprouts, kale, cauliflower and broccoli), are sulfur-containing phytochemicals derived from myrosinase (β-thioglucoside glucohydrolase) hydrolysis of glucosinolates (GLs) [85]. GLs coexist in the same plant, but in separate cells, with the myrosinase enzyme and they are also found within human bowel microflora [86,87]. After mechanical damage of cells, for example, predation/mastication by humans or animals, freeze-thaw injury, or plant pathogens, GLs undergo hydrolysis and release, apart from glucose and sulfate, several biologically active compounds, including ITCs, thiocyanates, and nitriles, depending on the hydrolytic conditions [88,89]. Overall, GLs display a structural homogeneity based on a β-D-glucopyranosyl unit and an *O*-sulfated anomeric (*Z*)-thiohydroximate function connected to a variable side chain depending on the amino acid metabolism of the plant species [90].

The beneficial effects of ITCs consumption have been known since the 1950s, as several studies have reported that regular consumption of Brassicaceae vegetables can contribute to reduce the risk of carcinogenesis and certain chronic diseases, such as cardiovascular diseases and neurodegenerative diseases [91]. In the last three years, ITCs were investigated in the prevention and treatment of cognitive diseases, due to their antioxidant and anti-amyloidogenic features. From a literature search in PubMed, by using the keywords "isothiocyanates and dementia" 23 papers were found, of which 20 papers were focused exclusively on the role of ITCs in AD, highlighting the emerging role of these phytochemicals in the field of dementia.

3.1. Sulforaphane

Among ITCs, *R*-sulforaphane (4*R*-1-isothiocyanato-4-(methylsulfinyl)butane; SFN) derived from the enzymatic action of myrosinase on the GL precursor glucoraphanin (GRA; (R_S)-4-methylsulfinylbutyl GL) [92] is the most extensively studied ITC in the course of the past two decades. The configuration of the sulfoxide stereogenic center in the GRA side chain was recently ascertained by NMR to be R_S, a configuration retained in the hydrolysis product *R*-sulforaphane (Figure 4) [93]. In the last decade, SFN has been proven to have neuroprotective activity in both *in vitro* and *in vivo* models of neurodegeneration due to their ability not only to address many targets, but also to modulate different pathways in neuronal cells [94–96]. It seems very likely that the beneficial effects of SFN could be mainly ascribed to its peculiar capacity to activate Nrf2/antioxidant response element (ARE) pathway [97]. In addition, many papers published about the biological properties of SFN in experimental models of neurodegeneration have demonstrated that this phytochemical is able to decrease NFκB translocation and consequent production of the main pro-inflammatory cytokines, oxidative species generation and to inhibit neuronal apoptotic death pathway [98–101].

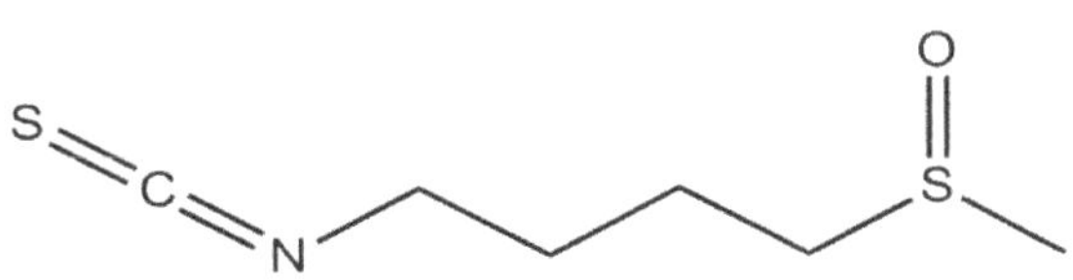

Figure 4. Molecular structure of sulforaphane.

According to these findings, Lee *et al.* [102] examined the protective effect and the molecular mechanism of SFN against Aβ-induced oxidative and apoptosis. SH-SY5Y cells pre-treated with SFN at different concentrations (1 μM, 2 μM, and 5 μM for 30 min) and exposed for 24 h to Aβ(25-35) showed a direct evidence that SFN protects SH-SY5Y cells from Aβ-induced toxicity through increasing cell viability as well as inhibiting the apoptotic cell death in a dose-dependent manner. Pre-treatment with SFN attenuated also JNK activation via inhibition of its phosphorylation and regulated the ratio of Bax to Bcl-2. Furthermore, it was observed that SFN reduced ROS production by upregulating the expression of antioxidant enzymes, including GCLC, NQO1 and HO-1 through the activation of the Nrf2 pathway. In addition, by using siRNA targeting Nrf2 expression, the same authors further demonstrated that the protective effect of SFN against Aβ-induced apoptotic cell death was mediated via Nrf2 activation [102].

Moreover, several studies performed on neuronal cell lines have shown that the neuroprotective effects of SFN against oxidative stress and Aβ-mediated cytotoxicity could be due in part to the regulation of the proteasome system [103–105]. Specifically, Park *et al.* [103] reported that SFN treatment protected Neuro2A and N1E115 murine neuronal cells from Aβ-induced oxidative damage and promoted also Aβ clearance, by enhancing the proteasome activity. Furthermore, they observed that the SFN protective effect was abolished by a specific inhibitor of the proteasome, suggesting that SFN protected cells from oxidative damage by increasing the expression of the Nrf2 pathway that in turn enhanced the expression of multiple subunits of the proteasome. Kwak *et al.* [106] reported that SFN protected Neuro2a cells from hydrogen peroxide-mediated cytotoxicity by promoting the proteasome activity via the up-regulation of the proteasome catalytic subunit, 26S. Similar results were obtained in another study performed by Gan *et al.* [104] in which SFN (10 and 7.5 μM) treatment on HeLa and COS-1 cells reduced the level of oxidized proteins and amyloid β by enhancing the proteasome activities through heat shock protein, Hsp27 activation. According to these results, it is likely that the induction of proteasome by SFN may facilitate the clearance of the Aβ aggregates, which leads to the improvement of protein folding in AD.

A study by Brandenburg *et al.* [107] suggested SFN as a good candidate for anti-inflammatory treatment of the central nervous system. Here, the authors demonstrated that SFN administration prevented the anti-inflammatory and pro-apoptotic response induced by LPS stimulation in primary rat microglia and in BV2 microglia cells. In particular, it was demonstrated that SFN reduced the expression of IL-1β, IL-6, and TNF-α and NO production from microglia in a dose-dependent manner through the inhibition of the NF-kB and activator protein-1 (AP-1). SFN was shown also to inhibit LPS-mediated phosphorylation and activation of pro-apoptotic ERK1/2 and JNK. Zhang *et al.* [108] proposed that SFN has potential application in AD therapeutics. SFN oral treatment (25 mg/kg) in mice with AD-like lesions (induced by combined administration of aluminum and D-galactose) reduced the cholinergic neuronal loss by lowering aluminum levels and ameliorated the cognitive impairment. In addition, it was proposed that SFN reduced brain aluminum cargo by accelerating blood aluminum excretion, and also in this model the antioxidative effect of SFN was attributed to its ability to activate the Nrf2 pathway. In a further study, Zhang and coauthors [109], using the same animal model and the same concentration of SFN, investigated the anti-amyloidogenic properties of SFN. They found that SFN administration reduced the numbers of Aβ plaques and caused a significant increase in carbonyl group levels as well as decreased the levels of GPx in the hippocampus and cerebral cortex areas. Since carbonyl formation is an important marker of protein oxidation, results from this study suggested that SFN could exert a protective effect against lipid peroxidation in AD mouse brain by restoring the endogenous antioxidant defenses.

The role of SFN in modulating the cholinergic system has been proven in mouse model of scopolamine-induced memory impairment [110]. In this study, it was demonstrated that oral treatment with SFN (10 or 50 mg/kg) exerted a significant neuroprotective effect on cholinergic deficit and cognitive impairment in mice. Of note, scopolamine is a non-selective muscarinic ACh receptor (mAChR) antagonist that mainly targets M1AChR and M2AChR, thereby impairing learning acquisition and short-term memory in rodents as well as in humans [111], and it was found that SFN improved the cholinergic system reactivity by increasing ACh and choline acetyltransferase

(ChAT) levels in the hippocampus and frontal cortex. AChE activity was decreased by SFN. Similar results were obtained in *in vitro* study. SFN (10 or 20 μM) treatment increased ACh level and showed protection in scopolamine-activated primary cortical neurons [110].

In a recent study, Dwivedi *et al.* [112] investigated the role of SFN in rats treated with Okadaic acid (OKA). OKA is an polyether toxins produced by marine microalgae which causes hyperphosphorylation of Tau and development of AD-like symptoms due to its property to inhibit phosphatase activity of PP1 and PP2A phosphatases [113]. The administration of SFN (5 and 10 mg/kg i.p.) in OKA-treated rats ameliorated the cognitive impairment by reducing the release of pro-oxidant species (ROS and nitrite), pro-inflammatory mediators and cytokines (NFκB, TNF-α and IL-10) and blocking neuronal cell death in the hippocampus and cerebral cortex of the OKA-treated rats. Furthermore, they observed that SFN increased Nrf2 expression as well as the expression of the downstream antioxidant enzymes, GCLC and HO-1. In the same study, It was demonstrated that the protective effects of SFN were abolished with Nrf2 siRNA treatment in a rat astrocytoma cell line (C6), suggested the possible Nrf2-dependent activation of cellular antioxidant machinery in SFN-mediated protection against OKA-induced memory loss in rats. Although current evidence indicates that SFN possesses several neuroprotective properties *in vivo* and *in vitro* (as showed in Table 5), clinical trials to test its efficacy in patients suffering from dementia have not yet been investigated.

Table 5. Preclinical studies of sulforaphane-mediated neuroprotective effects.

Model	SFN-Mediated Protective Effects	Proposed Mechanisms Involved	Up/Down	References
	In vitro			
Aβ-exposed SHSY5Y cells	anti-apoptotic antioxidative	JNK Nrf2	↓ ↑	[102]
Neuro 2A cells N1E115 cells	anti-amyloidogenic antioxidative	Nrf2	↑	[103]
Hela and COS-1 cells	antioxidative anti-amyloidogenic	Hsp27	↑	[104]
BV2 microglia cells	anti-inflammatory anti-apoptotic	NFκB, ERK1/2, JNK	↓	[107]
	In vivo			
Scopolamine-infused mice	improve scopolamine-induced memory impairment	ACh	↑	[110]
Rats treated with OKA	antioxidative anti-inflammatory	Nrf2	↑	[112]

3.2. Moringin

Recently, the attention of researchers has been focused on the study of the glycosylated isothiocyanate moringin (MG) or [4-(α-L-rhamnosyloxy)benzyl isothiocyanate; GMG-ITC], resulting from quantitative myrosinase-induced hydrolysis of glucomoringin (GMG) (4-(α-L-rhamnopyranosyloxy)benzyl GL), an uncommon member of the arylaliphatic GL class, which is present in fair amounts in vegetables belonging to the family *Moringaceae* (Figure 5) [114]. Growing in many tropical and equatorial areas and commonly known as "horse-radish tree", *Moringa oleifera* is the most widely distributed species in the genus Moringa [115]. MG has been shown to exert many beneficial activities, including anti-inflammatory as well as antioxidant effects, protecting against neurodegenerative disorders [114–118].

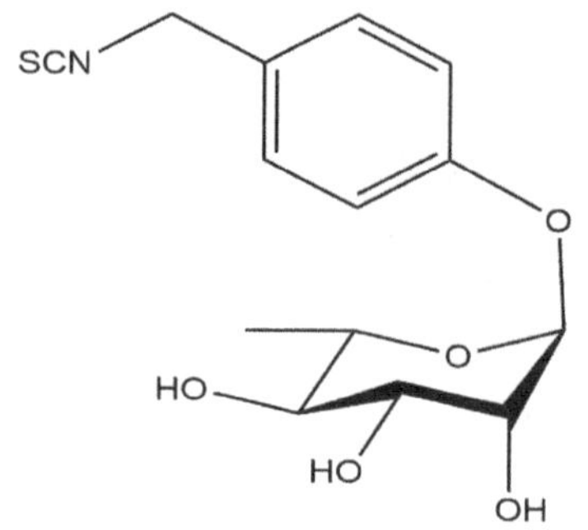

Figure 5. Molecular structure of moringin.

The neuroprotective effect of *M. oleifera* extracts was also investigated in animal models of age-related dementia. AD was induced in rats by bilateral intracerebroventricular administration of the cholinergic neurotoxin ethylcholine aziridinium (AF64A). AF64A-treated rats orally administered with *M. oleifera* leaves extract at doses of 100, 200, and 400 mg/kg for a period of 7 days before and 7 days after the AD induction improved spatial memory and neurodegeneration especially in CA1, CA2, CA3, and dentate gyrus of hippocampus areas. The effects produced by treatment with *M. oleifera* extract may occur partly via the decreased oxidative stress and the enhanced cholinergic function, as proven by reduction of MDA and AChE levels, and increase of SOD, CAT [119].

In addition, *M. oleifera* leaf extract ameliorates memory impairment via nootropic activity and provides notable antioxidants to counteract oxidative stress in rats infused with colchicine (15 μg). Several lines of evidence also suggest that chronic oral treatment with *M. oleifera* at different doses (50, 100, 150, 200, 250, 300 and 350 mg/kg) can alter electrical activity in the brain and the production of monoamines, including norepinephrine, dopamine and serotonin, involved in memory processing, thus ameliorating cognitive functions [120]. It was shown also that this extract increases SOD and CAT enzymatic activity as well as to decrease activity of lipid peroxidase in the cerebral cortex of AD rats by acting as free-radical scavenger [121]. The preclinical studies about the neuroprotective mechanisms of MG are summarized in Table 6.

Although these *in vitro* studies showed the neuroprotective effect of MG in dementia models, further *in vitro* and *in vivo* studies based on different dementia models are required to investigate the efficiency of MG in dementia, which may support to initiate clinical trials in dementia patients with MG treatment.

Table 6. Preclinical studies of moringin-mediated neuroprotective effects.

Model	MG-Mediated Protective Effects	Proposed Mechanisms Involved	Up/Down	References
	In vivo			
AF64A rats	antioxidative	SOD, CAT MDA, AChE	↑ ↓	[119]
Rats infused with colchicine	ameliorating cognitive functions	SOD, CAT	↑	[120]

4. Alkaloids

Alkaloids are a class of naturally occurring organic nitrogen-containing compounds extracted from several flowering plants such as the *Papaveraceae, Ranunculaceae, Solanaceae* and *Amaryllidaceae* [122–124]. Alkaloids represent a wide and ancient family of compounds with analgesic, antiasthmatic, antiarrhythmic, anticancer, antihypertensive, antipyretics, antibacterial and antihyperglycemic activities. Since the 1960s, the role of alkaloids in the field of dementia has been extensively investigated. The Food and Drug Administration (FDA) approval of the two alkaloid-based drugs, GAL and RIV, for AD treatment in the early 2000s has led to a renewed interest in alkaloids for dementia therapy. In addition, the intrinsic anticholinesterase activity found in alkaloid compounds makes them potential therapeutic agents for dementia.

In this review, we report some of the alkaloids that have shown beneficial effects in the treatment of dementia. Specifically, by a literature search in PubMed we found 61 papers for morphine, 84 and 220 papers for caffeine and nicotine, respectively, 123 papers for huperzine A, and 33 papers for berberine.

4.1. Rivastigmine

RIV (Figure 6G) is a synthetic analog derived from the natural alkaloid physostigmine, isolated from the poisonous seeds of *Physostigma venosum* (Calabar bean) belonging to the *Fabaceae* family [125]. RIV possesses a better therapeutic and safety profile than physostigmine. RIV is a reversible, non-competitive inhibitor of AChE [126]. In 2000 RIV (Exelon®) was approved by the FDA as a transdermal patch [127] to treat mild to moderate AD [128], and as of 2014, it has been used for the treatment of AD in more than 90 countries worldwide. Furthermore, from 2006 it has also been used for Parkinson's disease dementia (PDD) [129]. The transdermal patch formulation has shown fewer gastrointestinal side effects than the oral formulation and a higher tolerability rate that permits the administration OF higher doses of RIV in advanced stages of AD [130].

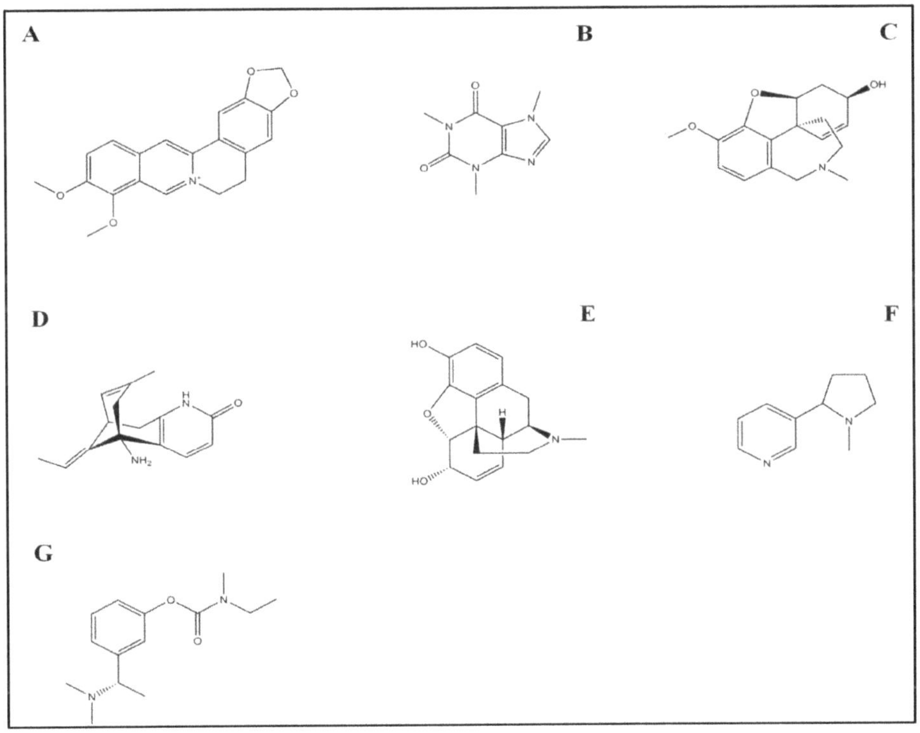

Figure 6. Chemical structures of some alkaloids: (**A**) berberine; (**B**) caffeine; (**C**) galantamine; (**D**) huperzine A; (**E**) morphine; (**F**) nicotine; (**G**) rivastigmine.

A recent Cochrane review [131] evaluated all controlled, double-blind, randomized clinical trials in which RIV was administered daily orally (6 to 12 mg) as well as transdermally (9.5 mg) in patients with AD for 12 weeks or more. The results of this study showed that RIV ameliorated the cognitive decline function and daily living in patients affected by mild to moderate AD compared with placebo, but did not induce any changes in behavior and in the clinical global assessment.

Of note, the transdermal patch as well as capsules showed comparable efficacy but the transdermal patch manifested fewer side effects than the capsules. Studies in recent years strongly support the efficacy of RIV in AD treatment. The Okayama Rivastigmine Study (ORS) carried out in 2015 [132] analyzed the clinical effects of RIV and donepezil in AD patients at 3, 6, and 12 months. According to this study, it is evident that RIV improved both cognitive and affective functions at 3 and 6 months, showed more benefits compared to donepezil. Ehret *et al.* [133] illustrated in a recent systematic review that AChEIs, including RIV, have consistent but modest effects even in late-phase trials. Additionally, Spalletta *et al.* [134] demonstrated that RIV treatment attenuated the frequency and severity of depressive episodes in patients with mild AD during a 6-month open-label observational study.

In addition to AD and PDD treatment, studies have also suggested a potential therapeutic role of RIV in VaD. In particular, a clinical study evaluated the effect of RIV on the cognitive performance of elderly subjects affected by different subtypes of VaD. After six months of treatment, it was demonstrated that RIV ameliorated the cognitive ability, particularly in patients affected by subcortical ischemic vascular dementia, a VaD subtype characterized by small vessel disease dementia [135]. Furthermore, Birks *et al.* [136], by analyzing different clinical trials, observed that RIV exhibited beneficial effects on vascular cognitive impairment, but it also showed a lot of adverse effects such as vomiting, nausea, diarrhea, anorexia and withdrawals. Although RIV has displayed beneficial effects in patients affected by DLB [137], a recent systematic review reported that RIV has greater risk of adverse events [138]. Moreover, RIV treatment in patients suffering from FTD reduced behavioral impairment and caregiver burden, but failed to prevent the cognitive impairment after 12-month of follow-up.

Overall, RIV is able to slow the cognitive decline in AD patients and some trend of efficacy in the management of behavioral symptoms associated with the disease, while in the other forms of dementia, it exhibits a greater risk of adverse effects.

4.2. Galantamine

GAL (Figure 6C) is a synthetic isoquinoline alkaloid, originally extracted in the 1950s from the bulbs and flowers of *Galanthus nivalis* L., belonging to the *Amaryllidaceae* family. GAL has been used in humans for decades as an anesthetic drug and to treat neuropathic pain. To date, after the first approval in Sweden in 2000, GAL (Reminyl®, Razadyne®) is prescribed in sustained-release capsules to treat mild to moderate AD in European Union as well as in the United States [109,139]. GAL has shown to be a selective, competitive and reversible AChE inhibitor. In particular, it is characterized by two pharmacological mechanisms by which it increases the acetylcholine concentration in the synapses and compensates the decline of cholinergic function in AD patients: (i) the inhibition of acetylcholine esterase and (ii) the allosteric modulation of the nicotinic cholinergic receptor [140].

During the 1990s, clinical studies were focused to investigate the therapeutic potential of GAL in AD patients and to evaluate its safety and efficacy in clinical practice. Particularly, it was demonstrated that GAL administration at 8–32 mg/day resulted in consistent symptomatic improvement of cognitive functions and activities of daily living in patients with mild to moderate AD over 3–6 months [139,141,142]. Also, it was found that GAL (24 mg/day) exerted a sustained effect for 12 months [143]. Richarz *et al.* [144] carried out an open-label trial for three years in order to assess long-term effectiveness of GAL in patients with mild AD. Results showed that after the first year of treatment, GAL improved cognition, behavior, and activities of daily living. Interestingly, after three years the beneficial effect of GAL on cognition was well maintained in AD patients, although a worsening in the general outcomes was recorded. Recently, a clinical study was performed to investigate the influence of cholinesterase inhibitors including GAL, RIV and donezepil on sleep pattern and sleep disturbance in 87 mild to moderate stage dementia patients [145]. In this study, GAL was proved to ameliorate sleep quality compared to treatment with RIV and donepezil, by evaluating the Pittsburgh Sleep Quality Index at the beginning and at the final assessment. Furthermore, GAL has displayed pleiotropic activity in experimental studies such as the ability to inhibit Aβ aggregation and cytotoxicity *in vitro* [146] and to prevent Aβ-induced oxidative stress [147], due to its scavenging properties [148,149].

Only a limited number of clinical studies have evaluated the therapeutic relevance of GAL in the other forms of dementia. In a randomized double-blind trial, Birks *et al.* [150] found that GAL treatment (at the dose of 16–24 mg/day) in VaD patients ameliorated the cognitive impairment and the global assessment, and showed good safety and tolerability [151]. However, gastrointestinal side-effects were observed in these patients. In another clinical study, Edwards *et al.* [152] tested GAL efficacy and safety in a cohort of 50 patients affected by DLB and found that GAL attenuated the neuropsychiatric symptoms associated with the disease such as hallucinations. Moreover, GAL-induced side effects were mild and transient. According to these findings, O'Brien *et al.* [153] affirmed that AChEIs, including GAL, can improve cognitive performance in DLB patients and suggested the application of AChEIs especially for the treatment of neuropsychiatric symptoms associated with DLB. Another open clinical trial evaluated the effect of GAL treatment for a period of 8 weeks in a cohort of patients affected by the two most common varieties of FTD: the behavioral variety FTD and the primary progressive aphasia. Results from this trial reported that GAL showed a trend of efficacy only in patients affected by the aphasic variety of FTD according to the clinical global impressions scale [154].

A recent meta-analysis [155] evaluated whether treatment with AChEIs could provide cognitive benefits in VaD patients. Here, it was found that patients treated with donepezil as well as with GAL showed relevant improvement in Alzheimer's Disease Assessment Scale-cognitive subscale (ADAS-cog) compared to the placebo group, but not in the Mini Mental State Examination (MMSE). Conversely, RIV treatment did not show any benefit on AD [155].

Overall, GAL has demonstrated to slow cognitive decline in AD patients and thus to be useful in the management of some behavioral symptoms. Furthermore, it has shown some efficacy in VaD, DLB and FTD patients. However, we assume that the achieved results in these forms of dementia need further validation.

4.3. Morphine

Morphine (MOR, Figure 6E) is a benzylisoquinoline alkaloid first isolated from *Papaver somniferum* about 200 years ago. MOR is considered an opiod compound as it targets the opioid receptors. Since the 1950s MOR is recognized as one of the leading analgesics for alleviating acute and chronic pain and it has been also administered in palliative care in the terminal stages of cancer [156]. MOR is also considered a narcotic drug, characterized by important side effects such as heavy sedation and physical dependence, and as such it was added to the list of narcotic drugs.

In the last years, literature data has reported that MOR possesses anti-amyloidogenic properties in experimental models of AD. MOR treatment in rat primary neuronal cultures as well as in APP/PS1 mice was shown to protect against Aβ toxicity by promoting the estradiol release from neurons and by up-regulating the Heat shock protein-70 (Hsp70), which in turn restores the proteasome activity impaired by Aβ [157]. In addition, Wang *et al.* [158] showed that MOR pre-treatment attenuated Aβ oligomers-induced neurotoxicity in primary cultured cortical neurons in a dose-dependent manner. This effect was shown to be dependent on activation of μ-opioid receptor and was mediated by reversal of Aβ oligomers-induced downregulation of mTOR signaling. The role of mTOR pathway has been widely investigated in the pathogenesis of AD. Indeed, mTOR signaling is involved in modulating long-lasting synaptic plasticity [159] and the consolidation of long-term learning and memory [160] processes, which are dramatically impaired during AD. These studies suggest opioid receptors as potential therapeutic targets for AD. To date, there are no relevant data reported in the literature on the use of MOR in the treatment of VaD or other forms of dementia.

MOR has also been evaluated in the management of dementia-related symptoms. In a randomized clinical trial in patients with moderate to severe AD, Husebo *et al.* [161] demonstrated that pain treatment with MOR seems to reduce agitation behaviors. Furthermore, the same group, in a previous clinical study, has observed that MOR administration in these patients could ameliorate mood symptoms including depression [162]. Although the preclinical results (summarized in Table 7) indicated that MOR could be protective against Aβ toxicity and clinical studies suggested that MOR may help to manage some AD symptoms, its sedative side effects could be a limiting factor for its potential application in the treatment of dementia.

Table 7. Preclinical studies of morphine-mediated neuroprotective effects.

Model	MOR-Mediated Protective Effects	Proposed Mechanisms Involved	Up/Down	References
	In vitro			
Aβ-exposed rat primary neurons	anti-amyloidogenic	Hsp70	↑	[157]
Aβ-primary cortical neurons	anti-amyloidogenic	mTOR	↓	[158]
	In vivo			
APP/PS1 double transgenic AD mice	anti-amyloidogenic	Hsp70	↑	[159]

4.4. Caffeine

Caffeine (CAF, 1,3,7-trimethylxanthine, Figure 6B) is a purine alkaloid isolated from coffee plants (*C. arabica* L.), present in high concentrations in beverages, including coffee, tea, soft drinks and chocolate. It is considered a non-selective antagonist of the adenosine A2A receptor [163]. Literature data regarding the role of CAF in several human diseases are still controversial. However, epidemiological and observational studies have suggested that habitual consumption of CAF can be associated with a decreased risk to develop Parkinson's disease [164–166], which encouraged other studies in the field of the neurological disorders.

Indeed, preclinical studies have proposed that CAF intake can prevent memory decline during aging and can reduce the risk to develop dementia and particularly AD [167–169]. In line with these findings, Laurent *et al.* [170] demonstrated that chronic CAF administration (10 months) through drinking water (0.3 g/L) in the THY-Tau22 transgenic mousemodel of progressive AD improved spatial memory performance in the Morris Water Maze test. In addition, CAF treatment significantly reduced hippocampal Tau phosphorylation and the respective proteolytic Tau fragments in THY-Tau22 mice, and these effects were paralleled by down-regulation of inflammatory mediators (TNF-α, GFAP and MAPK) and oxidative stress markers (Nrf2 and manganese-dependent superoxide dismutase (MnSOD)) [170]. In line with these findings, Arendash *et al.* [171] demonstrated that daily CAF administration (1.5 mg/mouse, corresponding to five cups of coffee/day in humans) for six weeks in drinking water decreased hippocampal Aβ levels by reducing the expression of PS1 and BACE-1in young Tg APP_{swe} mice. In the same study, the effect of CAF to reduce Aβ production was confirmed in N2a/APP_{swe} cells, where concentration-dependent reduction in both $A\beta_{1–40}$ and $A\beta_{1–42}$ was observed [171]. In another study, the same authors, using old $TgAPP_{swe}$ mice (aged 18–19 months), found similar results, demonstrated that CAF administration reduced Aβ burden and the memory impairment [172]. Han *et al.* [173] showed that low (0.75 mg/day) and high (1.5 mg/day) doses of CAF administered for eight weeks in APP/PS1 double transgenic mice ameliorated the spatial learning and memory abilities and increased the hippocampal expression of BDNF and its receptor, the tropomyosin receptor kinase B (TrkB), in a dose dependent manner. The role of BDNF and TrkB in the pathophysiology and cognitive deficits of AD has been well reported in previous studies [174] and it seems that the protective role of CAF against memory impairment in AD might be resulted from the activation of BDNF/TrkB signaling. Furthermore, in a rabbit model of sporadic AD induced by cholesterol-enriched diet, CAF administration (0.5 and 30 mg/day for 12 weeks in the drinking water) restored the increased levels of Aβ and phosphorylated Tau, and decreased the oxidative stress levels induced by cholesterol [175]. The summary of molecular mechanisms of CAF described earlier is listed in Table 8.

Table 8. Preclinical studies of caffeine-mediated neuroprotective effects.

Model	CAF-Mediated Protective Effects	Proposed Mechanisms Involved	Up/Down	References
	In vivo			
THY-Tau22 Transgenic mouse	anti-inflammatory antioxidative	TNF-α, GFAP, MAPK, Nrf2, MnSOD	↓ ↑	[170]
AD transgenic mouse model (Tg APP_{swe})	anti-amyloidogenic	PS1, BACE-1	↓	[171]
APP/PS1 double transgenic AD mice	anti-amyloidogenic	BDNF, TrkB	↑	[173]

The beneficial effects of CAF in AD progression and prevention have been evaluated in several clinical studies. In Maia and de Mendonça study [167] the association between CAF intake and AD risk was investigated by comparing AD patients, who had an average daily caffeine intake of 74 mg during the 20 years that preceded the diagnosis of AD, with the healthy controls who had an average daily CAF intake of 199 mg during the corresponding 20 years of their lifetimes. By logistic regression analysis it was found that the CAF intake during this period was inversely associated with AD. Similarly, another study reported that coffee drinkers (3–5 cups per day) at midlife had lower risk to develop dementia compared with those drinking no or only little coffee [176]. In another case-control study with two separated cohorts of elderly (65–88 years old), it was observed that high plasma CAF levels were associated with a reduced risk to develop dementia [169]. However, controversial results have also been documented in clinical trials. A latest meta-analysis of observational epidemiological studies found that there was no correlation associated between CAF intake and the risk of cognitive disorders [177].

Similarly, Gelber and colleagues [178] proved a lack of association between coffee intake and development or progression of cognitive impairment, overall dementia, AD, VaD, or moderate/high levels of the individual neuropathologic lesion types. Consequently, further clinical trials with longer follow-up periods are needed to investigate the relationship between CAF and AD development.

4.5. Nicotine

Nicotine (NIC, Figure 6F) is a pyrrolidine alkaloid isolated from tobacco (*Nicotiana tabacum* L.) leaf and it is also the main psychoactive component of tobacco smoke. Although smoking is associated with negative health effects, the pure form of NIC has been investigated by researchers as potential therapeutic agent in AD [179] since NIC is an allosteric modulator of the ACh nicotininc receptors (nAChRs). Indeed, a great amount of studies has reported that the activation of brain nAChRs can potentiate the cholinergic system, representing an important therapeutic target in AD [180–182]. According to these findings, NIC has shown a neuroprotective effect against Aβ toxicity and neuroinflammation [183]. Structural and *in vitro* studies demonstrated that NIC was able to break down preformed Aβ fibrils due to the ability of its *N*-methylpyrrolidine moieties to bind with the Aβ histidine residues, which exerted a neuroprotective effects [182,184].

In vivo chronic administration of NIC (2 mg/kg for 6 weeks) in AD rat model reduced BACE-1 expression and Aβ levels, attenuated the Aβ-induced memory and learning impairment and furthermore, prevented the decreased expression of the nicotinic receptors α_7- and α_4-nAChR induced by Aβ [185]. Moreover, in transgenic mice (aged 12 months) expressing neuron-specific enolase (NSE)-controlled APP_{swe}, low, middle, and high doses treatment of NIC for 6 months displayed an improvement in memory and increased the expression of nAchRα7 receptors [186]. Likewise, in another study, it has been demonstrated that male Wistar rats subjected to intermittent and repeated exposure of NIC (0.35 mg/kg every 12 h for 14 days) improved memory performance and increased the expression of choline acetyltransferase (ChAT), vesicular ACh transporter (VAChT) and NGF receptor,

TrkA [187]. Conversely, another study found that chronic NIC-treated-water supplementation in the transgenic AD mouse model (3xTg) increased the levels of nicotinic receptors that in turn increased Tau aggregation and phosphorylation state, which eventually exacerbated Tau pathology [188]. Similarly, a study of Deng *et al.* [189] reported that NIC did not improve cognitive impairment in rats Aβ-injected, and increased Aβ-induced Tau phosphorylation. Until now, the effects of NIC in VaD and in FTD have not been investigated. Ono *et al.* study [190] demonstrated that NIC inhibited *in vitro* α-Syn aggregation in a dose-dependent manner, suggested a protective role of NIC in DLB. The molecular mechanisms of NIC described earlier are summarized in Table 9.

Table 9. Preclinical studies of nicotine-mediated neuroprotective effects.

Model	NIC-Mediated Protective Effects	Proposed Mechanisms Involved	Up/Down	References
	In vivo			
AD rat model	anti-amyloidogenic	BACE-1	↓	[185]
AD transgenic mouse model (Tg APP_{swe})	anti-amyloidogenic	nAchRα7	↑	[186]
Male Wistar rats	improved memory performance	ChAT, VAChT NGF, TrkA	↑	[187]

The therapeutic value of NIC has been investigated in clinical trials. A double-blind, cross-over study reported that NIC transdermal patches, worn for 16 h a day at the following doses: 5 mg/day during week 1, 10 mg/day during week 2 and week 3 and 5 mg/day during week 4, improved only attentional performance in AD patients but not motor and memory abilities [191]. In addition, Newhouse *et al.* [192] demonstrated in a preliminary study that NIC therapy for six months through transdermal patches (15 mg/day) improved cognitive test performance in patients with mild cognitive impairment but did not ameliorate the clinical global impression. However, further clinical studies are required to have more data in order to assess the therapeutic relevance.

4.6. Huperzine A

Huperzine A (HupA, Figure 6D) is an alkaloid compound extracted from the Chinese herb *Huperzia serrata*. The beneficial effects of HupA were discovered centuries ago, when HupA was administered to treat different diseases such as fever, rheumatism, schizophrenia, contusions and myastenia gravis [193].

A review by Ma *et al.* [193], by collecting the data obtained from different clinical trials performed in China in AD patients (around 100,000), reported that HupA significantly improved memory deficits. The convincing results obtained about the efficacy of HupA have led to its approval in China for AD treatment in 1994 [194].

Furthermore, in the last decade, many *in vitro* and *in vivo* studies have elucidated the neuroprotective effects of HupA. Tang *et al.* [195] showed that HupA pre-treatment (10 μM) protected neuroblastoma cells SHSY5Y from hydrogen peroxide (H_2O_2)-induced toxicity in part by up-regulating the expression of NGF and its receptors $P75^{NTR}$ and TrkA and in part by activating the ERK/MAPK signal pathway, suppressing H_2O_2-induced apoptosis. Antioxidative property of HupA has been investigated in different cell lines exposed to Aβ-induced toxicity. HupA treatment increased the level of antioxidant enzymes, such as GPx and CAT, enhanced the level of ATP to improve the mitochondrial energy metabolism, and reduced ROS accumulation, cleaved-caspase-3 expression and nuclei fragmentation induced by Aβ toxicity [196–198]. HupA has shown a greater penetration ability to cross BBB [199] and higher AChE inhibitory effects compared to that of tacrine, donezepil and RIV drugs [200] in *in vivo* studies. Additionally, the neurogenesis effect of HupA has been observed in the subgranular zone of the hippocampus in adult mice, via MAPK/ERK signaling pathway activation [201]. Anti-amyloidogenic effects of HupA have been demonstrated in rats subjected to Aβ icv-infusion. Daily i.p. administration of HupA (0.1–0.2 mg/kg for 12 consecutive days) significantly ameliorated learning deficits. Furthermore, HupA reduced apoptosis by up-regulating the anti-apoptotic Bcl-2 and downregulating the expression of pro-apoptotic Bax and p53 [202]. Another study showed significant reduction of Aβ accumulation in HupA treated rats exposed to Aβ. In this study, the authors suggested that HupA might increase the activity of PKC, which stimulated the non-amyloidogenic pathway of APP formation. Similar PKC activation was noticed in mutant APP_{swe} ($HEK293_{swe}$) expressing HEK293 cells treated with HupA [203].

A summary of molecular mechanisms underlying HupA-induced antioxidative and anti-amyloidogenic effects discussed above is listed in Table 10. It has been demonstrated that, in dementia patients, HupA showed a selective inhibitory effect against AChE and increased the ACh level in the brain. Cognitive impairment was ameliorated by HupA treatment. In addition, HupA reduced the glutamate excitotoxicity by antagonising NMDA receptors [204]. As regard VaD, HupA was found to improve the cognitive function in a randomized double-blind clinical trial, performed on a cohort of patients with mild to moderate VaD [205], and confirmed also by a meta-analysis study [194]. However, a systematic Cochrane review reported controversial data about the efficacy of HupA in VaD patients [206].

Overall, HupA may represent one of the most interesting alkaloid candidates in dementia, since several clinical studies have demonstrated its efficacy in AD treatment and preclinical studies have highlited its neuroprotective features. Nevertheless, controversial evidence from the literature suggests that large scale clinical trials are required to validate the efficacy of HupA in dementia.

Table 10. Preclinical studies of huperzine A-mediated neuroprotective effects.

Model	HupA-Mediated Protective Effects	Proposed Mechanisms Involved	Up/Down	References
	In vitro			
SHSY5Y exposed to H_2O_2	antioxidative	NGF, $P75^{NTR}$, MAPK/ERK	↑	[195]
Aβ-exposed cell lines	antioxidative anti-amyloidogenic anti-apoptotic	GPx, CAT, ATP ROS Cleaved-caspase 3	↑ ↓	[196,197] [198]
Mutant APP_{swe} over expression in HEK293 cells	anti-amyloidogenic	PKC	↑	[203]
	In vivo			
Aβ-infused rats	anti-amyloidogenic	PKC	↑	[203]
Aβ-infused rats	neurogenesis	MAPK/ERK	↑	[201]
Aβ-infused rats	improved memory performance anti-apoptotic	Bax, p53	↓	[202]

4.7. Berberine

Berberine (BER, Figure 6A) is a natural isoquinoline alkaloid extracted from *Coptis chinensis* and other plants, which displays a lot of pharmacological benefits such as antioxidative [207], anti-inflammatory [208], neuroprotective, antitumor [209] and antimalarial [210]. Like HupA, BER has been used for centuries in Chinese herbal medicine to cure different kind of infections [211]. Since the 1970s BER has been widely investigated by researchers for its anti-tumor properties [212].

Recently, the attention of researchers has grown considerably with regard to the role of BER in dementia. It has been reported that BER acts on the central nervous system by crossing the BBB [213,214], where it increases the cholinergic transmission by inhibiting AchE and butyryl-cholinesterase (BChE) [215]. The role of BER in cholinergic transmission has been greatly explored in *in vitro* and *in vivo* models of AD [216,217]. BER could reduce Aβ production by enhancing the non-amyloidogenic pathway. Asai *et al.* [218] showed that BER treatment in APP_{swe} variant expressing human neuroglioma H4 cells significantly reduced the level of Aβ accumulation, in part by stimulating the α-secretase activity and in part by inhibiting the β-secretase, which resulted in a shift of APP processing towards non-amyloidogenic pathway. A similar reduction of β-secretase and Aβ synthesis was observed in HEK293-APP_{swe} cells treated with BER. This study suggested that BER-mediated ERK1/2 pathway activation may attenuate β-secretase and Aβ synthesis [219]. Moreover, BER administration in N2a/APP_{swe} cells inhibited Aβ generation and Tau hyperphosphorylation by modulating the Akt/GSK3β signaling pathway. Interestingly, BER administration for 4 months (25 mg/day) in AD transgenic mouse model (TgCRND8) reduced the learning deficits as well as ameliorated the long-term spatial memory impairment [43].

Antioxidative and anti-inflammatory effects of BER have also been investigated in *in vitro* model of AD. In normal rat primary astrocytes, BER treatment (10 μM) increased the HO-1 expression in a dose-dependent manner, by activating the PI3-kinase/Akt pathway [220]. In Aβ exposed murine microglia BV2 cells, BER treatment (5 μM) decreased the release of IL-6, monocyte chemoattractant protein-1 (MCP-1), iNOS, and COX-2, via inhibiting MAPK and NFκB signaling [221]. However, it is important to mention that some *in vitro* and *in vivo* studies have demonstrated the neurotoxic effects BER in PD model. Kwon *et al.* [222] observed that BER administration aggravated the 6-hydroxydopamine (6-OHDA)-induced cytotoxicity in PC12 cells and promoted *in vivo* degeneration of dopaminergic neuronal cells in the substantia nigra of OHDA-lesioned rats. In addition, BER treatment decreased the levels of dopamine, norepinephrine, 3,4-dihydroxy- phenylacetic acid (DOPAC) and homovanillic acid (HVA) in the striatum. The summary of molecular mechanisms underlying BER-induced antioxidative and anti-amyloidogenic effects discussed above is listed in Table 11.

Many clinical trials have reported the therapeutic effects of BER in patients with various diseases, such as type 2 diabetes [223] non-alcoholic fatty liver disease [224] and diarrhea-predominant irritable bowel syndrome [225]. However, its neuroprotective effects in dementia patients has yet to be demonstrated. Combined neuroprotective and neurotoxic effects obtained from preclinical studies with different models described earlier suggest the requirement of further evaluation of protective and adverse effects of BER in dementia models, which may assist to commence BER-based clinical trials in dementia patients.

Table 11. Preclinical studies of berberine-mediated neuroprotective effects.

Model	BER-Mediated Protective Effects	Proposed Mechanisms Involved	Up/Down	References
	In vitro			
Mutant APP_{swe} over expression in H4	anti-amyloidogenic	β-secretase	↓	[218]
Mutant APP_{swe} over expression in HEK293 cells	anti-amyloidogenic	β-secretase ERK1/2	↓ ↑	[219]
Mutant APP_{swe} over expression in Neuro 2A	anti-amyloidogenic	GSK3β	↓	[43]
rat primary astrocytes	antioxidative	PI3-kinase/Akt, HO-1	↑	[220]
Aβ-exposed microglia BV2 cells	anti-inflammatory	MAPK, NF-kB	↓	[220]
	In vivo			
AD transgenic mouse model (TgCRND8)	improved learning deficits and long-term spatial memory			[43]

5. Phytocannabinoids

Phytocannabinoids (pCBs) are lipid-soluble phytochemicals present in the plant *Cannabis sativa* L., used for a thousand years for both recreational and medicinal purposes [226]. pCBs are terpenophenol compounds, produced by the enzymatic condensation of a terpenic moiety (geranyl diphosphate) with a phenolic group (mainly olivetolic or divarinic acid) [227].

By a literature search in PubMed, we found that the application of pCBs in the treatment of human diseases has been developed in an exponential manner in the last decade. Particularly, by using the keywords "cannabinoids and dementia" 105 papers were found, of which 59 have been published from 2010 to 2016. Interestingly, the recent interest of researchers for cannabinoids is focused not only on their role in alleviating AD-related symptoms but also as potential neuroprotective compounds. Indeed, many Galenic formulations of two important pCBs, namely cannabidiol (CBD, Figure 7) and delta-9 tetrahydrocannabinol (Δ^9-THC) in different percentages are available in the market (Bedrocan®, Bedrobinol®, Bediol®, Bedrolite® and Bedica®).

Among pCBs, Δ^9-THC is the most widely investigated one, but the predominant psychotropic activity strongly limiting its therapeutic use as an isolated agent. Consequently, the therapeutic efficiency of CBD, a non-psychoactive compound, has been studied in central nervous system diseases. Most of the evidence supporting the potential therapeutic utility of CBD in AD have been obtained by using *in vitro* and *in vivo* models of dementia variety of AD-related changes.

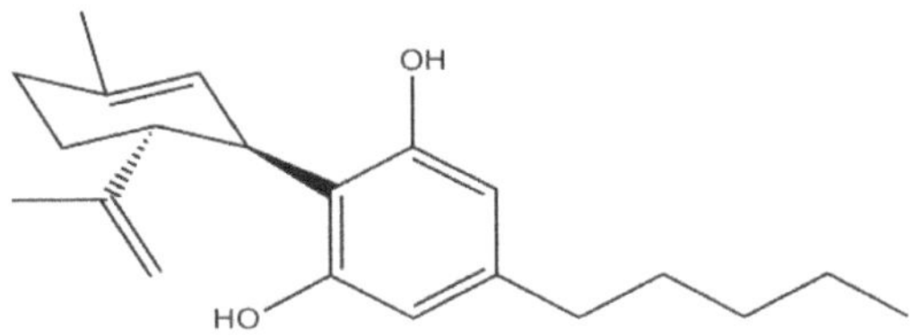

Figure 7. Molecular structure of cannabidiol.

Cannabidiol

An *in vitro* study demonstrated that treatment with CBD (10^{-7} to 10^{-5} M) inhibited hyper-phosphorylation of Tau protein in Aβ-stimulated PC12 neuronal cells via the reduction of the phosphorylated active form of GSK-3β, one of the known Tau kinases, that leads to rescue Wnt/β-catenin pathway and subsequent reduction of neuronal cell loss [228]. In a further study, the same authors showed that CBD treatment (10^{-6} to 10^{-4} M) reduced the expression of iNOS in Aβ-stimulated PC12 cells, by inhibiting the phosphorylation of MAPK, limiting the transcription of pro-inflammatory downstream genes and preventing the translocation of NFκB into the nucleus [229].

The evidence that CBD exerts a combination of neuroprotective, antioxidative and anti-apoptotic effects against Aβ-peptide toxicity was provided by Iuvone *et al.* study [230] which showed that CBD (10^{-7}–10^{-4} M) treatment in PC12 cells exposed to Aβ prevented ROS production, lipid peroxidation, and reduced apoptosis by down-regulating caspase 3 expression, DNA fragmentation and intracellular calcium concentration. Moreover, in similar conditions CBD reduced the levels of NO and iNOS, thus confirming its antioxidative properties [231]. In addition, both CBD and Δ^9-THC prevented the cell death in glutamate induced toxicity in rat cortical neurons, and this neuroprotection was mediated by NMDA, α-amino-3-hydroxy-5-methyl-4-isoxazolepropionic acid (AMPA) and kainate receptors [232]. Besides, CBD protected neuron cultures against hydroperoxide toxicity and showed about 30%–50% more efficacy against oxidative stress compared to other antioxidants such as α-tocopherol or ascorbate [232].

Scuderi *et al.* [233] investigated CBD as a possible modulating compound of APP in transfected human neuroblastoma SHSY5Y^{APP+} cells. They demonstrated that CBD treatment (10^{-9} to 10^{-6} M) induced the ubiquitination of APP protein, leading to a significant decrease in APP full length protein levels in SHSY5Y^{APP+} with the consequent decrease in Aβ production. Additionally, CBD promoted an increased survival of SHSY5Y^{APP+} cells, reduced apoptotic rate and increased the survival over long periods in culture. In line with these findings, the anti amyloidogenic, anti-inflammatory and antioxidant properties of CBD were also demonstrated in *in vivo* studies, supporting the consideration of a cannabis-based medicine as a potential therapy in AD. The role of PPARγ in the mediating anti-inflammatory and neuroprotective effects of CBD was examined in rat AD model. Specifically, it was demonstrated that administration of CBD (10 mg/kg, i.p.) in Aβ-injected rats, antagonized the Aβ-mediated release of pro-inflammatory molecules and cytokines (NO, IL-1β and TNF-α). However, by using a PPARγ antagonist, it was observed that CBD effect was completely suppressed, suggested that CBD activities are regulated by PPARγ [234].

In mice inoculated with human Aβ (1-42) peptide into the right dorsal hippocampus, CBD treatment (2.5 or 10 mg/kg^{-1}, i.p.) attenuated Aβ plaques formation, modulated iNOS expression, and decreased MAPK and NFκB levels. In this experiment, CBD suppressed the production of proinflammatory molecules, including IL-1β and NO, thus limiting the propagation of neuro-inflammation and oxidative stress, in a dose-dependent manner [235]. Martín-Moreno *et al.* [236] showed that subchronic and systemic administration of CBD (20 mg/kg for 3 weeks) as well as synthetic cannabinoid WIN 55,212-2 in Aβ-injected mice improved learning behavior. Furthermore, they demonstrated that CBD treatment modulate the microglial cell function and cytokine expression.

To date, the only commercially available preparation containing cannabinoids is Sativex® (GW Pharma, Ltd., Salisbury, Wiltshire, UK), an oral spray consists approximately 1:1 mixture of Δ^9-THC:CBD in an aromatized water-ethanol solution, approved for the treatment of spasticity and pain in some forms of multiple sclerosis (MS) [237]. In a recent work, Aso and coworkers [238] tested the therapeutic effects of the combination of Δ^9-THC + CBD (0.75 mg/kg each) in a APP/PS1 transgenic mouse which mimics the most common features of the disease, including cognitive impairment and several pathological alterations, such as Aβ deposition, dystrophic neurites, synaptic failure, mitochondrial dysfunction, and oxidative stress damage. They demonstrated that administration of the mixture of these two compounds in the early stage of the pathology reduced the expression of several cytokines and pro-inflammatory mediators in APP/PS1 transgenic mice, preserved memory and reduced learning impairment [238]. In addition, a considerable decrease in soluble Aβ (1–42) peptide levels and a change in plaques composition were observed in Δ^9-THC + CBD-treated APP/PS1 transgenic mice, due to a reduced microgliosis and expression of several cytokines and related molecules of neuro-inflammation [238]. In this study, the authors suggested that the combination of Δ^9-THC + CBD exhibits a better beneficial effect than each *Cannabis* component alone.

Moreover, the effects of pCBs on the regulation of cerebral blood flow may contribute to their potential benefits in AD. Several studies have proved that cannabinoids may cause vasodilation of brain blood vessels and consequently increase cerebral blood flow [239,240]. As decreased cerebral blood flow in AD contributes to the reduction of oxygen and nutrients in brain [8], it is possible that treatment with cannabinoids could improve cerebral perfusion. In this context, CBD was shown to reduce the infarct volume in animal models of focal or global cerebral ischemia, and since VaD is a consequence of brain ischemia, it was suggested that CBD may prevent VaD [241]. In mouse model of focal ischemia with middle cerebral artery (MCA) occlusion used for studying VaD, CBD treatment (3 mg/kg) before and 3 h after MCA occlusion reduced the infarct volume and increased cerebral blood flow. Furthermore, it was demonstrated that the neuroprotective effect of CBD was inhibited by a serotonin 5-hydroxytriptamine1A (5-HT1A) receptor antagonist (WAY100135), suggested that CBD prevented cerebral infarction though a serotonergic receptor-dependent mechanism [242]. The summary of molecular mechanisms underlying CBD discussed above is listed in Table 12.

Currently, there are few data regarding clinical effects of pCBs on human AD. A single, open-label, non-placebo controlled study performed in AD patients reported that dronabinol, derived from Δ^9-THC, has a beneficial role in reducing anorexia and improving behavior, like nocturnal motor activity and agitation [243]. Similarly, one clinical trial, including 15 patients suffering from AD showed a decreased severity of altered behavior and an increase in the body weight in AD patients after 6 weeks of treatment with dronabinol. Adverse effects associated with this treatment were limited to euphoria, somnolence and tiredness, but these effects did not warrant discontinuation of therapy [244]. Moreover, a systematic Cochrane review identified only one study that meets the criteria to assess the efficacy of cannabinoids to treat dementia [245]. However, since the data are insufficient, the effectiveness of cannabinoids in the improvement of behavior and other parameters of dementia patients are still unclear. Therefore, more controlled trials are needed to assess the effectiveness of pCBs in the treatment of dementia and even more for VaD and other dementia since there are still no clinical studies in these forms.

Table 12. Preclinical studies of cannabidiol-mediated neuroprotective effects.

Model	CBD-Mediated Protective Effects	Proposed Mechanisms Involved	Up/Down	References
Aβ-stimulated PC12 neuronal cells	anti-amyloidogenic	GSK3β Wnt/β-catenin	↓ ↑	[228]
Aβ-stimulated PC12 neuronal cells	antioxidative anti-apoptotic	ROS, iNOS, NO, Casp3	↓	[230,231]
rat cortical neurons exposed to toxic glutamate	antioxidative anti-apoptotic	NMDA, AMPA and kainate receptor toxicity	↓	[232]
SHSY5Y overexpressing APPswe	anti-amyloidogenic	PPARγ	↑	[233]
	In vivo			
Aβ-infused mice	anti-amyloidogenic antioxidative anti-inflammatory	iNOS, NO, MAPK, NFκB, IL-1β	↓	[235]
Aβ-injected rats	anti-inflammatory	PPARγ	↑	[234]

6. Conclusions

New drug candidates acting on multiple molecular targets for the treatment of dementia are urgently required. In this review, we aimed at elucidating the pleiotropic effects of some phytochemicals, belonging to the polyphenol, isothiocyanate, alkaloid and cannabinoid families, and their ability to target in parallel several pathological pathways involved in dementia.

Polyphenols have displayed antioxidative, anti-amyloidogenic and anti-inflammatory properties in preclinical studies, representing interesting candidates in the prevention and treatment of dementia. Nevertheless, clinical trials for therapeutic assessment of polyphenols in dementia patients have not shown encouraging data. Isothiocyanates have exhibited antioxidative properties in AD models, suggesting a potential role in dementia treatment. However, clinical studies to assess their efficacy are still missing.

Alkaloids have displayed a trend of efficacy in the management of behavioral symptoms associated with AD, but in parallel they have also shown side effects, such as toxicity or addiction properties. To date, among alkaloids, HupA is likely to be the most interesting candidate for dementia treatment.

CBD is one of the most promising cannabinoid family members, lacking psycoactive properties and characterized by antioxidative and anti-inflammatory features. However, clinical studies have not shown promising results.

Therefore, our opinion is that phytochemicals could represent an important resource in the development of new medications or as starting point to develop new synthetic analogs or alternatively, they can be associated to conventional therapies for dementia. However, an exhaustive amount of clinical evidence are missing or controversial, and new designed clinical trials are required to better understand their therapeutic or preventive potential in dementia.

Acknowledgments: This work has been supported by current research funds 2014 of IRCCS - Centro Neurolesi "Bonino-Pulejo" (Messina, Italy).

Author Contributions: Author (1) Rosaliana Libro has performed bibliographic researches and drafted the manuscript; Author (2) Sabrina Giacoppo revised isothiocyanates and phytocannabinoids section and also helped in revising the entire manuscript critically for important intellectual content; Author (3) Thangavelu Soundara Rajan revised polyphenols section and also helped in revising the entire manuscript critically for important intellectual content; Author (4) Placido Bramanti made substantial contributions to the conception and design of the study and revising the manuscript; Author (5) Emanuela Mazzon made substantial contributions to the conception and design of the study and revising the manuscript.

Abbreviations

The following abbreviations are used in this manuscript:

α-Syn	α-Synuclein
ACh	Acetylcholine
AChE	Acetylcholinesterase
AChEIs	Acetylcholinesterase inhibitors
AD	Alzheimer's disease
Akt	protein kinase B
AMPA	α-amino-3-hydroxy-5-methyl-4-isoxazolepropionic acid
AMPK	5′ adenosine monophosphate-activated protein kinase activated protein kinase
APP	Amyloid Precursor Protein
APP_{swe}	Swedish mutant of the Amyloid Precursor Protein
ARE	Antioxidant Responsive Element
Aβ	Amyloid beta
BACE-1	Beta-site amyloid precursor protein cleaving enzyme 1
BBB	Blood brain barrier
Bax	Bcl-2-associated X protein
BChE	Butyryl-cholinesterase
BER	Berberine
CAF	Caffeine
CBD	Cannabidiol
CCH	Chronic cerebral hypoperfusion
ChAT	Choline acetyltransferase
COX-2	Cyclooxygenase 2
CREB	cAMP-responsive element-binding protein
CUR	Curcumin
DLB	Dementia with Lewy bodies
EGCG	Epigallocatechin 3-Gallate
ERK	Extracellular-signal-regulated kinases
FDA	Food and Drug Administration
FTD	Frontotemporal Dementia
GAL	Galantamine
GCLC	Glutamate cysteine ligase
GFAP	Glial fibrillary acidic protein
GPx	Glutathione peroxidase
GSH	Glutathione
GSK3β	Glycogen synthase kinase 3 β
GST	glutathione-S-transferase
$HEK293_{swe}$	HEK293 cells trasnsfected with APP_{swe} variant
5-HT1A	5-hydroxytriptamine1A
HO-1	Heme oxygenase-1
Hsp	Heat shock protein
HupA	Huperzine A
icv	intracerebroventricular
icv-STZ	Intracerebroventricular administration of streptozocin
IL-1β	Interleukin-1beta
IL-6	Interleukin-6
iNOS	Inducible nitric oxide synthase
ITCs	Isothiocyanates
JNK	c-Jun N-terminal kinases
LPS	Lipopolysaccharide
MCP-1	Monocyte Chemoattractant Protein-1

MG	Moringin
MnSOD	Manganese-dependent Superoxide Dismutase
mTOR	Mammalian target of rapamycin
N2a/APP_{swe}	Neuro2a cells overexpressing mutant APP_{swe} gene
NFκB	Nuclear Factor Kappa B
NFTs	Neurofibrillary tangles
NIC	Nicotine
NMDA	*N*-methyl-D-aspartate
NO	Nitric oxide
NQO1	NAD(P)H:quinone oxidoreductase 1
Nrf2	Nuclear erythroid-2 related factor
OGD/R	Oxygen-Glucose Deprivation/Reoxygenation
OKA	Okadaic acid
pCBs	Phytocannabinoids
PDD	Parkinson's disease dementia
PGE2	Prostaglandin E2
PI3K	Phosphatidylinositol 3-Kinase
PKA	Protein kinase A
PKC	Protein kinase C
PPARγ	Proliferator-activated receptor gamma antagonist
PS1	Presenilin-1
PS2	Presenilin 2
RESV	Resveratrol
RIV	Rivastigmine
RNS	Reactive Nitrogen Species
ROS	Reactive Oxygen Species
SIRT-1	Sirtuin-1
SOD	Superoxide dismutase
TNF-α	Tumor Necrosis Factor-alpha
TrkA	Tropomyosin receptor kinase A
TrkB	Tropomyosin receptor kinase B
VAChT	Vesicular ACh transporter
VaD	Vascular Dementia
Δ^9-THC	Delta-9 tetrahydrocannabinol

References

1. World Health Organization. "WHO | Dementia". Available online: http://www.who.int/mediacentre/factsheets/fs362/en (accessed on 14 April 2016).
2. Raz, L.; Knoefel, J.; Bhaskar, K. The neuropathology and cerebrovascular mechanisms of dementia. *J. Cereb. Blood Flow Metab.* **2015**. [CrossRef] [PubMed]
3. Holmes, C. Dementia. *Medicine* **2012**, *40*, 628–631. [CrossRef]
4. Serrano-Pozo, A.; Frosch, M.P.; Masliah, E.; Hyman, B.T. Neuropathological alterations in Alzheimer disease. *Cold Spring Harb. Perspect. Med.* **2011**, *1*. [CrossRef] [PubMed]
5. Barage, S.H.; Sonawane, K.D. Amyloid cascade hypothesis: Pathogenesis and therapeutic strategies in Alzheimer's disease. *Neuropeptides* **2015**, *52*. [CrossRef] [PubMed]
6. Deardorff, W.J.; Feen, E.; Grossberg, G.T. The Use of Cholinesterase Inhibitors Across All Stages of Alzheimer's Disease. *Drugs Aging* **2015**, *32*, 537–547. [CrossRef] [PubMed]
7. Chu, L.W. Alzheimer's disease: Early diagnosis and treatment. *Hong Kong Med. J.* **2012**, *18*, 228–237. [PubMed]
8. Iadecola, C. The pathobiology of vascular dementia. *Neuron* **2013**, *80*, 844–866. [CrossRef] [PubMed]
9. Kwon, K.J.; Kim, M.K.; Lee, E.J.; Kim, J.N.; Choi, B.-R.; Kim, S.Y.; Cho, K.S.; Han, J.-S.; Kim, H.Y.; Shin, C.Y.; *et al.* Effects of donepezil, an acetylcholinesterase inhibitor, on neurogenesis in a rat model of vascular dementia. *J. Neurol. Sci.* **2014**, *347*, 66–77. [CrossRef] [PubMed]

10. O'Brien, J.T.; Thomas, A. Vascular dementia. *Lancet* **2015**, *386*, 1698–1706. [CrossRef]
11. Baba, M.; Nakajo, S.; Tu, P.H.; Tomita, T.; Nakaya, K.; Lee, V.M.; Trojanowski, J.Q.; Iwatsubo, T. Aggregation of alpha-synuclein in Lewy bodies of sporadic Parkinson's disease and dementia with Lewy bodies. *Am. J. Pathol.* **1998**, *152*, 879–884. [PubMed]
12. Higuchi, S.; Arai, H.; Matsushita, S.; Matsui, T.; Kimpara, T.; Takeda, A.; Shirakura, K. Mutation in the alpha-synuclein gene and sporadic Parkinson's disease, Alzheimer's disease, and dementia with Lewy bodies. *Exp. Neurol.* **1998**, *153*, 164–166. [CrossRef] [PubMed]
13. Mao, P. Oxidative Stress and Its Clinical Applications in Dementia. *J. Neurodegener. Dis.* **2013**. [CrossRef] [PubMed]
14. Valera, E.; Masliah, E. Combination therapies: The next logical Step for the treatment of synucleinopathies? *Mov. Disord.* **2016**, *31*, 225–234. [CrossRef] [PubMed]
15. Jicha, G.A. Medical management of frontotemporal dementias: The importance of the caregiver in symptom assessment and guidance of treatment strategies. *J. Mol. Neurosci.* **2011**, *45*, 713–723. [PubMed]
16. Howes, L.G. Cardiovascular effects of drugs used to treat Alzheimer's disease. *Drug Saf.* **2014**, *37*, 391–395. [CrossRef] [PubMed]
17. Kröger, E.; Mouls, M.; Wilchesky, M.; Berkers, M.; Carmichael, P.-H.; van Marum, R.; Souverein, P.; Egberts, T.; Laroche, M.-L. Adverse Drug Reactions Reported With Cholinesterase Inhibitors: An Analysis of 16 Years of Individual Case Safety Reports from VigiBase. *Ann. Pharmacother.* **2015**, *49*, 1197–1206. [CrossRef] [PubMed]
18. Ghosh, D.; Scheepens, A. Vascular action of polyphenols. *Mol. Nutr. Food Res.* **2009**, *53*, 322–331. [CrossRef] [PubMed]
19. Tsao, R. Chemistry and biochemistry of dietary polyphenols. *Nutrients* **2010**, *2*, 1231–1246. [CrossRef] [PubMed]
20. Vauzour, D. Effect of flavonoids on learning, memory and neurocognitive performance: Relevance and potential implications for Alzheimer's disease pathophysiology. *J. Sci. Food Agric.* **2014**, *94*, 1042–1056. [CrossRef] [PubMed]
21. Dai, J.; Mumper, R.J. Plant phenolics: Extraction, analysis and their antioxidant and anticancer properties. *Molecules* **2010**, *15*, 7313–7352. [CrossRef] [PubMed]
22. Baraboui, V.A.; Medovar, B.I. Anti-radiation and anti-oxidation properties of some polyphenols. *Ukr. Biokhim. Zhurnal* **1963**, *35*, 924–930.
23. Hur, J.-M.; Hyun, M.-S.; Lim, S.-Y.; Lee, W.-Y.; Kim, D. The combination of berberine and irradiation enhances anti-cancer effects via activation of p38 MAPK pathway and ROS generation in human hepatoma cells. *J. Cell. Biochem.* **2009**, *107*, 955–964. [CrossRef] [PubMed]
24. Mukhtar, H.; Ahmad, N. Tea polyphenols: Prevention of cancer and optimizing health. *Am. J. Clin. Nutr.* **2000**, *71*, 1698S–1702S. [PubMed]
25. Vita, J.A. Polyphenols and cardiovascular disease: Effects on endothelial and platelet function. *Am. J. Clin. Nutr.* **2005**, *81*, 292S–297S. [PubMed]
26. Albarracin, S.L.; Stab, B.; Casas, Z.; Sutachan, J.J.; Samudio, I.; Gonzalez, J.; Gonzalo, L.; Capani, F.; Morales, L.; Barreto, G.E. Effects of natural antioxidants in neurodegenerative disease. *Nutr. Neurosci.* **2012**, *15*. [CrossRef] [PubMed]
27. Ngoungoure, V.L.N.; Schluesener, J.; Moundipa, P.F.; Schluesener, H. Natural polyphenols binding to amyloid: A broad class of compounds to treat different human amyloid diseases. *Mol. Nutr. Food Res.* **2015**, *59*, 8–20. [CrossRef] [PubMed]
28. Vauzour, D.; Vafeiadou, K.; Rodriguez-Mateos, A.; Rendeiro, C.; Spencer, J.P.E. The neuroprotective potential of flavonoids: A multiplicity of effects. *Genes Nutr.* **2008**, *3*, 115–126. [CrossRef] [PubMed]
29. Hatcher, H.; Planalp, R.; Cho, J.; Torti, F.M.; Torti, S.V. Curcumin: From ancient medicine to current clinical trials. *Cell. Mol. Life Sci.* **2008**, *65*, 1631–1652. [CrossRef] [PubMed]
30. Ganguli, M.; Chandra, V.; Kamboh, M.I.; Johnston, J.M.; Dodge, H.H.; Thelma, B.K.; Juyal, R.C.; Pandav, R.; Belle, S.H.; DeKosky, S.T. Apolipoprotein E polymorphism and Alzheimer disease: The Indo-US Cross-National Dementia Study. *Arch. Neurol.* **2000**, *57*, 824–830. [CrossRef] [PubMed]
31. Kim, J.; Lee, H.J.; Lee, K.W. Naturally occurring phytochemicals for the prevention of Alzheimer's disease. *J. Neurochem.* **2010**, *112*, 1415–1430. [CrossRef] [PubMed]
32. Cole, G.M.; Teter, B.; Frautschy, S.A. Neuroprotective effects of curcumin. *Adv. Exp. Med. Biol.* **2007**, *595*, 197–212. [PubMed]

33. Waseem, M.; Parvez, S. Neuroprotective activities of curcumin and quercetin with potential relevance to mitochondrial dysfunction induced by oxaliplatin. *Protoplasma* **2016**, *253*, 417–430. [CrossRef] [PubMed]
34. Priyadarsini, K.I. Chemical and structural features influencing the biological activity of curcumin. *Curr. Pharm. Des.* **2013**, *19*, 2093–2100. [CrossRef] [PubMed]
35. Chin, D.; Huebbe, P.; Pallauf, K.; Rimbach, G. Neuroprotective properties of curcumin in Alzheimer's disease—Merits and limitations. *Curr. Med. Chem.* **2013**, *20*, 3955–3985. [CrossRef] [PubMed]
36. Baum, L.; Ng, A. Curcumin interaction with copper and iron suggests one possible mechanism of action in Alzheimer's disease animal models. *J. Alzheimers Dis.* **2004**, *6*, 367–377; discussion 443–449. [PubMed]
37. Jin, C.-Y.; Lee, J.-D.; Park, C.; Choi, Y.-H.; Kim, G.-Y. Curcumin attenuates the release of pro-inflammatory cytokines in lipopolysaccharide-stimulated BV2 microglia. *Acta Pharmacol. Sin.* **2007**, *28*, 1645–1651. [CrossRef] [PubMed]
38. Shi, X.; Zheng, Z.; Li, J.; Xiao, Z.; Qi, W.; Zhang, A.; Wu, Q.; Fang, Y. Curcumin inhibits Aβ-induced microglial inflammatory responses *in vitro*: Involvement of ERK1/2 and p38 signaling pathways. *Neurosci. Lett.* **2015**, *594*, 105–110. [CrossRef] [PubMed]
39. Lim, G.P.; Chu, T.; Yang, F.; Beech, W.; Frautschy, S.A.; Cole, G.M. The Curry Spice Curcumin Reduces Oxidative Damage and Amyloid Pathology in an Alzheimer Transgenic Mouse. *J. Neurosci.* **2001**, *21*, 8370–8377. [PubMed]
40. Rinwa, P.; Kaur, B.; Jaggi, A.S.; Singh, N. Involvement of PPAR-gamma in curcumin-mediated beneficial effects in experimental dementia. *Naunyn Schmiedebergs Arch. Pharmacol.* **2010**, *381*, 529–539. [CrossRef] [PubMed]
41. Landreth, G.; Jiang, Q.; Mandrekar, S.; Heneka, M. PPARγ agonists as therapeutics for the treatment of Alzheimer's disease. *Neurotherapeutics* **2008**, *5*, 481–489. [CrossRef] [PubMed]
42. Park, S.-Y.; Kim, H.-S.; Cho, E.-K.; Kwon, B.-Y.; Phark, S.; Hwang, K.-W.; Sul, D. Curcumin protected PC12 cells against beta-amyloid-induced toxicity through the inhibition of oxidative damage and tau hyperphosphorylation. *Food Chem. Toxicol.* **2008**, *46*, 2881–2887. [CrossRef] [PubMed]
43. Durairajan, S.S.K.; Liu, L.-F.; Lu, J.-H.; Chen, L.-L.; Yuan, Q.; Chung, S.K.; Huang, L.; Li, X.-S.; Huang, J.-D.; Li, M. Berberine ameliorates β-amyloid pathology, gliosis, and cognitive impairment in an Alzheimer's disease transgenic mouse model. *Neurobiol. Aging* **2012**, *33*, 2903–2919. [CrossRef] [PubMed]
44. Lu, X.; Deng, Y.; Yu, D.; Cao, H.; Wang, L.; Liu, L.; Yu, C.; Zhang, Y.; Guo, X.; Yu, G. Histone acetyltransferase p300 mediates histone acetylation of PS1 and BACE1 in a cellular model of Alzheimer's disease. *PLoS ONE* **2014**, *9*, e103067. [CrossRef] [PubMed]
45. Yanagisawa, D.; Ibrahim, N.F.; Taguchi, H.; Morikawa, S.; Hirao, K.; Shirai, N.; Sogabe, T.; Tooyama, I. Curcumin derivative with the substitution at C-4 position, but not curcumin, is effective against amyloid pathology in APP/PS1 mice. *Neurobiol. Aging* **2015**, *36*, 201–210. [CrossRef] [PubMed]
46. Wang, C.; Zhang, X.; Teng, Z.; Zhang, T.; Li, Y. Downregulation of PI3K/Akt/mTOR signaling pathway in curcumin-induced autophagy in APP/PS1 double transgenic mice. *Eur. J. Pharmacol.* **2014**, *740*, 312–320. [CrossRef] [PubMed]
47. Wang, P.; Su, C.; Li, R.; Wang, H.; Ren, Y.; Sun, H.; Yang, J.; Sun, J.; Shi, J.; Tian, J.; Jiang, S. Mechanisms and effects of curcumin on spatial learning and memory improvement in APPswe/PS1dE9 mice. *J. Neurosci. Res.* **2014**, *92*, 218–231. [CrossRef] [PubMed]
48. Garcia-Alloza, M.; Borrelli, L.A.; Rozkalne, A.; Hyman, B.T.; Bacskai, B.J. Curcumin labels amyloid pathology *in vivo*, disrupts existing plaques, and partially restores distorted neurites in an Alzheimer mouse model. *J. Neurochem.* **2007**, *102*, 1095–1104. [CrossRef] [PubMed]
49. Duron, E.; Hanon, O. Vascular risk factors, cognitive decline, and dementia. *Vasc. Health Risk Manag.* **2008**, *4*, 363–381. [PubMed]
50. Tian, M.; Zhang, X.; Wang, L.; Li, Y. Curcumin induces ABCA1 expression and apolipoprotein A-I-mediated cholesterol transmembrane in the chronic cerebral hypoperfusion aging rats. *Am. J. Chin. Med.* **2013**, *41*, 1027–1042. [CrossRef] [PubMed]
51. Zhao, H.; Li, Z.; Wang, Y.; Zhang, Q. Hippocampal expression of synaptic structural proteins and phosphorylated cAMP response element-binding protein in a rat model of vascular dementia induced by chronic cerebral hypoperfusion. *Neural Regen. Res.* **2012**, *7*, 821–826. [PubMed]
52. Li, H.; Wang, J.; Wang, P.; Rao, Y.; Chen, L. Resveratrol Reverses the Synaptic Plasticity Deficits in a Chronic Cerebral Hypoperfusion Rat Model. *J. Stroke Cerebrovasc. Dis.* **2015**, *25*, 122–128. [CrossRef] [PubMed]

53. Baum, L.; Lam, C.W.K.; Cheung, S.K.-K.; Kwok, T.; Lui, V.; Tsoh, J.; Lam, L.; Leung, V.; Hui, E.; Ng, C.; *et al.* Six-month randomized, placebo-controlled, double-blind, pilot clinical trial of curcumin in patients with Alzheimer disease. *J. Clin. Psychopharmacol.* **2008**, *28*, 110–113. [CrossRef] [PubMed]
54. Ringman, J.M.; Frautschy, S.A.; Teng, E.; Begum, A.N.; Bardens, J.; Beigi, M.; Gylys, K.H.; Badmaev, V.; Heath, D.D.; Apostolova, L.G.; *et al.* Oral curcumin for Alzheimer's disease: Tolerability and efficacy in a 24-week randomized, double blind, placebo-controlled study. *Alzheimers Res. Ther.* **2012**, *4*. [CrossRef] [PubMed]
55. Hishikawa, N.; Takahashi, Y.; Amakusa, Y.; Tanno, Y.; Tuji, Y.; Niwa, H.; Murakami, N.; Krishna, U.K. Effects of turmeric on Alzheimer's disease with behavioral and psychological symptoms of dementia. *Ayu* **2012**, *33*, 499–504. [CrossRef] [PubMed]
56. Brondino, N.; Re, S.; Boldrini, A.; Cuccomarino, A.; Lanati, N.; Barale, F.; Politi, P. Curcumin as a Therapeutic Agent in Dementia: A Mini Systematic Review of Human Studies. *Sci. World J.* **2014**, *2014*. [CrossRef] [PubMed]
57. Hu, S.; Maiti, P.; Ma, Q.; Zuo, X.; Jones, M.R.; Cole, G.M.; Frautschy, S.A. Clinical development of curcumin in neurodegenerative disease. *Expert Rev. Neurother.* **2015**, *15*, 629–637. [CrossRef] [PubMed]
58. Li, F.; Gong, Q.; Dong, H.; Shi, J. Resveratrol, a neuroprotective supplement for Alzheimer's disease. *Curr. Pharm. Des.* **2012**, *18*, 27–33. [CrossRef] [PubMed]
59. Wang, Q.; Xu, J.; Rottinghaus, G.E.; Simonyi, A.; Lubahn, D.; Sun, G.Y.; Sun, A.Y. Resveratrol protects against global cerebral ischemic injury in gerbils. *Brain Res.* **2002**, *958*, 439–447. [CrossRef]
60. Rege, S.D.; Geetha, T.; Griffin, G.D.; Broderick, T.L.; Babu, J.R. Neuroprotective effects of resveratrol in Alzheimer disease pathology. *Front. Aging Neurosci.* **2014**, *6*. [CrossRef] [PubMed]
61. Mokni, M.; Elkahoui, S.; Limam, F.; Amri, M.; Aouani, E. Effect of resveratrol on antioxidant enzyme activities in the brain of healthy rat. *Neurochem. Res.* **2007**, *32*, 981–987. [CrossRef] [PubMed]
62. Kim, Y.A.; Lim, S.-Y.; Rhee, S.-H.; Park, K.Y.; Kim, C.-H.; Choi, B.T.; Lee, S.J.; Park, Y.-M.; Choi, Y.H. Resveratrol inhibits inducible nitric oxide synthase and cyclooxygenase-2 expression in beta-amyloid-treated C6 glioma cells. *Int. J. Mol. Med.* **2006**, *17*, 1069–1075. [PubMed]
63. Jang, J.-H.; Surh, Y.-J. Protective effect of resveratrol on beta-amyloid-induced oxidative PC12 cell death. *Free Radic. Biol. Med.* **2003**, *34*, 1100–1110. [CrossRef]
64. Han, Y.-S.; Zheng, W.-H.; Bastianetto, S.; Chabot, J.-G.; Quirion, R. Neuroprotective effects of resveratrol against beta-amyloid-induced neurotoxicity in rat hippocampal neurons: Involvement of protein kinase C. *Br. J. Pharmacol.* **2004**, *141*, 997–1005. [CrossRef] [PubMed]
65. Racchi, M.; Mazzucchelli, M.; Pascale, A.; Sironi, M.; Govoni, S. Role of protein kinase Calpha in the regulated secretion of the amyloid precursor protein. *Mol. Psychiatry* **2003**, *8*, 209–216. [CrossRef] [PubMed]
66. Cai, Z.; Yan, L.-J.; Li, K.; Quazi, S.H.; Zhao, B. Roles of AMP-activated protein kinase in Alzheimer's disease. *Neuromol. Med.* **2012**, *14*. [CrossRef] [PubMed]
67. Vingtdeux, V.; Giliberto, L.; Zhao, H.; Chandakkar, P.; Wu, Q.; Simon, J.E.; Janle, E.M.; Lobo, J.; Ferruzzi, M.G.; Davies, P.; *et al.* AMP-activated protein kinase signaling activation by resveratrol modulates amyloid-beta peptide metabolism. *J. Biol. Chem.* **2010**, *285*, 9100–9113. [CrossRef] [PubMed]
68. Braidy, N.; Jayasena, T.; Poljak, A.; Sachdev, P.S. Sirtuins in cognitive ageing and Alzheimer's disease. *Curr. Opin. Psychiatry* **2012**, *25*, 226–230. [CrossRef] [PubMed]
69. Porquet, D.; Casadesús, G.; Bayod, S.; Vicente, A.; Canudas, A.M.; Vilaplana, J.; Pelegrí, C.; Sanfeliu, C.; Camins, A.; Pallàs, M.; *et al.* Dietary resveratrol prevents Alzheimer's markers and increases life span in SAMP8. *Age* **2013**, *35*, 1851–1865. [CrossRef] [PubMed]
70. Porquet, D.; Griñán-Ferré, C.; Ferrer, I.; Camins, A.; Sanfeliu, C.; del Valle, J.; Pallàs, M. Neuroprotective role of trans-resveratrol in a murine model of familial Alzheimer's disease. *J. Alzheimers Dis.* **2014**, *42*, 1209–1220. [PubMed]
71. Ma, X.; Sun, Z.; Liu, Y.; Jia, Y.; Zhang, B.; Zhang, J. Resveratrol improves cognition and reduces oxidative stress in rats with vascular dementia. *Neural Regen. Res.* **2013**, *8*, 2050–2059. [PubMed]
72. Ozacmak, V.H.; Sayan-Ozacmak, H.; Barut, F. Chronic treatment with resveratrol, a natural polyphenol found in grapes, alleviates oxidative stress and apoptotic cell death in ovariectomized female rats subjected to chronic cerebral hypoperfusion. *Nutr. Neurosci.* **2015**. [CrossRef] [PubMed]
73. Sun, Z.-K.; Ma, X.-R.; Jia, Y.-J.; Liu, Y.-R.; Zhang, J.-W.; Zhang, B.-A. Effects of resveratrol on apoptosis in a rat model of vascular dementia. *Exp. Ther. Med.* **2014**, *7*, 843–848. [CrossRef] [PubMed]

74. Lonze, B.E.; Ginty, D.D. Function and Regulation of CREB Family Transcription Factors in the Nervous System. *Neuron* **2002**, *35*, 605–623. [CrossRef]
75. Davinelli, S.; Sapere, N.; Zella, D.; Bracale, R.; Intrieri, M.; Scapagnini, G. Pleiotropic protective effects of phytochemicals in Alzheimer's disease. *Oxid. Med. Cell. Longev.* **2012**, *2012*. [CrossRef] [PubMed]
76. Na, H.-K.; Surh, Y.-J. Modulation of Nrf2-mediated antioxidant and detoxifying enzyme induction by the green tea polyphenol EGCG. *Food Chem. Toxicol.* **2008**, *46*, 1271–1278. [CrossRef] [PubMed]
77. Cheng-Chung Wei, J.; Huang, H.-C.; Chen, W.-J.; Huang, C.-N.; Peng, C.-H.; Lin, C.-L. Epigallocatechin gallate attenuates amyloid β-induced inflammation and neurotoxicity in EOC 13.31 microglia. *Eur. J. Pharmacol.* **2015**, *770*, 16–24. [CrossRef] [PubMed]
78. Kim, S.-J.; Jeong, H.-J.; Lee, K.-M.; Myung, N.-Y.; An, N.-H.; Yang, W.M.; Park, S.K.; Lee, H.-J.; Hong, S.-H.; Kim, H.-M.; *et al.* Epigallocatechin-3-gallate suppresses NF-kappaB activation and phosphorylation of p38 MAPK and JNK in human astrocytoma U373MG cells. *J. Nutr. Biochem.* **2007**, *18*, 587–596. [CrossRef] [PubMed]
79. Dragicevic, N.; Smith, A.; Lin, X.; Yuan, F.; Copes, N.; Delic, V.; Tan, J.; Cao, C.; Shytle, R.D.; Bradshaw, P.C. Green tea epigallocatechin-3-gallate (EGCG) and other flavonoids reduce Alzheimer's amyloid-induced mitochondrial dysfunction. *J. Alzheimers Dis.* **2011**, *26*, 507–521. [PubMed]
80. Biasibetti, R.; Tramontina, A.C.; Costa, A.P.; Dutra, M.F.; Quincozes-Santos, A.; Nardin, P.; Bernardi, C.L.; Wartchow, K.M.; Lunardi, P.S.; Gonçalves, C.-A. Green tea (−)epigallocatechin-3-gallate reverses oxidative stress and reduces acetylcholinesterase activity in a streptozotocin-induced model of dementia. *Behav. Brain Res.* **2013**, *236*, 186–193. [CrossRef] [PubMed]
81. Lee, J.W.; Lee, Y.K.; Ban, J.O.; Ha, T.Y.; Yun, Y.P.; Han, S.B.; Oh, K.W.; Hong, J.T. Green tea (−)-epigallocatechin-3-gallate inhibits beta-amyloid-induced cognitive dysfunction through modification of secretase activity via inhibition of ERK and NF-kappaB pathways in mice. *J. Nutr.* **2009**, *139*, 1987–1993. [CrossRef] [PubMed]
82. Liu, M.; Chen, F.; Sha, L.; Wang, S.; Tao, L.; Yao, L.; He, M.; Yao, Z.; Liu, H.; Zhu, Z.; *et al.* (−)-Epigallocatechin-3-gallate ameliorates learning and memory deficits by adjusting the balance of TrkA/p75NTR signaling in APP/PS1 transgenic mice. *Mol. Neurobiol.* **2014**, *49*, 1350–1363. [CrossRef] [PubMed]
83. Lambert, J.D.; Kennett, M.J.; Sang, S.; Reuhl, K.R.; Ju, J.; Yang, C.S. Hepatotoxicity of high oral dose (−)-epigallocatechin-3-gallate in mice. *Food Chem. Toxicol.* **2010**, *48*, 409–416. [CrossRef] [PubMed]
84. Mazzanti, G.; Menniti-Ippolito, F.; Moro, P.A.; Cassetti, F.; Raschetti, R.; Santuccio, C.; Mastrangelo, S. Hepatotoxicity from green tea: A review of the literature and two unpublished cases. *Eur. J. Clin. Pharmacol.* **2009**, *65*, 331–341. [CrossRef] [PubMed]
85. Fahey, J.W.; Zalcmann, A.T.; Talalay, P. The chemical diversity and distribution of glucosinolates and isothiocyanates among plants. *Phytochemistry* **2001**, *56*, 5–51. [CrossRef]
86. Conaway, C.C.; Getahun, S.M.; Liebes, L.L.; Pusateri, D.J.; Topham, D.K.; Botero-Omary, M.; Chung, F.L. Disposition of glucosinolates and sulforaphane in humans after ingestion of steamed and fresh broccoli. *Nutr. Cancer* **2000**, *38*, 168–178. [CrossRef] [PubMed]
87. Song, L.; Thornalley, P.J. Effect of storage, processing and cooking on glucosinolate content of Brassica vegetables. *Food Chem. Toxicol.* **2007**, *45*, 216–224. [CrossRef] [PubMed]
88. Abdull Razis, A.F.; Bagatta, M.; de Nicola, G.R.; Iori, R.; Ioannides, C. Up-regulation of cytochrome P450 and phase II enzyme systems in rat precision-cut rat lung slices by the intact glucosinolates, glucoraphanin and glucoerucin. *Lung Cancer* **2011**, *71*, 298–305. [CrossRef] [PubMed]
89. Fimognari, C.; Nüsse, M.; Cesari, R.; Iori, R.; Cantelli-Forti, G.; Hrelia, P. Growth inhibition, cell-cycle arrest and apoptosis in human T-cell leukemia by the isothiocyanate sulforaphane. *Carcinogenesis* **2002**, *23*, 581–586. [CrossRef] [PubMed]
90. Hanschen, F.S.; Lamy, E.; Schreiner, M.; Rohn, S. Reactivity and stability of glucosinolates and their breakdown products in foods. *Angew. Chem. Int. Ed. Engl.* **2014**, *53*, 11430–11450. [CrossRef] [PubMed]
91. Dinkova-Kostova, A.T.; Kostov, R.V. Glucosinolates and isothiocyanates in health and disease. *Trends Mol. Med.* **2012**, *18*, 337–347. [CrossRef] [PubMed]
92. De Nicola, G.R.; Rollin, P.; Mazzon, E.; Iori, R. Novel gram-scale production of enantiopure R-sulforaphane from Tuscan black kale seeds. *Molecules* **2014**, *19*, 6975–6986. [CrossRef] [PubMed]

93. Vergara, F.; Wenzler, M.; Hansen, B.G.; Kliebenstein, D.J.; Halkier, B.A.; Gershenzon, J.; Schneider, B. Determination of the absolute configuration of the glucosinolate methyl sulfoxide group reveals a stereospecific biosynthesis of the side chain. *Phytochemistry* **2008**, *69*, 2737–2742. [CrossRef] [PubMed]

94. De Figueiredo, S.M.; Binda, N.S.; Nogueira-Machado, J.A.; Vieira-Filho, S.A.; Caligiorne, R.B. The antioxidant properties of organosulfur compounds (sulforaphane). *Recent Pat. Endocr. Metab. Immune Drug Discov.* **2015**, *9*, 24–39. [CrossRef] [PubMed]

95. Giacoppo, S.; Galuppo, M.; Montaut, S.; Iori, R.; Rollin, P.; Bramanti, P.; Mazzon, E. An overview on neuroprotective effects of isothiocyanates for the treatment of neurodegenerative diseases. *Fitoterapia* **2015**, *106*, 12–21. [CrossRef] [PubMed]

96. Tarozzi, A.; Angeloni, C.; Malaguti, M.; Morroni, F.; Hrelia, S.; Hrelia, P. Sulforaphane as a potential protective phytochemical against neurodegenerative diseases. *Oxid. Med. Cell. Longev.* **2013**, *2013*. [CrossRef] [PubMed]

97. Jazwa, A.; Rojo, A.I.; Innamorato, N.G.; Hesse, M.; Fernández-Ruiz, J.; Cuadrado, A. Pharmacological targeting of the transcription factor Nrf2 at the basal ganglia provides disease modifying therapy for experimental parkinsonism. *Antioxid. Redox Signal.* **2011**, *14*, 2347–2360. [CrossRef] [PubMed]

98. Giacoppo, S.; Galuppo, M.; Iori, R.; de Nicola, G.R.; Bramanti, P.; Mazzon, E. The protective effects of bioactive (RS)-glucoraphanin on the permeability of the mice blood-brain barrier following experimental autoimmune encephalomyelitis. *Eur. Rev. Med. Pharmacol. Sci.* **2014**, *18*, 194–204. [PubMed]

99. Galuppo, M.; Giacoppo, S.; de Nicola, G.R.; Iori, R.; Mazzon, E.; Bramanti, P. RS-Glucoraphanin bioactivated with myrosinase treatment counteracts proinflammatory cascade and apoptosis associated to spinal cord injury in an experimental mouse model. *J. Neurol. Sci.* **2013**, *334*, 88–96. [CrossRef] [PubMed]

100. Giacoppo, S.; Galuppo, M.; Iori, R.; de Nicola, G.R.; Cassata, G.; Bramanti, P.; Mazzon, E. Protective role of (RS)-glucoraphanin bioactivated with myrosinase in an experimental model of multiple sclerosis. *CNS Neurosci. Ther.* **2013**, *19*, 577–584. [CrossRef] [PubMed]

101. Galuppo, M.; Iori, R.; de Nicola, G.R.; Bramanti, P.; Mazzon, E. Anti-inflammatory and anti-apoptotic effects of (RS)-glucoraphanin bioactivated with myrosinase in murine sub-acute and acute MPTP-induced Parkinson's disease. *Bioorg. Med. Chem.* **2013**, *21*, 5532–5547. [CrossRef] [PubMed]

102. Lee, C.; Park, G.H.; Lee, S.-R.; Jang, J.-H. Attenuation of β-amyloid-induced oxidative cell death by sulforaphane via activation of NF-E2-related factor 2. *Oxid. Med. Cell. Longev.* **2013**, *2013*. [CrossRef] [PubMed]

103. Park, H.-M.; Kim, J.-A.; Kwak, M.-K. Protection against amyloid beta cytotoxicity by sulforaphane: Role of the proteasome. *Arch. Pharm. Res.* **2009**, *32*, 109–115. [CrossRef] [PubMed]

104. Gan, N.; Wu, Y.-C.; Brunet, M.; Garrido, C.; Chung, F.-L.; Dai, C.; Mi, L. Sulforaphane activates heat shock response and enhances proteasome activity through up-regulation of Hsp27. *J. Biol. Chem.* **2010**, *285*, 35528–35536. [CrossRef] [PubMed]

105. Sherman, M.Y.; Goldberg, A.L. Cellular defenses against unfolded proteins: A cell biologist thinks about neurodegenerative diseases. *Neuron* **2001**, *29*, 15–32. [CrossRef]

106. Kwak, M.-K.; Cho, J.-M.; Huang, B.; Shin, S.; Kensler, T.W. Role of increased expression of the proteasome in the protective effects of sulforaphane against hydrogen peroxide-mediated cytotoxicity in murine neuroblastoma cells. *Free Radic. Biol. Med.* **2007**, *43*, 809–817. [CrossRef] [PubMed]

107. Brandenburg, L.-O.; Kipp, M.; Lucius, R.; Pufe, T.; Wruck, C.J. Sulforaphane suppresses LPS-induced inflammation in primary rat microglia. *Inflamm. Res.* **2010**, *59*, 443–450. [CrossRef] [PubMed]

108. Zhang, R.; Zhang, J.; Fang, L.; Li, X.; Zhao, Y.; Shi, W.; An, L. Neuroprotective effects of sulforaphane on cholinergic neurons in mice with Alzheimer's disease-like lesions. *Int. J. Mol. Sci.* **2014**, *15*, 14396–14410. [CrossRef] [PubMed]

109. Zhang, R.; Miao, Q.-W.; Zhu, C.-X.; Zhao, Y.; Liu, L.; Yang, J.; An, L. Sulforaphane ameliorates neurobehavioral deficits and protects the brain from amyloid β deposits and peroxidation in mice with Alzheimer-like lesions. *Am. J. Alzheimers Dis. Other Demen.* **2015**, *30*, 183–191. [CrossRef] [PubMed]

110. Lee, S.; Kim, J.; Seo, S.G.; Choi, B.-R.; Han, J.-S.; Lee, K.W.; Kim, J. Sulforaphane alleviates scopolamine-induced memory impairment in mice. *Pharmacol. Res.* **2014**, *85*, 23–32. [CrossRef] [PubMed]

111. Molchan, S.E.; Martinez, R.A.; Hill, J.L.; Weingartner, H.J.; Thompson, K.; Vitiello, B.; Sunderland, T. Increased cognitive sensitivity to scopolamine with age and a perspective on the scopolamine model. *Brain Res. Brain Res. Rev.* *17*, 215–226.

112. Dwivedi, S.; Rajasekar, N.; Hanif, K.; Nath, C.; Shukla, R. Sulforaphane Ameliorates Okadaic Acid-Induced Memory Impairment in Rats by Activating the Nrf2/HO-1 Antioxidant Pathway. *Mol. Neurobiol.* **2015**. [CrossRef] [PubMed]
113. Kamat, P.K.; Rai, S.; Swarnkar, S.; Shukla, R.; Nath, C. Molecular and cellular mechanism of okadaic acid (OKA)-induced neurotoxicity: A novel tool for Alzheimer's disease therapeutic application. *Mol. Neurobiol.* **2014**, *50*, 852–865. [CrossRef] [PubMed]
114. Abdull Razis, A.F.; Ibrahim, M.D.; Kntayya, S.B. Health benefits of *Moringa oleifera*. *Asian Pac. J. Cancer Prev.* **2014**, *15*, 8571–8576. [CrossRef] [PubMed]
115. Bennett, R.N.; Mellon, F.A.; Foidl, N.; Pratt, J.H.; Dupont, M.S.; Perkins, L.; Kroon, P.A. Profiling glucosinolates and phenolics in vegetative and reproductive tissues of the multi-purpose trees *Moringa oleifera* L. (horseradish tree) and *Moringa stenopetala* L. *J. Agric. Food Chem.* **2003**, *51*, 3546–3553. [CrossRef] [PubMed]
116. Galuppo, M.; Giacoppo, S.; de Nicola, G.R.; Iori, R.; Navarra, M.; Lombardo, G.E.; Bramanti, P.; Mazzon, E. Antiinflammatory activity of glucomoringin isothiocyanate in a mouse model of experimental autoimmune encephalomyelitis. *Fitoterapia* **2014**, *95*, 160–174. [CrossRef] [PubMed]
117. Galuppo, M.; Giacoppo, S.; Iori, R.; de Nicola, G.R.; Milardi, D.; Bramanti, P.; Mazzon, E. 4(α-L-rhamnosyloxy)-benzyl isothiocyanate, a bioactive phytochemical that defends cerebral tissue and prevents severe damage induced by focal ischemia/reperfusion. *J. Biol. Regul. Homeost. Agents* **2015**, *29*, 343–356. [PubMed]
118. Giacoppo, S.; Galuppo, M.; de Nicola, G.R.; Iori, R.; Bramanti, P.; Mazzon, E. 4(α-L-rhamnosyloxy)-benzyl isothiocyanate, a bioactive phytochemical that attenuates secondary damage in an experimental model of spinal cord injury. *Bioorg. Med. Chem.* **2015**, *23*, 80–88. [CrossRef] [PubMed]
119. Sutalangka, C.; Wattanathorn, J.; Muchimapura, S.; Thukham-Mee, W. *Moringa oleifera* mitigates memory impairment and neurodegeneration in animal model of age-related dementia. *Oxid. Med. Cell. Longev.* **2013**, *2013*. [CrossRef] [PubMed]
120. Ganguly, R.; Guha, D. Alteration of brain monoamines & EEG wave pattern in rat model of Alzheimer's disease & protection by *Moringa oleifera*. *Indian J. Med. Res.* **2008**, *128*, 744–751. [PubMed]
121. Ganguly, R.; Hazra, R.; Ray, K.; Guha, D. Effect of *Moringa oleifera* in Experimental Model of Alzheimer's Disease: Role of Antioxidants. *Ann. Neurosci.* **2005**, *12*, 33–36. [CrossRef]
122. Preininger, V.; Thakur, R.S.; Santavý, F. Isolation and chemistry of alkaloids from plants of the family Papaveraceae LXVII: *Corydalis cava* (L.) Sch. et K. (*C. tuberosa* DC). *J. Pharm. Sci.* **1976**, *65*, 294–296. [CrossRef] [PubMed]
123. Schläger, S.; Dräger, B. Exploiting plant alkaloids. *Curr. Opin. Biotechnol.* **2015**, *37*, 155–164. [CrossRef] [PubMed]
124. Mukherjee, P.K.; Satheeshkumar, N.; Venkatesh, P.; Venkatesh, M. Lead finding for acetyl cholinesterase inhibitors from natural origin: Structure activity relationship and scope. *Mini Rev. Med. Chem.* **2011**, *11*, 247–262. [CrossRef] [PubMed]
125. Konrath, E.L.; Passos, C.; Dos, S.; Klein, L.C.; Henriques, A.T. Alkaloids as a source of potential anticholinesterase inhibitors for the treatment of Alzheimer's disease. *J. Pharm. Pharmacol.* **2013**, *65*, 1701–1725. [CrossRef] [PubMed]
126. Mehta, M.; Adem, A.; Sabbagh, M. New acetylcholinesterase inhibitors for Alzheimer's disease. *Int. J. Alzheimers. Dis.* **2012**, *2012*. [CrossRef] [PubMed]
127. Kurz, A.; Farlow, M.; Lefèvre, G. Pharmacokinetics of a novel transdermal rivastigmine patch for the treatment of Alzheimer's disease: A review. *Int. J. Clin. Pract.* **2009**, *63*, 799–805. [CrossRef] [PubMed]
128. Schneider, S.L. A critical review of cholinesterase inhibitors as a treatment modality in Alzheimer's disease. *Dialogues Clin. Neurosci.* **2000**, *2*, 111–128.
129. Cummings, J.; Winblad, B. A rivastigmine patch for the treatment of Alzheimer's disease and Parkinson's disease dementia. *Expert Rev. Neurother.* **2007**, *7*, 1457–1463. [CrossRef] [PubMed]
130. Boot, B.P. Comprehensive treatment of dementia with Lewy bodies. *Alzheimers. Res. Ther.* **2015**, *7*. [CrossRef] [PubMed]
131. Birks, J.S.; Chong, L.Y.; Grimley Evans, J. Rivastigmine for Alzheimer's disease. *Cochrane Database Syst. Rev.* **2015**, *9*. [CrossRef]

132. Matsuzono, K.; Sato, K.; Kono, S.; Hishikawa, N.; Ohta, Y.; Yamashita, T.; Deguchi, K.; Nakano, Y.; Abe, K. Clinical Benefits of Rivastigmine in the Real World Dementia Clinics of the Okayama Rivastigmine Study (ORS). *J. Alzheimers. Dis.* **2015**, *48*, 757–763. [CrossRef] [PubMed]
133. Ehret, M.J.; Chamberlin, K.W. Current Practices in the Treatment of Alzheimer Disease: Where is the Evidence After the Phase III Trials? *Clin. Ther.* **2015**, *37*, 1604–1616. [CrossRef] [PubMed]
134. Spalletta, G.; Gianni, W.; Giubilei, F.; Casini, A.R.; Sancesario, G.; Caltagirone, C.; Cravello, L. Rivastigmine patch ameliorates depression in mild AD: Preliminary evidence from a 6-month open-label observational study. *Alzheimer Dis. Assoc. Disord.* **2013**, *27*, 289–291. [CrossRef] [PubMed]
135. Servello, A.; Andreozzi, P.; Bechini, F.; de Angelis, R.; Pontecorvo, M.L.; Vulcano, A.; Cerra, E.; Vigliotta, M.T.; Artini, M.; Selan, L.; *et al.* Effect of AChE and BuChE inhibition by rivastigmin in a group of old-old elderly patients with cerebrovascular impairment (SIVD type). *Minerva Med.* **2014**, *105*, 167–174. [PubMed]
136. Birks, J.; McGuinness, B.; Craig, D. Rivastigmine for vascular cognitive impairment. *Cochrane Database Syst. Rev.* **2013**, *5*. [CrossRef]
137. Ringman, J.M.; Cummings, J.L. Current and emerging pharmacological treatment options for dementia. *Behav. Neurol.* **2006**, *17*, 5–16. [CrossRef] [PubMed]
138. Stinton, C.; McKeith, I.; Taylor, J.-P.; Lafortune, L.; Mioshi, E.; Mak, E.; Cambridge, V.; Mason, J.; Thomas, A.; O'Brien, J.T. Pharmacological Management of Lewy Body Dementia: A Systematic Review and Meta-Analysis. *Am. J. Psychiatry* **2015**, *172*, 731–742. [CrossRef] [PubMed]
139. Heinrich, M.; Lee Teoh, H. Galanthamine from snowdrop—The development of a modern drug against Alzheimer's disease from local Caucasian knowledge. *J. Ethnopharmacol.* **2004**, *92*, 147–162. [CrossRef] [PubMed]
140. Koola, M.M.; Buchanan, R.W.; Pillai, A.; Aitchison, K.J.; Weinberger, D.R.; Aaronson, S.T.; Dickerson, F.B. Potential role of the combination of galantamine and memantine to improve cognition in schizophrenia. *Schizophr. Res.* **2014**, *157*, 84–89. [CrossRef] [PubMed]
141. Wilcock, G.K.; Lilienfeld, S.; Gaens, E. Efficacy and safety of galantamine in patients with mild to moderate Alzheimer's disease: Multicentre randomised controlled trial. Galantamine International-1 Study Group. *BMJ* **2000**, *321*, 1445–1449. [CrossRef] [PubMed]
142. Schneider, L.S.; Mangialasche, F.; Andreasen, N.; Feldman, H.; Giacobini, E.; Jones, R.; Mantua, V.; Mecocci, P.; Pani, L.; Winblad, B.; *et al.* Clinical trials and late-stage drug development for Alzheimer's disease: An appraisal from 1984 to 2014. *J. Intern. Med.* **2014**, *275*, 251–283. [CrossRef] [PubMed]
143. Miranda, L.F.J.R.; Gomes, K.B.; Silveira, J.N.; Pianetti, G.A.; Byrro, R.M.D.; Peles, P.R.H.; Pereira, F.H.; Santos, T.R.; Assini, A.G.; Ribeiro, V.; *et al.* Predictive factors of clinical response to cholinesterase inhibitors in mild and moderate Alzheimer's disease and mixed dementia: A one-year naturalistic study. *J. Alzheimers Dis.* **2015**, *45*, 609–620. [PubMed]
144. Richarz, U.; Gaudig, M.; Rettig, K.; Schauble, B. Galantamine treatment in outpatients with mild Alzheimer's disease. *Acta Neurol. Scand.* **2014**, *129*, 382–392. [CrossRef] [PubMed]
145. Naharci, M.I.; Ozturk, A.; Yasar, H.; Cintosun, U.; Kocak, N.; Bozoglu, E.; Tasci, I.; Doruk, H. Galantamine improves sleep quality in patients with dementia. *Acta Neurol. Belg.* **2015**, *115*, 563–568. [CrossRef] [PubMed]
146. Matharu, B.; Gibson, G.; Parsons, R.; Huckerby, T.N.; Moore, S.A.; Cooper, L.J.; Millichamp, R.; Allsop, D.; Austen, B. Galantamine inhibits beta-amyloid aggregation and cytotoxicity. *J. Neurol. Sci.* **2009**, *280*, 49–58. [CrossRef] [PubMed]
147. Melo, J.B.; Sousa, C.; Garção, P.; Oliveira, C.R.; Agostinho, P. Galantamine protects against oxidative stress induced by amyloid-beta peptide in cortical neurons. *Eur. J. Neurosci.* **2009**, *29*, 455–464. [CrossRef] [PubMed]
148. Tsvetkova, D.; Obreshkova, D.; Zheleva-Dimitrova, D.; Saso, L. Antioxidant activity of galantamine and some of its derivatives. *Curr. Med. Chem.* **2013**, *20*, 4595–4608. [CrossRef] [PubMed]
149. Ezoulin, M.J.M.; Ombetta, J.-E.; Dutertre-Catella, H.; Warnet, J.-M.; Massicot, F. Antioxidative properties of galantamine on neuronal damage induced by hydrogen peroxide in SK-N-SH cells. *Neurotoxicology* **2008**, *29*, 270–277. [CrossRef] [PubMed]
150. Birks, J.; Craig, D. Galantamine for vascular cognitive impairment. *Cochrane Database Syst. Rev.* **2013**, *4*. [CrossRef]
151. Auchus, A.P.; Brashear, H.R.; Salloway, S.; Korczyn, A.D.; de Deyn, P.P.; Gassmann-Mayer, C. Galantamine treatment of vascular dementia: A randomized trial. *Neurology* **2007**, *69*, 448–458. [CrossRef] [PubMed]

152. Edwards, K.; Royall, D.; Hershey, L.; Lichter, D.; Hake, A.; Farlow, M.; Pasquier, F.; Johnson, S. Efficacy and safety of galantamine in patients with dementia with Lewy bodies: A 24-week open-label study. *Dement. Geriatr. Cogn. Disord.* **2007**, *23*, 401–405. [CrossRef]
153. O'Brien, J.T.; Burns, A. Clinical practice with anti-dementia drugs: A revised (second) consensus statement from the British Association for Psychopharmacology. *J. Psychopharmacol.* **2011**, *25*, 997–1019. [CrossRef] [PubMed]
154. Kertesz, A.; Morlog, D.; Light, M.; Blair, M.; Davidson, W.; Jesso, S.; Brashear, R. Galantamine in frontotemporal dementia and primary progressive aphasia. *Dement. Geriatr. Cogn. Disord.* **2008**, *25*, 178–185. [CrossRef] [PubMed]
155. Chen, Y.-D.; Zhang, J.; Wang, Y.; Yuan, J.-L.; Hu, W.-L. Efficacy of Cholinesterase Inhibitors in Vascular Dementia: An Updated Meta-Analysis. *Eur. Neurol.* **2016**, *75*, 132–141. [CrossRef] [PubMed]
156. Schug, S.A.; Zech, D.; Dörr, U. Cancer pain management according to WHO analgesic guidelines. *J. Pain Symptom Manag.* **1990**, *5*, 27–32. [CrossRef]
157. Cui, J.; Wang, Y.; Dong, Q.; Wu, S.; Xiao, X.; Hu, J.; Chai, Z.; Zhang, Y. Morphine protects against intracellular amyloid toxicity by inducing estradiol release and upregulation of Hsp70. *J. Neurosci.* **2011**, *31*, 16227–16240. [CrossRef] [PubMed]
158. Wang, Y.; Wang, Y.-X.; Liu, T.; Law, P.-Y.; Loh, H.H.; Qiu, Y.; Chen, H.-Z. μ-Opioid receptor attenuates Aβ oligomers-induced neurotoxicity through mTOR signaling. *CNS Neurosci. Ther.* **2015**, *21*, 8–14. [CrossRef] [PubMed]
159. Swiech, L.; Perycz, M.; Malik, A.; Jaworski, J. Role of mTOR in physiology and pathology of the nervous system. *Biochim. Biophys. Acta* **2008**, *1784*, 116–132. [CrossRef] [PubMed]
160. Parsons, R.G.; Gafford, G.M.; Helmstetter, F.J. Translational control via the mammalian target of rapamycin pathway is critical for the formation and stability of long-term fear memory in amygdala neurons. *J. Neurosci.* **2006**, *26*, 12977–12983. [CrossRef] [PubMed]
161. Husebo, B.S.; Ballard, C.; Cohen-Mansfield, J.; Seifert, R.; Aarsland, D. The response of agitated behavior to pain management in persons with dementia. *Am. J. Geriatr. Psychiatry* **2014**, *22*, 708–717. [CrossRef] [PubMed]
162. Husebo, B.S.; Ballard, C.; Sandvik, R.; Nilsen, O.B.; Aarsland, D. Efficacy of treating pain to reduce behavioural disturbances in residents of nursing homes with dementia: Cluster randomised clinical trial. *BMJ* **2011**, *343*. [CrossRef] [PubMed]
163. Haller, S.; Rodriguez, C.; Moser, D.; Toma, S.; Hofmeister, J.; Sinanaj, I.; van de Ville, D.; Giannakopoulos, P.; Lovblad, K.-O. Acute caffeine administration impact on working memory-related brain activation and functional connectivity in the elderly: A BOLD and perfusion MRI study. *Neuroscience* **2013**, *250*, 364–371. [CrossRef] [PubMed]
164. Palacios, N.; Gao, X.; McCullough, M.L.; Schwarzschild, M.A.; Shah, R.; Gapstur, S.; Ascherio, A. Caffeine and risk of Parkinson's disease in a large cohort of men and women. *Mov. Disord.* **2012**, *27*, 1276–1282. [CrossRef] [PubMed]
165. Ross, G.W.; Abbott, R.D.; Petrovitch, H.; Morens, D.M.; Grandinetti, A.; Tung, K.H.; Tanner, C.M.; Masaki, K.H.; Blanchette, P.L.; Curb, J.D.; *et al.* Association of coffee and caffeine intake with the risk of Parkinson disease. *JAMA* **2000**, *283*, 2674–2679. [CrossRef] [PubMed]
166. Ascherio, A.; Zhang, S.M.; Hernán, M.A.; Kawachi, I.; Colditz, G.A.; Speizer, F.E.; Willett, W.C. Prospective study of caffeine consumption and risk of Parkinson's disease in men and women. *Ann. Neurol.* **2001**, *50*, 56–63. [CrossRef] [PubMed]
167. Maia, L.; de Mendonça, A. Does caffeine intake protect from Alzheimer's disease? *Eur. J. Neurol.* **2002**, *9*, 377–382. [CrossRef] [PubMed]
168. Ritchie, K.; Carrière, I.; de Mendonca, A.; Portet, F.; Dartigues, J.F.; Rouaud, O.; Barberger-Gateau, P.; Ancelin, M.L. The neuroprotective effects of caffeine: A prospective population study (the Three City Study). *Neurology* **2007**, *69*, 536–545. [CrossRef] [PubMed]
169. Cao, C.; Loewenstein, D.A.; Lin, X.; Zhang, C.; Wang, L.; Duara, R.; Wu, Y.; Giannini, A.; Bai, G.; Cai, J.; *et al.* High Blood caffeine levels in MCI linked to lack of progression to dementia. *J. Alzheimers Dis.* **2012**, *30*, 559–572. [PubMed]

170. Laurent, C.; Eddarkaoui, S.; Derisbourg, M.; Leboucher, A.; Demeyer, D.; Carrier, S.; Schneider, M.; Hamdane, M.; Müller, C.E.; Buée, L.; *et al.* Beneficial effects of caffeine in a transgenic model of Alzheimer's disease-like tau pathology. *Neurobiol. Aging* **2014**, *35*, 2079–2090. [CrossRef] [PubMed]
171. Arendash, G.W.; Schleif, W.; Rezai-Zadeh, K.; Jackson, E.K.; Zacharia, L.C.; Cracchiolo, J.R.; Shippy, D.; Tan, J. Caffeine protects Alzheimer's mice against cognitive impairment and reduces brain beta-amyloid production. *Neuroscience* **2006**, *142*, 941–952. [CrossRef] [PubMed]
172. Arendash, G.W.; Mori, T.; Cao, C.; Mamcarz, M.; Runfeldt, M.; Dickson, A.; Rezai-Zadeh, K.; Tane, J.; Citron, B.A.; Lin, X.; *et al.* Caffeine reverses cognitive impairment and decreases brain amyloid-beta levels in aged Alzheimer's disease mice. *J. Alzheimers Dis.* **2009**, *17*, 661–680. [PubMed]
173. Han, K.; Jia, N.; Li, J.; Yang, L.; Min, L.-Q. Chronic caffeine treatment reverses memory impairment and the expression of brain BNDF and TrkB in the PS1/APP double transgenic mouse model of Alzheimer's disease. *Mol. Med. Rep.* **2013**, *8*, 737–740. [PubMed]
174. Nagahara, A.H.; Merrill, D.A.; Coppola, G.; Tsukada, S.; Schroeder, B.E.; Shaked, G.M.; Wang, L.; Blesch, A.; Kim, A.; Conner, J.M.; *et al.* Neuroprotective effects of brain-derived neurotrophic factor in rodent and primate models of Alzheimer's disease. *Nat. Med.* **2009**, *15*, 331–337. [CrossRef] [PubMed]
175. Prasanthi, J.R.P.; Dasari, B.; Marwarha, G.; Larson, T.; Chen, X.; Geiger, J.D.; Ghribi, O. Caffeine protects against oxidative stress and Alzheimer's disease-like pathology in rabbit hippocampus induced by cholesterol-enriched diet. *Free Radic. Biol. Med.* **2010**, *49*, 1212–1220. [CrossRef] [PubMed]
176. Eskelinen, M.H.; Ngandu, T.; Tuomilehto, J.; Soininen, H.; Kivipelto, M. Midlife coffee and tea drinking and the risk of late-life dementia: A population-based CAIDE study. *J. Alzheimers Dis.* **2009**, *16*, 85–91. [PubMed]
177. Kim, Y.-S.; Kwak, S.M.; Myung, S.-K. Caffeine intake from coffee or tea and cognitive disorders: A meta-analysis of observational studies. *Neuroepidemiology* **2015**, *44*, 51–63. [CrossRef] [PubMed]
178. Gelber, R.P.; Petrovitch, H.; Masaki, K.H.; Ross, G.W.; White, L.R. Coffee intake in midlife and risk of dementia and its neuropathologic correlates. *J. Alzheimers Dis.* **2011**, *23*, 607–615. [PubMed]
179. Picciotto, M.R.; Zoli, M. Nicotinic receptors in aging and dementia. *J. Neurobiol.* **2002**, *53*, 641–655. [CrossRef] [PubMed]
180. Echeverria, V.; Yarkov, A.; Aliev, G. Positive modulators of the $\alpha 7$ nicotinic receptor against neuroinflammation and cognitive impairment in Alzheimer's disease. *Prog. Neurobiol.* **2016**. [CrossRef] [PubMed]
181. Kihara, T.; Shimohama, S.; Sawada, H.; Kimura, J.; Kume, T.; Kochiyama, H.; Maeda, T.; Akaike, A. Nicotinic receptor stimulation protects neurons against beta-amyloid toxicity. *Ann. Neurol.* **1997**, *42*, 159–163. [CrossRef] [PubMed]
182. Ono, K.; Hasegawa, K.; Yamada, M.; Naiki, H. Nicotine breaks down preformed Alzheimer's beta-amyloid fibrils *in vitro*. *Biol. Psychiatry* **2002**, *52*, 880–886. [CrossRef]
183. Buckingham, S.D.; Jones, A.K.; Brown, L.A.; Sattelle, D.B. Nicotinic acetylcholine receptor signalling: Roles in Alzheimer's disease and amyloid neuroprotection. *Pharmacol. Rev.* **2009**, *61*, 39–61. [CrossRef] [PubMed]
184. Moore, S.A.; Huckerby, T.N.; Gibson, G.L.; Fullwood, N.J.; Turnbull, S.; Tabner, B.J.; El-Agnaf, O.M.A.; Allsop, D. Both the D-(+) and L-(−) enantiomers of nicotine inhibit Abeta aggregation and cytotoxicity. *Biochemistry* **2004**, *43*, 819–826. [CrossRef] [PubMed]
185. Srivareerat, M.; Tran, T.T.; Salim, S.; Aleisa, A.M.; Alkadhi, K.A. Chronic nicotine restores normal Aβ levels and prevents short-term memory and E-LTP impairment in Aβ rat model of Alzheimer's disease. *Neurobiol. Aging* **2011**, *32*, 834–844. [CrossRef] [PubMed]
186. Shim, S.B.; Lee, S.H.; Chae, K.R.; Kim, C.K.; Hwang, D.Y.; Kim, B.G.; Jee, S.W.; Lee, S.H.; Sin, J.S.; Bae, C.J.; *et al.* Nicotine leads to improvements in behavioral impairment and an increase in the nicotine acetylcholine receptor in transgenic mice. *Neurochem. Res.* **2008**, *33*, 1783–1788. [CrossRef] [PubMed]
187. Hernandez, C.M.; Terry, A. V Repeated nicotine exposure in rats: Effects on memory function, cholinergic markers and nerve growth factor. *Neuroscience* **2005**, *130*, 997–1012. [CrossRef] [PubMed]
188. Oddo, S.; Caccamo, A.; Green, K.N.; Liang, K.; Tran, L.; Chen, Y.; Leslie, F.M.; LaFerla, F.M. Chronic nicotine administration exacerbates tau pathology in a transgenic model of Alzheimer's disease. *Proc. Natl. Acad. Sci. USA* **2005**, *102*, 3046–3051. [CrossRef] [PubMed]
189. Deng, J.; Shen, C.; Wang, Y.-J.; Zhang, M.; Li, J.; Xu, Z.-Q.; Gao, C.-Y.; Fang, C.-Q.; Zhou, H.-D. Nicotine exacerbates tau phosphorylation and cognitive impairment induced by amyloid-beta 25-35 in rats. *Eur. J. Pharmacol.* **2010**, *637*, 83–88. [CrossRef] [PubMed]

190. Ono, K.; Hirohata, M.; Yamada, M. Anti-fibrillogenic and fibril-destabilizing activity of nicotine *in vitro*: Implications for the prevention and therapeutics of Lewy body diseases. *Exp. Neurol.* **2007**, *205*, 414–424. [CrossRef] [PubMed]
191. White, H.K.; Levin, E.D. Chronic transdermal nicotine patch treatment effects on cognitive performance in age-associated memory impairment. *Psychopharmacology* **2004**, *171*, 465–471. [CrossRef] [PubMed]
192. Newhouse, P.; Kellar, K.; Aisen, P.; White, H.; Wesnes, K.; Coderre, E.; Pfaff, A.; Wilkins, H.; Howard, D.; Levin, E.D. Nicotine treatment of mild cognitive impairment: A 6-month double-blind pilot clinical trial. *Neurology* **2012**, *78*, 91–101. [CrossRef] [PubMed]
193. Ma, X.; Tan, C.; Zhu, D.; Gang, D.R.; Xiao, P. Huperzine A from Huperzia species—An ethnopharmacolgical review. *J. Ethnopharmacol.* **2007**, *113*, 15–34. [CrossRef] [PubMed]
194. Xing, S.-H.; Zhu, C.-X.; Zhang, R.; An, L. Huperzine a in the treatment of Alzheimer's disease and vascular dementia: A meta-analysis. *Evid. Based Complement. Altern. Med.* **2014**, *2014*. [CrossRef] [PubMed]
195. Tang, L.-L.; Wang, R.; Tang, X.-C. Huperzine A protects SHSY5Y neuroblastoma cells against oxidative stress damage via nerve growth factor production. *Eur. J. Pharmacol.* **2005**, *519*, 9–15. [CrossRef] [PubMed]
196. Xiao, X.Q.; Wang, R.; Han, Y.F.; Tang, X.C. Protective effects of huperzine A on beta-amyloid(25-35) induced oxidative injury in rat pheochromocytoma cells. *Neurosci. Lett.* **2000**, *286*, 155–158. [CrossRef]
197. Gao, X.; Tang, X.C. Huperzine A attenuates mitochondrial dysfunction in beta-amyloid-treated PC12 cells by reducing oxygen free radicals accumulation and improving mitochondrial energy metabolism. *J. Neurosci. Res.* **2006**, *83*, 1048–1057. [CrossRef] [PubMed]
198. Xiao, X.Q.; Zhang, H.Y.; Tang, X.C. Huperzine A attenuates amyloid beta-peptide fragment 25-35-induced apoptosis in rat cortical neurons via inhibiting reactive oxygen species formation and caspase-3 activation. *J. Neurosci. Res.* **2002**, *67*, 30–36. [CrossRef] [PubMed]
199. Wang, R.; Yan, H.; Tang, X. Progress in studies of huperzine A, a natural cholinesterase inhibitor from Chinese herbal medicine. *Acta Pharmacol. Sin.* **2006**, *27*. [CrossRef] [PubMed]
200. Wang, H.; Tang, X.C. Anticholinesterase effects of huperzine A, E2020, and tacrine in rats. *Zhongguo Yao Li Xue Bao* **1998**, *19*, 27–30. [PubMed]
201. Ma, T.; Gong, K.; Yan, Y.; Zhang, L.; Tang, P.; Zhang, X.; Gong, Y. Huperzine A promotes hippocampal neurogenesis *in vitro* and *in vivo*. *Brain Res.* **2013**, *1506*, 35–43. [CrossRef] [PubMed]
202. Wang, R.; Zhang, H.Y.; Tang, X.C. Huperzine A attenuates cognitive dysfunction and neuronal degeneration caused by beta-amyloid protein-(1-40) in rat. *Eur. J. Pharmacol.* **2001**, *421*, 149–156. [CrossRef]
203. Zhang, H.Y.; Yan, H.; Tang, X.C. Huperzine A enhances the level of secretory amyloid precursor protein and protein kinase C-alpha in intracerebroventricular beta-amyloid-(1-40) infused rats and human embryonic kidney 293 Swedish mutant cells. *Neurosci. Lett.* **2004**, *360*, 21–24. [CrossRef] [PubMed]
204. Yang, G.; Wang, Y.; Tian, J.; Liu, J.-P. Huperzine A for Alzheimer's disease: A systematic review and meta-analysis of randomized clinical trials. *PLoS ONE* **2013**, *8*, e74916. [CrossRef] [PubMed]
205. Xu, Z.-Q.; Liang, X.-M.; Wu, J.; Zhang, Y.-F.; Zhu, C.-X.; Jiang, X.-J. Treatment with Huperzine A improves cognition in vascular dementia patients. *Cell Biochem. Biophys.* **2012**, *62*, 55–58. [CrossRef] [PubMed]
206. Hao, Z.; Liu, M.; Liu, Z.; Lv, D. Huperzine A for vascular dementia. *Cochrane Database Syst. Rev.* **2009**. [CrossRef]
207. Racková, L.; Májeková, M.; Kost'álová, D.; Stefek, M. Antiradical and antioxidant activities of alkaloids isolated from *Mahonia aquifolium*. Structural aspects. *Bioorg. Med. Chem.* **2004**, *12*, 4709–4715. [CrossRef] [PubMed]
208. Küpeli, E.; Koşar, M.; Yeşilada, E.; Hüsnü, K.; Başer, C. A comparative study on the anti-inflammatory, antinociceptive and antipyretic effects of isoquinoline alkaloids from the roots of Turkish Berberis species. *Life Sci.* **2002**, *72*, 645–657. [CrossRef]
209. Kettmann, V.; Kosfálová, D.; Jantová, S.; Cernáková, M.; Drímal, J. *In vitro* cytotoxicity of berberine against HeLa and L1210 cancer cell lines. *Pharmazie* **2004**, *59*, 548–551. [PubMed]
210. Tran, Q.L.; Tezuka, Y.; Ueda, J.; Nguyen, N.T.; Maruyama, Y.; Begum, K.; Kim, H.-S.; Wataya, Y.; Tran, Q.K.; Kadota, S. *In vitro* antiplasmodial activity of antimalarial medicinal plants used in Vietnamese traditional medicine. *J. Ethnopharmacol.* **2003**, *86*, 249–252. [CrossRef]
211. Han, J.; Lin, H.; Huang, W. Modulating gut microbiota as an anti-diabetic mechanism of berberine. *Med. Sci. Monit.* **2011**, *17*, RA164–RA167. [CrossRef] [PubMed]

212. Shvarev, I.F.; Tsetlin, A.L. Anti-blastic properties of berberine and its derivatives. *Farmakol. Toksikol.* **1972**, *35*, 73–75. [PubMed]
213. Wang, X.; Wang, R.; Xing, D.; Su, H.; Ma, C.; Ding, Y.; Du, L. Kinetic difference of berberine between hippocampus and plasma in rat after intravenous administration of Coptidis rhizoma extract. *Life Sci.* **2005**, *77*, 3058–3067. [CrossRef] [PubMed]
214. Kulkarni, S.K.; Dhir, A. Berberine: A plant alkaloid with therapeutic potential for central nervous system disorders. *Phytother. Res.* **2010**, *24*, 317–324. [CrossRef] [PubMed]
215. Su, T.; Xie, S.; Wei, H.; Yan, J.; Huang, L.; Li, X. Synthesis and biological evaluation of berberine-thiophenyl hybrids as multi-functional agents: Inhibition of acetylcholinesterase, butyrylcholinesterase, and Aβ aggregation and antioxidant activity. *Bioorg. Med. Chem.* **2013**, *21*, 5830–5840. [CrossRef] [PubMed]
216. Huang, M.; Chen, S.; Liang, Y.; Guo, Y. The Role of Berberine in the Multi-Target Treatment of Senile Dementia. *Curr. Top. Med. Chem.* **2016**, *16*, 867–873. [CrossRef] [PubMed]
217. Kim, M.H.; Kim, S.-H.; Yang, W.M. Mechanisms of action of phytochemicals from medicinal herbs in the treatment of Alzheimer's disease. *Planta Med.* **2014**, *80*, 1249–1258. [PubMed]
218. Asai, M.; Iwata, N.; Yoshikawa, A.; Aizaki, Y.; Ishiura, S.; Saido, T.C.; Maruyama, K. Berberine alters the processing of Alzheimer's amyloid precursor protein to decrease Abeta secretion. *Biochem. Biophys. Res. Commun.* **2007**, *352*, 498–502. [CrossRef] [PubMed]
219. Zhu, F.; Wu, F.; Ma, Y.; Liu, G.; Li, Z.; Sun, Y.; Pei, Z. Decrease in the production of β-amyloid by berberine inhibition of the expression of β-secretase in HEK293 cells. *BMC Neurosci.* **2011**, *12*. [CrossRef] [PubMed]
220. Chen, J.-H.; Huang, S.-M.; Tan, T.-W.; Lin, H.-Y.; Chen, P.-Y.; Yeh, W.-L.; Chou, S.-C.; Tsai, C.-F.; Wei, I.-H.; Lu, D.-Y. Berberine induces heme oxygenase-1 up-regulation through phosphatidylinositol 3-kinase/AKT and NF-E2-related factor-2 signaling pathway in astrocytes. *Int. Immunopharmacol.* **2012**, *12*, 94–100. [CrossRef] [PubMed]
221. Jia, L.; Liu, J.; Song, Z.; Pan, X.; Chen, L.; Cui, X.; Wang, M. Berberine suppresses amyloid-beta-induced inflammatory response in microglia by inhibiting nuclear factor-kappaB and mitogen-activated protein kinase signalling pathways. *J. Pharm. Pharmacol.* **2012**, *64*, 1510–1521. [CrossRef] [PubMed]
222. Kwon, I.H.; Choi, H.S.; Shin, K.S.; Lee, B.K.; Lee, C.K.; Hwang, B.Y.; Lim, S.C.; Lee, M.K. Effects of berberine on 6-hydroxydopamine-induced neurotoxicity in PC12 cells and a rat model of Parkinson's disease. *Neurosci. Lett.* **2010**, *486*, 29–33. [CrossRef] [PubMed]
223. Yin, J.; Xing, H.; Ye, J. Efficacy of berberine in patients with type 2 diabetes mellitus. *Metabolism* **2008**, *57*, 712–717. [CrossRef] [PubMed]
224. Yan, H.-M.; Xia, M.-F.; Wang, Y.; Chang, X.-X.; Yao, X.-Z.; Rao, S.-X.; Zeng, M.-S.; Tu, Y.-F.; Feng, R.; Jia, W.-P.; *et al.* Efficacy of Berberine in Patients with Non-Alcoholic Fatty Liver Disease. *PLoS ONE* **2015**, *10*, e0134172. [CrossRef] [PubMed]
225. Chen, C.; Tao, C.; Liu, Z.; Lu, M.; Pan, Q.; Zheng, L.; Li, Q.; Song, Z.; Fichna, J. A Randomized Clinical Trial of Berberine Hydrochloride in Patients with Diarrhea-Predominant Irritable Bowel Syndrome. *Phytother. Res.* **2015**, *29*, 1822–1827. [CrossRef] [PubMed]
226. Russo, E.; Guy, G.W. A tale of two cannabinoids: The therapeutic rationale for combining tetrahydrocannabinol and cannabidiol. *Med. Hypotheses* **2006**, *66*, 234–246. [CrossRef] [PubMed]
227. Giacoppo, S.; Mandolino, G.; Galuppo, M.; Bramanti, P.; Mazzon, E. Cannabinoids: New promising agents in the treatment of neurological diseases. *Molecules* **2014**, *19*, 18781–18816. [CrossRef] [PubMed]
228. Esposito, G.; de Filippis, D.; Carnuccio, R.; Izzo, A.A.; Iuvone, T. The marijuana component cannabidiol inhibits beta-amyloid-induced tau protein hyperphosphorylation through Wnt/beta-catenin pathway rescue in PC12 cells. *J. Mol. Med.* **2006**, *84*, 253–258. [CrossRef] [PubMed]
229. Esposito, G.; de Filippis, D.; Maiuri, M.C.; de Stefano, D.; Carnuccio, R.; Iuvone, T. Cannabidiol inhibits inducible nitric oxide synthase protein expression and nitric oxide production in beta-amyloid stimulated PC12 neurons through p38 MAP kinase and NF-kappaB involvement. *Neurosci. Lett.* **2006**, *399*, 91–95. [CrossRef] [PubMed]
230. Iuvone, T.; Esposito, G.; Esposito, R.; Santamaria, R.; di Rosa, M.; Izzo, A.A. Neuroprotective effect of cannabidiol, a non-psychoactive component from *Cannabis sativa*, on beta-amyloid-induced toxicity in PC12 cells. *J. Neurochem.* **2004**, *89*, 134–141. [CrossRef] [PubMed]

231. Esposito, G.; de Filippis, D.; Steardo, L.; Scuderi, C.; Savani, C.; Cuomo, V.; Iuvone, T. CB1 receptor selective activation inhibits beta-amyloid-induced iNOS protein expression in C6 cells and subsequently blunts tau protein hyperphosphorylation in co-cultured neurons. *Neurosci. Lett.* **2006**, *404*, 342–346. [CrossRef] [PubMed]
232. Hampson, A.J.; Grimaldi, M.; Lolic, M.; Wink, D.; Rosenthal, R.; Axelrod, J. Neuroprotective antioxidants from marijuana. *Ann. N. Y. Acad. Sci.* **2000**, *899*, 274–282. [CrossRef] [PubMed]
233. Scuderi, C.; Steardo, L.; Esposito, G. Cannabidiol promotes amyloid precursor protein ubiquitination and reduction of beta amyloid expression in SHSY5YAPP+ cells through PPARγ involvement. *Phytother. Res.* **2014**, *28*, 1007–1013. [CrossRef] [PubMed]
234. Esposito, G.; Scuderi, C.; Valenza, M.; Togna, G.I.; Latina, V.; de Filippis, D.; Cipriano, M.; Carratù, M.R.; Iuvone, T.; Steardo, L. Cannabidiol reduces Aβ-induced neuroinflammation and promotes hippocampal neurogenesis through PPARγ involvement. *PLoS ONE* **2011**, *6*, e28668. [CrossRef] [PubMed]
235. Esposito, G.; Scuderi, C.; Savani, C.; Steardo, L.; de Filippis, D.; Cottone, P.; Iuvone, T.; Cuomo, V. Cannabidiol *in vivo* blunts beta-amyloid induced neuroinflammation by suppressing IL-1beta and iNOS expression. *Br. J. Pharmacol.* **2007**, *151*, 1272–1279. [CrossRef] [PubMed]
236. Martín-Moreno, A.M.; Reigada, D.; Ramírez, B.G.; Mechoulam, R.; Innamorato, N.; Cuadrado, A.; de Ceballos, M.L. Cannabidiol and other cannabinoids reduce microglial activation *in vitro* and *in vivo*: Relevance to Alzheimer's disease. *Mol. Pharmacol.* **2011**, *79*, 964–973. [CrossRef] [PubMed]
237. Vaney, C.; Heinzel-Gutenbrunner, M.; Jobin, P.; Tschopp, F.; Gattlen, B.; Hagen, U.; Schnelle, M.; Reif, M. Efficacy, safety and tolerability of an orally administered cannabis extract in the treatment of spasticity in patients with multiple sclerosis: A randomized, double-blind, placebo-controlled, crossover study. *Mult. Scler.* **2004**, *10*, 417–424. [CrossRef] [PubMed]
238. Aso, E.; Sánchez-Pla, A.; Vegas-Lozano, E.; Maldonado, R.; Ferrer, I. Cannabis-based medicine reduces multiple pathological processes in AβPP/PS1 mice. *J. Alzheimers Dis.* **2015**, *43*, 977–991. [PubMed]
239. Iring, A.; Ruisanchez, É.; Leszl-Ishiguro, M.; Horváth, B.; Benkő, R.; Lacza, Z.; Járai, Z.; Sándor, P.; di Marzo, V.; Pacher, P.; *et al.* Role of endocannabinoids and cannabinoid-1 receptors in cerebrocortical blood flow regulation. *PLoS ONE* **2013**, *8*, e53390. [CrossRef] [PubMed]
240. Wagner, J.A.; Járai, Z.; Bátkai, S.; Kunos, G. Hemodynamic effects of cannabinoids: Coronary and cerebral vasodilation mediated by cannabinoid CB(1) receptors. *Eur. J. Pharmacol.* **2001**, *423*, 203–210. [CrossRef]
241. Walther, S.; Halpern, M. Cannabinoids and Dementia: A Review of Clinical and Preclinical Data. *Pharmaceuticals* **2010**, *3*, 2689–2708. [CrossRef]
242. Mishima, K.; Hayakawa, K.; Abe, K.; Ikeda, T.; Egashira, N.; Iwasaki, K.; Fujiwara, M. Cannabidiol prevents cerebral infarction via a serotonergic 5-hydroxytryptamine1A receptor-dependent mechanism. *Stroke* **2005**, *36*, 1077–1082. [CrossRef] [PubMed]
243. Walther, S.; Mahlberg, R.; Eichmann, U.; Kunz, D. Delta-9-tetrahydrocannabinol for nighttime agitation in severe dementia. *Psychopharmacology* **2006**, *185*, 524–528. [CrossRef] [PubMed]
244. Volicer, L.; Stelly, M.; Morris, J.; McLaughlin, J.; Volicer, B.J. Effects of dronabinol on anorexia and disturbed behavior in patients with Alzheimer's disease. *Int. J. Geriatr. Psychiatry* **1997**, *12*, 913–919. [CrossRef]
245. Krishnan, S.; Cairns, R.; Howard, R. Cannabinoids for the treatment of dementia. *Cochrane Database Syst. Rev.* **2009**. [CrossRef]

11

Curcumin and Resveratrol in the Management of Cognitive Disorders: What is the Clinical Evidence?

Gabriela Mazzanti * and Silvia Di Giacomo

Department of Physiology and Pharmacology, Sapienza—University of Rome, P.le Aldo Moro 5, 00185 Rome, Italy; silvia.digiacomo@uniroma1.it

* Correspondence: gabriela.mazzanti@uniroma1.it

Academic Editor: Derek J. McPhee

Abstract: A growing body of in vitro and in vivo evidences shows a possible role of polyphenols in counteracting neurodegeneration: curcumin and resveratrol are attractive substances in this regard. In fact, epidemiological studies highlight a neuroprotective effect of turmeric (rhizome of *Curcuma longa* L.), the main source of curcumin. Moreover, the consumption of red wine, the main source of resveratrol, has been related to a lower risk of developing dementia. In this review, we analyzed the published clinical trials investigating curcumin and resveratrol in the prevention or treatment of cognitive disorders. The ongoing studies were also described, in order to give an overview of the current search on this topic. The results of published trials (five for curcumin, six for resveratrol) are disappointing and do not allow to draw conclusions about the therapeutic or neuroprotective potential of curcumin and resveratrol. These compounds, being capable of interfering with several processes implicated in the early stages of dementia, could be useful in preventing or in slowing down the pathology. To this aim, an early diagnosis using peripheral biomarkers becomes necessary. Furthermore, the potential preventive activity of curcumin and resveratrol should be evaluated in long-term exposure clinical trials, using preparations with high bioavailability and that are well standardized.

Keywords: polyphenols; curcumin; turmeric; resveratrol; grape wine; dementia; Alzheimer; cognitive disorders; clinical trials

---

1. Introduction

Growing evidence suggests that polyphenols have potential health-promoting properties. In fact, these compounds have been associated to pleiotropic biological effects: they are known to behave as potent antioxidants, as direct radical scavengers in the lipid peroxidation, and to interact with a number of signalling targets involved in biological processes, such as carcinogenesis and inflammation [1]. Due to their multiple biological activities, polyphenols have been described as cardio-protective, anti-cancer, anti-microbial, and hepato-protective agents [2]. Evidence also suggests that polyphenols can counteract neurodegeneration so having a possible role in preventing or treating cognitive disorders and neurodegenerative diseases, particularly dementia.

Dementia is a multifactorial syndrome that affects memory, thinking, language, behavior and ability to perform everyday activities. According to the World Alzheimer Report [3], today, dementia affects over 46 million people worldwide and this number is estimated to increase to 131.5 million by 2050 due to increased expectation of life and an aging population [3]. The most common form of dementia is Alzheimer disease (AD) that possibly contributes to 60%–70% of cases, with a greater proportion in the higher age ranges [4]. AD is a multifactorial disease with genetic (70%) and environmental (30%) causes. The familial early-onset form of AD is caused by mutations in genes APP (amyloid precursor protein), PSEN1 (Presenilin 1) and PSEN2 (Presenilin 2). The APOE gene is responsible for the sporadic form of the disease [5]. The pathology initiates in the hippocampus brain region that is involved in memory and learning, then affects the entire brain. Major pathological features of AD include the accumulation of extracellular amyloid plaques and fibrils, intracellular neurofibrillary tangles, as well as chronic inflammation, an abnormal increase of oxidative stress and disruption of cholinergic transmission, including reduced acetylcholine levels in the basal forebrain. The neurodegenerative process leads to synaptic damage, neuronal loss accompanied by astrogliosis and microglial cell proliferation, ultimately leading to brain dysfunction and marked atrophy in susceptible regions of the brain, such as the hippocampus, amygdale and basal forebrain [6–9].

Amyloid plaques, also known as "senile plaques", originate from the amyloid beta (Aβ) peptide, following up its aberrant cleavage by β-secretase, of the transmembrane protein amyloid precursor protein (APP), whose function is unclear but thought to be involved in neuronal development. Aβ monomers aggregate into soluble oligomers and coalesce to form fibrils insoluble deposited outside neurons in dense formations, the amyloid plaques, in less dense aggregates as diffuse plaques, and sometimes in the walls of small blood vessels in the brain. Small Aβ oligomers (40 and 42 amino-acids) are particularly toxic to neurons causing membrane damage, Ca^{2+} leakage, oxidative damage, disruptions to insulin signaling pathways and synaptic function, and mitochondrial dysfunction [8,10]. Abnormal Aβ accumulation may be associated with disruption in cholinergic neurotransmission and initiate inflammatory mechanisms that produce reactive oxygen species (ROS). Abnormal release of neurotransmitters such as glutamate contributes to neuronal death and inflammation [11].

In AD, abnormal aggregation of the tau protein (P-tau), a microtubule-associated protein expressed in neurons, is also observed. P-tau acts to stabilize microtubules in the cell cytoskeleton. Like most microtubule-associated proteins, tau protein is normally regulated by phosphorylation; in AD patients, hyperphosphorylated P-tau accumulates as paired helical filaments that in turn aggregate into masses inside nerve cell bodies known as neurofibrillary tangles (NFTs), the other key pathological hallmark of AD [6,12].

There is a direct evidence for free radical oxidative damage in brain of patients with AD [13]. Oxidative stress is associated with various aspects of AD such as metabolic, mitochondrial, metal, and cell cycle abnormalities [14]. Dysregulation of metal homeostasis can lead to the binding of these metal ions to Aβ and acceleration of Aβ aggregation [15]. Oxidative stress is evidenced by lipid peroxidation end products, formation of toxic peroxides, alcohols, free carbonyl, and oxidative modifications in nuclear and mitochondrial DNA [16].

Neuroinflammation is also involved in the complex cascade leading to AD pathology and symptoms. It has been shown that AD is associated with increased levels of cycloxygenase 1 and 2 and of prostaglandins, release of cytokines and chemokines, acute phase reaction, astrocytosis and microgliosis [17]. These pro-inflammatory factors may induce degeneration of normal neurons through upregulation of nuclear factor-κB, mitogen-activated protein kinase, and c-Jun N-terminal kinase [18].

Finally, in patients with AD epigenetic alterations such as changes in DNA methylation, histone modifications, or changes in miRNA expression have been reported. Histone acetyltransferases (HATs) and histone deacetylases (HDACs) promote histone post-translational modifications, which lead to an epigenetic alteration in gene expression. Aberrant regulation of HATs and HDACs in neuronal cells results in pathological consequences such as neurodegeneration [19–21].

In summary, AD appears to be a complex and multifactorial disorder in which extracellular Aβ and intraneuronal hyperphosphorylated tau protein are the hallmark neuropathological features, along with oxidative stress and inflammation. Actually, no current effective disease-modifying treatments are available. Moreover, as Aβ-induced changes are believed to occur a long time before the impairment of cognitive function appears, so strategies to stop or to slow the progression of the disease are of greater importance as is an early diagnosis. Owing to the particular multifactorial nature of the disease, a novel approach consists in evaluating substances having multi-target mechanisms, such as polyphenols. Curcumin and resveratrol are naturally occurring polyphenols of emerging interest in this field (Figure 1). They show close similarity with the presence of several phenolic groups as well as unsaturated carbon chains. Moreover, they share similar biosynthetic pathways in spite of having different biological origins, being 4-hydroxycinnamic acid of the shikimate pathway their starting compound [22]. Curcumin and resveratrol share also other biological properties such as anticancer properties, in which they exert synergistic effects [23,24].

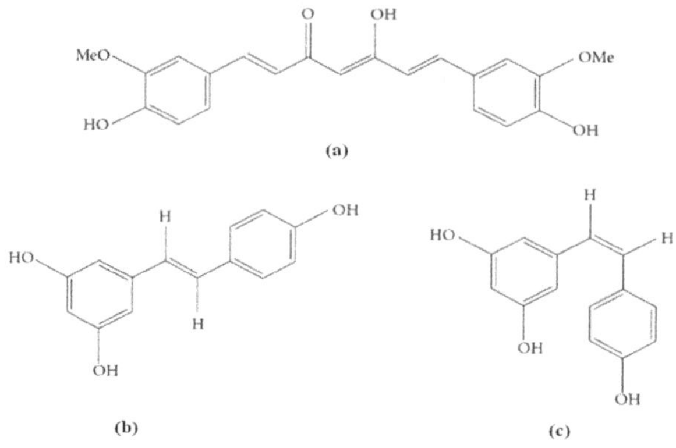

Figure 1. Chemical structures of (**a**) curcumin; (**b**) *trans*-resveratrol and (**c**) *cis*-resveratrol.

Despite the huge number of pharmacological studies on the potential beneficial effects of curcumin and resveratrol on cognitive disorders, very few of the studies have investigated their efficacy in humans. The present review is aimed not so much at establishing the effectiveness of curcumin and resveratrol in treating cognitive disorder, but rather to give an overview of the studies conducted or in progress using these substances and, possibly, to offer food for thought useful to better directing future research.

2. Mechanism of Neuroprotective Action of Curcumin and Resveratrol

Curcumin (1,7-bis(4-hydroxy-3-methoxyphenyl)-1,6-heptadiene-2,5-dione) is a polyphenolic compound obtained by turmeric, the dried rhizome of *Curcuma longa* L. (Fam. Zingiberaceae). Turmeric is the spice that gives curry its yellow color. It has been used in India for thousands of years as a food flavoring and preservative, and as a herbal remedy [8,25]. It is known in traditional medicine for its antiinflammatory, antioxidant, anticarcinogenic, hepatoprotective, cardioprotective, vasodilator, hypoglycemic, and anti-arthritic properties [26]. Turmeric has also been reputed to possess neuroprotective effects [27,28]; in fact, a lower prevalence of AD has been observed in Indian people, who regularly consume turmeric as a part of curry [29–31]. Moreover, some epidemiological studies support a link between dietary curry consumption and improved cognitive performance in elderly populations [32]. It is believed that the properties of turmeric are mainly due to its curcumin content [26].

Resveratrol (3,5,4′-trihydroxystilbene) belongs to a family of polyphenolic compounds known as stilbenes, a group of widespread plant secondary metabolites. Resveratrol is also one of the phytoalexins, a group of low-molecular-mass substances with antimicrobial activity, produced by plants as a defence response to some exogenous stimuli, such as UV radiation, chemical stressors, and particularly, microbial infections [33]. Sources of resveratrol in human diet are mainly peanuts, pistachios, berries and grapes; however, the most important dietary source of resveratrol is red wine [34]. The compound exists in two isomeric forms, the *trans*-isomer occurs in the berry skins of most grape cultivars, and its synthesis is stimulated by UV light, injury, and fungal infection. *Cis*-isomer is produced by UV irradiation of the *trans*-isomer; it is generally absent or only slightly detectable in grapes but originates from its *trans*-isomer during vinification, so both forms are present in variable amounts in commercial wines [33,35]. Most research on resveratrol concerns the *trans*-isomer owing to its natural presence in grapes and its greater stability [36].

The research interest in the therapeutic relevance of resveratrol has originated from its association with the "French Paradox" in the early 1990s [37]. It has been reported that the consumption of red wine on a regular basis may be related to a lower risk of developing dementia, such as AD and vascular dementia [38]. Orgogozo et al. [39] have shown a positive correlation between a moderate consumption of red wine and a decreased incidence of dementia. This protective effect is most likely due to the presence in wine of phenolic compounds, in particular resveratrol [1,33].

The neuroprotective potential of curcumin and resveratrol has been highlighted by in vitro and in vivo studies in which the compounds seem to slow down the progression of AD by multiple mechanisms. Both compounds possess anti-amyloidogenic effects. Curcumin has been shown to inhibit the formation and extension of neurotoxic Aβ fibrils, and to destabilize preformed Aβ fibrils [40,41]. A recent study conducted by Fu and coworkers [42] found that curcumin interacts with the *N*-terminus of $A\beta_{1\text{-}42}$ monomers and prevents the enlargement of oligomers from 1–2 nm to 3–5 nm. In another study, it was found that curcumin induces significant conformational changes in the Asp-23-Lys-28 salt bridge region and near the $A\beta_{1\text{-}42}$ C terminus. Mithu et al. [43] also showed, by using electron microscopy, that curcumin was able to disrupt the $A\beta_{1\text{-}42}$ fibrils architecture. Furthermore, the preventive administration of curcumin in Sprague-Dawley rats infused with $A\beta_{40}$ and $A\beta_{42}$ to induce neurodegeneration and Aβ deposits improved memory function [44]. These results were confirmed by a later study carried out by Ahmed et al. [45] who demonstrated that curcumin increased the expression levels of genes involved in synaptic plasticity, such as synaptophysin. More recently, Belviranli et al. [46] found that supplementation with curcumin for 12 days in aged female rat improves spatial memory. Also, resveratrol is reported to reduce the level of secreted or intracellular Aβ peptides by modulating the proteasome [47]. It may act indirectly by selectively stimulating the proteasomal degradation of critical regulators of Aβ clearance. The protective effect of resveratrol was also associated with the activation of protein kinase C, which stimulates α-secretase enzyme and consequently the non-amyloidogenic pathway, resulting in a reduction in the Aβ production [48]. In addition, a direct action of resveratrol towards Aβ plaques was also observed. In fact, it was shown to directly interact with Aβ peptides by inhibiting and destabilizing the formation of $A\beta_{1\text{-}42}$ fibrils [49]. Conversely, Granzotto and Zatta [50] reported that resveratrol was unable to prevent Aβ fibril formation in human neuroblastoma cells exposed to Aβ suggesting that resveratrol acts not through anti-aggregative pathways but mainly via its scavenging properties.

Curcumin and resveratrol have potent antioxidant activity that could have a role in preventing neurodegeneration in AD [51]. Cognitive deficits were shown to be associated with higher levels of reactive oxygen (ROS) and nitrogen species (RNS). Moreover, it seems that oxidative stress precedes the formation of senile plaques [52]. The brain possesses a relative deficiency of antioxidant systems and is very prone to oxidative imbalance and consequently to oxidative damage. The source of oxidant species in the AD brain may include unbound transition metals, damaged mitochondria and Aβ peptides themselves [51]. In vitro studies showed that curcumin scavenges nitric oxide (NO) radicals and protects the brain from lipid peroxidation [53]. It also prevents the DNA-oxidative damage by scavenging the hydroxyl radicals [54]. Curcumin was shown to bind Cu^{2+} and Fe^{2+} ions, which are involved in the exacerbation of Aβ aggregation and in the subsequent oxidative damage in the AD brain [55]. Recently, these results were confirmed by Banerjee [56], which demonstrated that curcumin is able to give complexes with Cu^{2+} and/or Zn^{2+} and consequently to inhibit the formation of β-sheet-rich Aβ protofibrils from less structured oligomers. Curcumin also activates glutathione S-transferase [57], partially restores glutathione content in the brain [58], and induces the antioxidant enzyme heme oxygenase-1 (HO-1), which has been shown to increase tolerance of the brain to stresses [59]. González-Reyes et al. [60] showed that the pre-treatment of cerebellar granule neurons of rats with curcumin effectively increased the HO-1 expression and GSH levels, by inducing nuclear factor (erythroid-derived 2)-like 2 (Nrf2) translocation into the nucleus. Besides, in vivo studies showed the ability of curcumin to reduce the brain levels of oxidized proteins containing carbonyl groups [41]. Begum et al. [61] observed a lower protein oxidation in the curcumin-treated Tg2576 mice and suggested that the dienone bridge, present in the chemical structure of curcumin, is necessary for this. In an in vivo study conducted by Belviranli et al. [46], a decrease of MDA levels in brain tissue was observed after curcumin supplementation. Also, resveratrol may block oxidative stress involved in the pathogenesis of AD. It scavenges free radicals, protects neurons and microglia [62,63] and attenuates Aβ-induced intracellular ROS accumulation [64]. Kwon et al. [65] found that the treatment of a murine HT22 hippocampal cell line with resveratrol attenuated ROS production and mitochondrial membrane-potential disruption; moreover, it restored the normal levels of GSH depleted by the $A\beta_{1-42}$. It is known that beta amyloid induces production of radical oxygen species and oxidative stress in neuronal cells, which in turn upregulates BACE-1 expression and beta amyloid levels, thereby propagating oxidative stress and increasing neuronal injury. Resveratrol is able to attenuate Aβ-induced intracellular ROS accumulation [64,66]. It also induces the up-regulation of cellular antioxidants (i.e., glutathione) and the gene expression of phase 2 enzymes, protects against oxidative and electrophilic injury [67], and, like curcumin, it potentiates the HO-1 pathway [68]. Chronic administration of this compound also significantly reduces the elevated levels of malondialdehyde in rats [69,70].

Another important pathological hallmark of AD is represented by brain inflammation. Inflammatory mediators such as cytokines and chemokines released by activated cells (microglia, astrocytes, macrophages and lymphocytes) contribute to the neuronal damage and enhance Aβ formation [71]. Curcumin has been reported to regulate inflammatory responses by suppressing the activity of the transcription factors, nuclear factor kappa-light-chain-enhancer of activated B cells (NF-κB) and activator protein-1 [72–74]. Additionally, curcumin blocks the induction of inducible nitric oxide synthase (iNOS) and inhibits lipoxygenase and cyclooxygenase-2 (COX-2) [72–74]. In vitro and in vivo studies also showed that it inhibits TNF-α, IL-1, -2, -6, -8, and -12 [75,76]. Resveratrol as well was shown to interfere with the neuroinflammatory process [77]. Particularly, it suppresses the activation of astrocytes and microglia [63,78,79], TNF-α and NO production by inhibiting NF-κB activation and p38 mitogen-activated protein kinase (MAPK) phosphorylation [79,80]. Resveratrol also blocks the expression of COX-2 and iNOS [81]. In a recent study carried out by Huang and coworkers [82], resveratrol treatment was shown to reverse the Aβ-induced iNOS overexpression. This compound is also able to reduce the expression of prostaglandin E synthase-1 [63]. Furthermore, the anti-inflammatory effects of resveratrol are due to the inhibition of TNF-α, IL-1β, and IL-6 expression [80,83], and STAT1 and STAT3 phosphorylation [84].

At last, the interference with epigenetic mechanisms has also been ascribed to curcumin and resveratrol. Epigenetic mechanisms modulate gene expression patterns without affecting the DNA sequence. Gene expression can be activated or silenced via epigenetic regulations; so, epigenetic changes may mediate the differences in risk for certain diseases [85]. Recently, it has been shown that curcumin is a potent inhibitor of histone acetyltransferases (HAT) [86] and DNA methyltransferase (DNMT1) [87]. These enzymes control the expression of genes involved in AD pathogenesis [88]. DNA methylation and histone post-translational modifications are crucial for synaptic plasticity, learning, memory, neuronal survival [89] and repair [90]. Also, resveratrol is able to inhibit DNMT activity [87] and to induce histone post-translational modifications. Indeed, it contributes to improvement of cognitive functions by activating SIRT1, a member of nicotinamide adenine dinucleotide (NAD+)-dependent deacetylases family [91,92].

3. Methods

A systematic research of the literature was carried out on PubMed, MedlinePlus and Google Scholar databases using the key words: curcumin, curcuminoids, turmeric, *Curcuma longa*, resveratrol, grapes, stilbenes, and wine. Each term was matched with the key words: neurodegenerative disorders, cognitive impairment, cognitive disorders, cognitive function, memory, learning, brain disease, dementia, Alzheimer, neuroprotection, and clinical trials. Furthermore, in order to find ongoing studies on curcumin and resveratrol in cognitive disorders, some accessible databases on clinical trials [93,94] were examined, using the methodology described above. No time or language restrictions were applied to the search strategy.

As yet stated, the aim of present review was to give an overview of the studies conducted or in progress using these substances, so all studies identified (both published and ongoing) in which curcumin and resveratrol are used in prevention, in treatment and in diagnosis of cognitive disorders, were selected and included in the review. Some studies carried out to evaluate the capability of the substances to increase the cerebral blood flow were included too, because this parameter is associated with improved cognitive performance [95]. Published studies were retrieved and carefully analyzed, also to acquire further relevant references. Ongoing studies were carefully examined and described, too.

4. Results

Our search identified five published studies for curcumin and six for resveratrol, along with 10 ongoing clinical trials on curcumin and nine on resveratrol. Following, the results of published studies will be described along with the characteristics of the ongoing ones (Tables 1 and 2).

4.1. Curcumin

Baum et al. [96] carried out a six-month randomized, double blind, placebo-controlled clinical trial on 34 Chinese patients of both sexes, ≥50 years old, with progressive decline in memory and cognitive function for 6 months, and diagnosis of probable or possible AD, to examine the curcumin safety and effects on biochemical parameters and cognitive function. Subjects received curcumin 1 g/day or 4 g/day; they were also given an additional treatment consisting in 120 mg/day of standardized gingko leaf extract. Patients treated with anticoagulant or antiplatelet agents or with bleeding risk factors were excluded. The main outcome measures were the Mini-Mental Status Examination (MMSE) score at baseline and at 6 months, plasma isoprostanes iPF2α-III and serum Aβ (at 0, 1, and 6 months); plasma levels of curcumin and its metabolites were also measured. No significant differences in MMSE score between treatments (1 g/day and 4 g/day) and placebo were observed, and neither was a reduction in serum Aβ_{40} levels nor differences in plasma isoprostanes iPF2α-III found. Plasma levels of curcuminoids, measured at 1 month, did not differ significantly between 1 g/day and 4 g/day groups so they were pooled and the results were as follows (in nanomolar): 250 $\pm$ 80 curcumin, 150 $\pm$ 50 demetoxycurcumin, 90 $\pm$ 30 bisdemetoxycurcumin, 440 $\pm$ 100 tetrahydrocurcumin. No differences in adverse events between curcumin groups and placebo were reported.

Ringman et al. [97] performed a randomized, double blind, placebo-controlled clinical trial on 36 subjects with mild-to-moderate AD. Patients were treated with Curcumin C3 Complex® (95% curcuminoids with curcumin 70%–80%, demethoxycurcumin 15%–25%, bisdemethoxycurcumin 2.5%–6.5%) at 2 g/day or 4 g/day for 24 weeks with an open-label extension to 48 weeks. Other medications such as acetylcholinesterase inhibitors and memantine were allowed, instead antioxidant, anticoagulant or antiplatelet drugs, including *Ginkgo biloba*, were not allowed. The purpose of the study was to acquire data on safety and tolerability and preliminary data on efficacy with regard to cognition, by measuring the incidence of adverse events, changes in clinical laboratory tests and Alzheimer's Disease Assessment Scale-Cognitive (ADAS-Cog) subscale, Neuropsychiatric Inventory (NPI), Alzheimer's Disease Co-operative Study-Activities of Daily Living (ADCS-ADL), MMSE score, plasma levels of A$\beta_{1\text{-}40}$ and A$\beta_{1\text{-}42}$, cerebrospinal fluid levels of A$\beta_{1\text{-}42}$, t-tau, p-tau181 and F_2-isoprostanes. Plasma levels of curcumin and its metabolites were also measured. No significant differences between curcumin and placebo in ADAS-Cog, NPI, ADCS-ADL or MMSE score were registered, as well as no differences between treatment groups in biomarker efficacy measures. Plasma levels of native curcumin and tetrahydrocurcumin, measured at a 24-week visit and 3 h after medication, were 7.76 $\pm$ 3.23 and 3.73 $\pm$ 2.0 ng/mL, respectively. The levels of glucuronidated curcumin and tetrahydrocurcumin were 96.05 $\pm$ 26 ng/mL and 298.2 $\pm$ 140.04 ng/mL. Levels of native curcumin were undetectable in the cerebrospinal fluid. Curcumin was generally well tolerated. On the whole, authors were unable to demonstrate clinical or biochemical evidence of curcumin efficacy against AD.

Table 1. Clinical trials on the effects of curcumin on cognitive function.

Reference and/or ID (Location)	Study Design Phase	Curcumin Preparation and Dose [Other Medication]	Duration	Subjects *n* Age Disorder/Status	Primary Purpose	Main Results	Adverse Events	Status
Baum et al. [96] (Hong Kong, China) NCT00164749	R, DB, PC NR	Curcumin 1 or 4 g/day (standardized ginkgo extract 120 mg/day)	6 months	34 ≥50 years Probable or possible AD	Effect in AD	No significant differences between curcumin and PL	No differences between curcumin and PL	Published
Ringman et al. [97] (Westwood, CA, USA) NCT00099710	R, DB, PC Phase 2	Curcumin C3 Complex® 2 or 4 g/day (1.9 or 3.8 g/day curcuminoids) [a] (AchE-Is and memantine)	24 weeks with an open-label extension to 48 weeks	36 ≥49 years Mild-to-moderate AD	Safety and efficacy with regard to cognition	No significant differences between curcumin and PL	No significant differences between curcumin and PL	Published
Hishikawa et al. [98] (Kariya, Japan)	Single cases	Turmeric 764 mg/day (curcumin 100 mg/day) (Yokukansan 2/3 subjects; donezepil 3/3)	12 weeks	3 79–83–84 years Progressive dementia	Effect on some symptoms of AD	Improvement in behavioral symptoms and quality of life	NR	Published
Cox et al. [99] (Melbourne, Australia) ACTRN12612001027808	R, DB, PC Phase 3/Phase 4	Longvida® Optimized Curcumin 400 mg (80 mg curcumin)	4 weeks	60 60–85 years Healthy	Effect on cognitive function	Improvement of cognitive functions	Treatment was well tolerated	Published
Rainey-Smith et al. [100] (Jondalup, Australia) ACTRN12611000437965	R, DB, PC	BCM-95®CG (Biocurcumax™) 1500 mg/day (1320 mg/day curcuminoids)	12 months	160 40–90 years Healthy	Prevention of cognitive decline	No changes in cognitive performance	Gastrointestinal complaints in 23 subjects	Published
NCT00595582 [101] Shreveport, LA, USA	Open-label NR	Curcumin 5.4 g/day (bioperine)	24 months	10 55–85 years MCI or mild AD	Effect on MCI or mild AD	None patient terminated the study	Two patients showed dyspepsia	Terminated
NCT01001637 [102] (Mumbai, Maharashtra, India)	R, DB, PC Phase 2	Longvida® 4 or 6 g/day	2 months	26 50–80 years Probable AD	Safety and effect on AD	-------	-------	Unknown
NCT01383161 [103] (Los Angeles, CA, USA)	R, DB, PC Phase 2	Theracurmin™ 2.79 g/day (180 mg/day curcumin)	18 months	132 50–90 years MCI	Effect on age-related cognitive impairment	-------	-------	Active, not recruiting
NCT01811381 [104] (Los Angeles, CA, USA)	R, DB, PC Phase 2	Longvida Curcumin® (800 mg/day of curcumin)	12 months	80 55–90 years MCI	Effect of curcumin alone or combined with yoga on AD	-------	-------	Recruiting
ACTRN12616000484448 [105] (Hawthorn, Australia)	R, DB, PC Phase 3/Phase 4	Longvida® Optimized Curcumin 400 mg/day (80–90 mg curcumin)	12 weeks	80 50–85 years Healthy	Effects on cognition, mood and well-being	-------	-------	Not yet recruiting

Table 1. *Cont.*

Reference and/or ID (Location)	Study Design Phase	Curcumin Preparation and Dose [Other Medication]	Duration	Subjects *n* Age Disorder/Status	Primary Purpose	Main Results	Adverse Events	Status
ACTRN12613000681752 [106] (NSW, Australia)	R, DB, PC Phase 2	Curcumin (Biocurcumax™): from 500 mg/day then 1 g/day then 1.5 g/day onwards	12 months	100 65–90 years Healthy but at high risk of AD	Prevention of AD	-------	-------	Recruiting
ACTRN12614001024639 [107] (sub study of ACTRN12613000681752) [106] (NSW, Australia)	R, B, PC Phase 2	Curcumin 1.5 g/day	3–6 months	48 65–90 years Healthy and MCI	Influence on the expression of inflammatory genetic markers	-------	-------	Not yet recruiting
ACTRN12613000367741 [108] (Nedlands, Australia)	Open study, not randomized Phase 2	Curcumin 20 gm/day (Vitamin E 500 IU/day)	7 days	40 ≥50 years AD, MCI, and healthy	Earlier detection of AD	-------	-------	Not yet recruiting
ACTRN12615000465550 [109] (Nedlands, Australia)	Open study, not randomised, unblended Phase 2/Phase 3	Longvida® 20 g/day (4 g/day curcumin) (Vitamin E 500 IU/day for 8 days)	7 days	100 ≥50 years Healthy and MCI	Earlier detection of AD	-------	-------	Recruiting
ACTRN12615000677505 [110] (Nedlands, Australia)	Open study, not randomised, Phase 2	Longvida® 20 g/day (containing 4 g curcumin)for 7 days (Vitamin E 500 IU/day for 8 days)	7 days	40 40–60 years Healthy	Earlier detection of AD	-------	-------	Not yet recruiting

[a] 95% curcuminoids with curcumin 70%–80%, demethoxycurcumin 15%–25%, bisdemethoxycurcumin 2.5%–6.5%. ID, Identifier; NR, Not Reported; R, randomized; DB, double blind; B, blind; PC, placebo controlled; AD, Alzheimer disease; PL, placebo; AchE-Is, Acethylcholinesterase inhibitors; MCI, Mild Cognitive Impairment; AEs, adverse events; SAEs, serious adverse events.

Table 2. Clinical trials on the effects of resveratrol on cognitive function.

Reference or ID (Location)	Study Design	Resveratrol Preparation and Dose [Other Medication]	Duration	Subjects *n* Age Disorder/Status	Purpose Outcome Measures	Main Results	Adverse Events	Status
Kennedy et al. [111] (Newcastle upon Tyne, UK)	R, DB, PC, CO	*Trans*-resveratrol from Biotivia Bioceuticals (Vienna, Austria) 250 mg or 500 mg	21 days	24 18–25 years Healthy 9 further subjects underwent bioavailability assessment	To investigate the ability to modulate mental function and increase cerebral blood flow	Cognitive function not affected. Increase in cerebral flow	Not assessed	Published
Wong et al. [112] (Adelaide, Australia) ACTRN12611000060943	R, DB, PC, CO	Resvida (resveratrol 75 mg/day)	12 weeks	28 45–70 years Obese but otherwise healthy	Effects of resveratrol on circulatory function and cognitive performance in obese adults	Increase of circulatory function. No effects on blood pressure, arterial compliance, and cognitive function	Resveratrol appears safe and well tolerated	Published
Witte et al. [113] (Berlin, Germany)	R, DB, PC,	Resveratrol 200 mg/day in a formula with quercetin	26 weeks	46 50–80 years Healthy overweight	To investigate the ability to enhance cognitive performance	Significant retention of memory, significant increase of hyppocampal FC, improvement of glucose metabolism	Not assessed	Published
Wightman et al. [114] (Newcastle upon Tyne, UK)	R, DB, PC, CO	*Trans*-resveratrol 250 mg/day or *trans*-resveratrol 250 mg/day with 20 mg piperine	21 days	23 19–34 years Healthy 6 healthy men underwent bioavailability assessment	To assess if piperine affects the efficacy and bioavailability of resveratrol	Piperine henances the effect of resveratrol on cerebral blood flow but not the cognitive performance and bioavailability	Not assessed	Published
Turner et al. [115] (Georgetown, USA) NCT01504854	R, DB, PC, MC Phase 2	Resveratrol 500 mg/day with dose excalation by 500 mg increments ending with 2 g/day	52 weeks	119 >49 years Mild-to-moderate AD	To assess safety and efficacy	Decrease of CSF and plasma Aβ_{40} levels. No significant effects on cognitive score	Resveratrol appears safe and well tolerated	Published
Wong et al. [116] ACTRN12614000891628 (Newcastle, Australia)	R, DB, PC, CO Phase 2	Resvida 75 mg/day, 150 mg/day, 300 mg/day	4 weeks	36 40–80 years Type 2 diabetes mellitus	Improvement of cerebrovascular responsiveness	Increase of cerebrovascular responsiveness	None	Published
NCT00743743 [117] (Milwaukee, WI, USA)	R, DB, PC Phase 3	Longevinex brand resveratrol supplement (resveratrol 215 mg/day)	52 weeks	50 50–90 years Mild-to-moderate AD on standard therapy	Effects on cognitive and global functioning	-------	-------	Withdrawn prior to enrollment
NCT00678431 [118] (Bronx, NY, USA)	R, DB, PC Phase 3	Resveratrol with glucose and malate	12 months	27 50–90 years Mild-to-moderate AD	To assess the ability to slow the progression of AD	Not available	Not available	Completed in June 2011

Table 2. *Cont.*

Reference or ID (Location)	Study Design	Resveratrol Preparation and Dose [Other Medication]	Duration	Subjects *n* Age Disorder/Status	Purpose Outcome Measures	Main Results	Adverse Events	Status
NCT01126229 [119] (Gainesville, FL, USA)	R, DB, PC Phase 1	Resveratrol 300 mg/day or 1000 mg/day	12 weeks	32 ≥65 years old	To assess the longer-term safety (3 months) and efficacy on age-related health conditions	Not available	Resveratrol appears safe and well tolerated [120]	Completed in December 2012
NCT01794351 [121] (Newcastle upon Tyne, UK)	R, DB, PC, CO	*Trans*-resveratrol 500 mg in unique dose	14 days	50 18–35 years Healthy	To assess the potential cognitive enhancement	Not available	-------	Completed in December 2012
NCT01219244 [122] (Berlin, Germany)	R, DB, PC Phase 4	Resveratrol or omega-3 supplementation or caloric restriction	6 months	330 50–80 years MCI	Effects on brain functions	-------	-------	Recruiting
NCT01766180 [123] (Lutherville, MD, USA)	R, DB, PC	ResVida (resveratrol 150 mg/day) alone or associated with Fruitflow [a]-II 150 mg/day	3 months	80 50–80 years Subjects with memory impairment	Efficacy in treating memory problems	-------	-------	Recruiting
NCT02621554 [124] (Leipzig, Germany)	R, DB, PC Phase 2/Phase 3	Resveratrol (dose not reported)	12 months	60 ≥50 years Healthy or with subjective memory complaints	Effects on memory and on brain structures and functions	-------	-------	Recruiting
NCT02502253 [125] (Baltimore, MD, USA)	R, DB Phase 1	Bioactive Dietary Polyphenol Preparation (BDPP) at low, moderate and high dose	4 months	48 55–85 years MCI	Safety and efficacy in treating mild cognitive impairment and prediabetes	-------	-------	Recruiting
ACTRN12611001288910 [126] (Hawthorn, Australia)	R, DB, PC, CO Phase 1/Phase 2	100mg of grape derived resveratrol in 100ml red wine	8 days (washout 7 days)	20 ≥65years Healthy	To assess the effect of resveratrol in red wine on cognitive function in older adults	-------	-------	Recruitment completed

[a] tomato extract. ID, Identifier; AD, Alzheimer disease; MCI, Mild Cognitive Impairment; R, randomized; DB, double blind; PC, placebo controlled; CO, cross over; MC, multicenter; FC, functional connectivity; CSF, Cerebrospinal fluid.

Hishikawa et al. [98] reported three cases of patients (79, 83, and 84 years old, respectively) with AD whose behavioral symptoms were improved remarkably as a result of turmeric treatment. Patients received turmeric 764 mg/day (curcumin 100 mg/day) for more than 1 year. After 12 weeks of treatment, all three patients experienced a reduction ($\geq$50%) of the Japanese version of Neuropsychiatric Inventory-brief Questionnaire (NPI-Q) score and the burden of caregivers was reduced (38%–86%), too. Particularly, agitation, apathy, anxiety, and irritability symptoms were relieved. One patient also increased his MMSE score from 12/30 to 17/30, improving calculation, concentration, transcription of the figure, and spontaneous writing. Of note, two patients were on donepezil treatment before starting curcumin.

Cox and colleagues [99] performed a randomized, double-bind, placebo controlled, phase 3/4 trial in healthy older subjects using Longvida® Optimized Curcumin, in dose of 400 mg, containing approximately 80 mg curcumin in a solid lipid formulation. Participants (aged 60–85 years) were randomly assigned to either curcumin (n = 30) or placebo (n = 30) treatment groups. The acute (1 and 3 h after a single dose), chronic (4 weeks) and acute-on-chronic (1 and 3 h after single dose following chronic treatment) effects of curcumin preparation on cognitive function, mood and blood biomarkers were examined. The authors reported significantly improved performance in sustained attention and working memory tasks, compared with placebo, one hour after administration of curcumin. Following chronic treatment, working memory and mood (general fatigue and change in state calmness, contentedness and fatigue induced by psychological stress) were significantly improved. A significant acute-on-chronic treatment effect on alertness and contentedness was also observed. Curcumin was associated with significant reduction of total and LDL cholesterol levels. Curcumin treatment was well tolerated and did not significantly impact any of the examined hematological safety measures.

A recent randomized, double-bind, placebo controlled trial (ACTRN12611000437965) was carried out on healthy older adults, to evaluate the potential efficacy of BCM-95®CG (Biocurcumax™), a standardised extract of *Curcuma longa* L. (88% curcuminoids and 7% volatile oil), in preventing cognitive decline [100]. One hundred and sixty healthy subjects (40–90 years aged) were selected for the study and randomly divided into two groups: an experimental group, taking Biocurcumax™ 1500 mg/day (1 capsule 500 mg three times a day), and a control group, taking a placebo (roasted rice powder). Sixty four subjects (23 in the placebo group and 41 in the curcumin group) did not complete the study for various reasons (ineligibility to remain in the study, suspect adverse reaction, intervention non-compliance, etc.) so 96 participants were included in the final analysis. The study lasted 12 months during which subjects were evaluated at the baseline and at the 6- and 12-months follow-ups. Mood was assessed by administration of the Depression Anxiety Stress Scale (DASS) [127]. Cognitive measures were obtained by a battery of cognitive tests for general cognitive function (MoCA) [128], verbal fluency, percentual motor speed, psychomotor speed, working memory, executive functions and visual memory. Blood pressure and weight were checked at baseline and every 3 months. No differences were observed in all clinical measures as well as for cognitive measures except for a significant interaction between time and treatment group in the MoCA test that, however, was due to a decline in general cognitive function of the placebo group at 6 months that was not observed in curcumin treatment group.

Besides the published ones, a number of studies of curcumin supplementation in healthy older people or in patients with Mild Cognitive Impairment (MCI) or AD are still underway or completed but results are not yet available.

A clinical trial (NCT00595582) [101] aimed at determining the efficacy of curcumin in the treatment of MCI or mild AD has been registered at the U.S. National Institutes of Health. Ten subjects (both sexes, $\geq$55 years old) already enrolled in another study (NCT00243451) [129] have been included in this clinical trial. They had to receive 5.4 g/day of curcumin in combination with bioperine, to improve curcumin bioavailability, for 24 months. Primary outcome was to determine if curcumin had an effect on neuropsychological scores, while determining if curcumin impacted the metabolic lesions found in patients who had MCI or might develop MCI was the secondary outcome. Unfortunately, none of the patients terminated the study. In particular, two out of 10 interrupted the study because of adverse effects (dyspepsia).

Another randomized, double-blind, placebo-controlled phase 2 study (NCT01001637) [102] has been designated to evaluate the efficacy and safety of the high-bioavailability curcumin formulation (Longvida®) in AD. The study planned to enrol 26 patients (both sexes $\geq$50 years old) with AD, who had to be treated with placebo, 4 g/day or 6 g/day of curcumin supplementation for 2 months. The main outcomes were to determine if curcumin formulation affects cognitive function in Alzheimer's patients, based on mental exams, and blood concentrations of Aβ. The recruitment status of this study is unknown.

A larger phase 2 clinical trial (NCT01383161) [103] has been designed to determine the effects of the curcumin supplement on age-related cognitive impairment, after 18 months' treatment. The investigators will study 132 subjects with MCI (aged 50–90 years), which will be randomly assigned to placebo or curcumin group (six 465 mg Theracurmin™ capsules/day, containing 30 mg of curcumin each). The main outcomes will be a change in cognitive testing results, in level of inflammatory markers in blood, and in the amount of brain amyloid protein. This study is ongoing, but is not recruiting participants.

Additionally, a randomized, double-blind, placebo-controlled phase 2 study (NCT01811381) [104] will evaluate the clinical benefits of curcumin alone or in combination with yoga in 80 individuals with MCI, 55–90 years old. For the first 6 months of the study, subjects will take either 800 mg of curcumin (Longvida® formulation) or placebo, before meals. Over the second 6 months of study, the curcumin and placebo groups will be further divided into groups receiving training in either aerobic or non-aerobic yoga (attendance at 2 classes of 1 h duration and 2 home practices of 30 min duration per week) to determine the synergism between curcumin supplementation and aerobic exercise. Primary outcome will be to determine if curcumin (first six month period), alone or associated to aerobic yoga (second six month period), reduces the levels of blood biomarkers for MCI. Secondary outcome will be to evaluate imaging changes in all subjects and adverse events. This study is currently recruiting participants.

Several clinical trials are also underway in Australia. The randomized, double-blind, placebo-controlled, phase 3/4 clinical trial ACTRN12616000484448 [105] will soon start to recruit participants. This study will investigate the effects of 12 weeks of treatment with a bioavailability enhanced curcumin supplement on cognitive function, mood and wellbeing in healthy older adults (n = 80; aged 50–85 years). Participants will receive 400 mg of Longvida® Optimized Curcumin (containing about 80–90 mg curcumin) daily. The study will also evaluate the effects of curcumin on cardiovascular function and a range of blood markers of health, to better understand how cognitive and mood benefits might be achieved. In a subset of participants, the effects of curcumin on brain function will be explored by functional Magnetic Resonance Imaging (fMRI). Finally, the study will investigate whether genetic differences can influence the effects of curcumin.

Another randomized, double-blind, placebo-controlled, phase 2 study (ACTRN12613000681752) [106] is in progress in Australia. This clinical trial will investigate the role of curcumin in preventing AD. Participants (n = 100; 65–90 years old) assessed as at high risk of AD will be assigned to placebo or curcumin (Biocurcumax™) group. The latter will receive 500 mg daily of curcumin for 2 weeks, progressing to 500 mg twice daily (1000 mg/daily) for another 2 weeks, then 500 mg three times daily, (1500 mg) until the end of the study (12 months). Primarily, the ability of Biocurcumax to positively alter AD-related blood biomarker profiles compared with placebo will be investigated, secondarily the possible increase in brain glucose utilisation, as measured by FDG-PET, and the correlation with the improvement in cognitive functioning will be studied. Currently, the recruitment of participants is in progress. Present clinical trial includes also a sub study (ACTRN12614001024639) [107], which will be performed in 48 subjects (24 healthy older people and 24 with MCI) to examine the influence of curcumin on expression of inflammatory genetic markers, by measuring associated proteins in the blood, and on existing lifestyle patterns including sleep, activity levels and nutrition.

In addition, three clinical trials have been designed to assess the possible use of curcumin in the early diagnosis of AD. It has been proposed, in fact, that beta-amyloid plaques may first appear in the retina, at the back of the eye, before they are detectable in the brain. Curcumin has molecular and optical properties that allow to image amyloid plaques using a specialized eye camera, and hence to detect Alzheimer's disease earlier. In these open, not randomized phase 2 or phase 2/3 studies, all groups receive the same intervention, i.e., 20 g of Longvida® (equivalent to 4 g of curcumin) along with Vitamin E supplement capsules, equivalent to 500 IU daily, for seven consecutive days; participants will be asked to have eye imaging done before and after taking curcumin for 7 days. The trial ACTRN12613000367741 [108] includes three groups of subjects: with AD, with MCI and healthy controls. The association between retinal imaging and brain amyloid imaging will be determined in AD and in MCI in comparison with the healthy controls. The second diagnosis trial (ACTRN12615000465550) [109] is recruiting subjects with MCI and healthy controls. Participants must have completed curcumin based fluorescence retinal imaging under the ACTRN12613000367741 study (parent study) [108] within the previous 21 months. The primary endpoint will be to evaluate the ability to detect changes over time in retinal Aβ plaque burden, and at this aim the results from participants with MCI will be compared with the results from the healthy controls and, in addition, with the participants' results from the parent study. Finally, ACTRN12615000677505 [110] has been designed to investigate the presence/absence of retinal amyloid plaques in a middle-aged control cohort (40–60 years). Furthermore, the comparison between retinal Aβ protein plaque burden with brain Aβ protein plaque burden will be done. Currently, the present study is not recruiting subjects.

4.2. *Resveratrol*

Six studies, aimed at evaluating the effects of resveratrol on cognitive function in humans, were retrieved (see Table 2).

In 2010, Kennedy et al. [111] performed a randomized double-blind, placebo-controlled, crossover study to investigate the possibility that single oral doses of resveratrol modulate mental function and increase cerebral blood flow (CBF) in the frontal cortex of healthy humans. Cognitive performance was measured by a battery of tasks and the cerebral blood flow in the prefrontal cortex was detected by Near-Infrared Spectroscopy (NIRS), during the tasks. The 24 subjects enrolled (age 18–25 years) received three single dose treatments: placebo, 250 mg *trans*-resveratrol, and 500 mg *trans*-resveratrol. The bioavailability of resveratrol and its metabolites (resveratrol glucuronide and resveratrol sulfate) at time points relevant to the CBF/cognitive task assessment, were also evaluated in a separate cohort of 9 healthy young adults. The 500 mg resveratrol supplementation significantly increased CBF and hemoglobin status in the period of 45–81 min following administration. Also, the 250 mg resveratrol dose increased CBF compared to placebo, although in a lesser extent and at fewer time points than the higher dose, suggesting that resveratrol improves CBF in a dose-dependent manner. The peak plasma levels after treatment with 250 and 500 mg of trans-resveratrol were 5.65 ng/mL and 14.4 ng/mL respectively; at the same doses, peak plasma levels of *trans*-resveratrol glucuronide were about 30 ng/mL and 200 ng/mL, respectively, while those of *trans*-resveratrol sulfate were about 300 ng/mL and 750 ng/mL, respectively. Despite increased blood flow in both treatment groups, resveratrol did not enhance cognitive function.

A further randomized, double-blind, placebo controlled, crossover clinical trial has been designed to evaluate the effects of resveratrol on circulatory function and cognitive performance in obese adults [112]. Twenty-eight subjects of both sexes (40–75 years old), obese but otherwise healthy, were enrolled. Participants were randomized to consume a capsule containing either 75 mg of resveratrol (resVida) or a color-matched placebo daily for 6 weeks. Then, participants were crossed over to an alternate dose for another 6 weeks. The assessments were done at baseline, at week 6, and at week 12. Moreover, following the assessments in week 6 and 12, participants consumed a single additional dose of the supplement and further assessments were performed 1 h after consumption. The primary outcome was to measure the degree of change in vasodilator function assessed by flow mediated dilatation (FMD) in the brachial artery. Secondary outcomes were the ability to maintain attention and concentration during the test (measured by the Stroop test), supine blood pressure, heart rate and arterial compliance. Resveratrol supplementation was found to be well tolerated and induced a 23% increase in FMD compared with placebo. Moreover, a single dose of resveratrol (75 mg) following chronic resveratrol supplementation resulted in an acute FMD response 35% greater than placebo. However, blood pressure, arterial compliance, and all components of the Stroop Color-Word Test were unaffected by chronic resveratrol supplementation.

Witte and colleagues in 2014 [113] carried out a double-blind placebo-controlled study aimed to assess the ability of resveratrol, given over 26 weeks, to enhance the cognitive performance. Forty-six overweight older adults (50–80 years old) were recruited and randomly divided in: treatment group, receiving 200 mg/day of resveratrol in a formulation with quercetin (320 mg) to increase its bioavailability and control group, receiving placebo. Memory retention was evaluated by a battery of tasks; volume, microstructure, and functional connectivity of the hippocampus were explored by magnetic resonance imaging (MRI). Further anthropometric measures were: glucose and lipid metabolism, inflammation, neurotrophic factors, and vascular parameters. Resveratrol supplementation induced retention of memory and improved the functional connectivity between hippocampus and frontal, parietal, and occipital areas, in healthy older overweight adults compared with placebo. The changes in resting-state functional connectivity networks of the hippocampus after resveratrol intake were linked with behavioral improvements. Also, glucose metabolism was improved and this may account for some of the beneficial effects of resveratrol on neuronal function. Finally, a significant reduction of body fat and increases in leptin compared with placebo was observed.

In 2014, Wightman et al. [114] performed a randomized, double-blind, placebo controlled, cross-over study investigating the effects of 250 mg resveratrol administered alone or co-supplemented with 20 mg piperine. The aim was to ascertain whether piperine is able to enhance the bioefficacy of resveratrol with regard to CBF and cognitive performance in a cohort of 23 healthy adults (age 19–34 years). Plasma concentrations of resveratrol were also measured in a separate cohort of 6 male adults, to investigate whether bioavailability correlated with bioefficacy. Participants were given placebo, *trans*-resveratrol (250 mg) and *trans*-resveratrol with 20 mg piperine on separate days, at least a week apart. Whereas 250 mg of orally administered *trans*-resveratrol had no significant effects on overall CBF during the performance of cognitively demanding tasks, co-administration of the same dose of resveratrol with 20 mg piperine resulted in significantly increased CBF for the duration of the 40 min post-dose task period. Cognitive function, mood and blood pressure were not affected. In subjects treated with resveratrol alone plasma concentrations of total resveratrol metabolites ranged from 2 to 18.2 μM. Resveratrol 3-*O*-sulphate was the major metabolite, contributing 59%–81% of total metabolites. The 4′-*O*-glucuronide and the 3-*O*-glucuronide forms made roughly equal contribution to the remaining metabolites. No significant differences were observed in the plasma concentrations of resveratrol in subjects receiving resveratrol plus piperine, so suggesting that piperine increases the efficacy of resveratrol on CBF by potentiating its vasorelaxant properties. Despite the piperine-mediated potentiation of CBF during task performance, no effects were found on cognitive performance.

Another randomized, placebo-controlled, double-blind, multicenter 52-week phase 2 trial of resveratrol in individuals with mild-to-moderate AD was conducted between June 2012 and March 2014 to assess the safety and efficacy of resveratrol [115]. Participants (n = 119, >49 years old) were recruited and randomly divided in placebo group and resveratrol group (500 mg orally once daily with dose escalation by 500 mg increments every 13 weeks, ending with 1000 mg twice daily). Pharmacokinetic studies were performed on a subset (n = 15) at baseline and weeks 13, 26, 39, and 52. The trial showed that resveratrol, also at the higher oral dose, was safe and well-tolerated. In fact, the most common AEs were nausea and diarrhea, but their frequency was similar to placebo. In the treatment group, weight loss was also highlighted. The levels of $A\beta_{40}$ in the cerebrospinal fluid (CSF) and plasma declined more in the placebo group than the resveratrol-treated group with a significant difference at week 52 (note that $A\beta_{40}$ levels decline as dementia advances). No effects of drug treatment were found on plasma $A\beta_{42}$, CSF $A\beta_{42}$, CSF tau, CSF phospho-tau 181, hippocampal volume, entorhinal cortex thickness, MMSE score, Clinical Dementia Rating (CDR) score, ADAS-cog score, NPI score, and glucose or insulin metabolism. Plasma levels of resveratrol and its metabolites at 45 weeks were approximately: resveratrol 22 ng/mL, 3-*O*-glucuronidated resveratrol 3800 ng/mL, 4-*O*-glucuronidated resveratrol 5000 ng/mL, sulphated resveratrol 7400 ng/mL. The levels in CSF were approximately: resveratrol 0.45 ng/mL, 3-*O*-glucuronidated resveratrol 8.5 ng/mL, 4-*O*-glucuronidated resveratrol 12 ng/mL, sulphated resveratrol 13 ng/mL. The altered CSF $A\beta_{40}$ path and the pharmacokinetic data suggest that the drug penetrates the blood–brain barrier to have central effects; however, the authors concluded that this result must be interpreted with caution, because although it is suggestive of CNS effects, it does not indicate benefit.

Recently, Wong et al. [116] carried out a randomized, double blind, placebo controlled, crossover clinical trial (registered as ACTRN12614000891628) to evaluate the effect of resveratrol supplementation on cerebrovascular function, in adults with a diagnosis of type 2 diabetes mellitus (T2DM). To manage T2DM, volunteers were using diet or exercise alone, or oral hypoglycemic agents. Enrolled participants (38 subjects of both sexes 40–80 years old) were randomly allocated to receive placebo or the resveratrol supplement Resvida™, at doses of 75 mg, 150 mg, or 300 mg, taken as a single dose during four intervention visits that took place at seven day intervals over 4 weeks. The main outcome was to determine the most effective dose of resveratrol to improve the cerebral vasodilator responsiveness (CVR) to hypercapnia in the middle cerebral artery, using Transcranial Doppler ultrasound. Effect of resveratrol on CVR in the posterior cerebral artery was the secondary outcome. Cerebral blood flow velocities were also measured. Any symptom of illness appearing during the trial was recorded. Thirty six participants concluded the study, while two withdrew their consent to participate before the first intervention visit. Resveratrol consumption significantly increased CVR in the middle cerebral artery at all tested doses with maximum improvement being observed with the lowest dose. CVR in the posterior cerebral artery was increased only at 75 mg. No adverse events occurred during the intervention.

Interestingly, several clinical trials evaluating the efficacy of resveratrol, alone or in combination with other supplements, in AD or MCI, are currently at various stages of completion. A randomized, double-blind, placebo-controlled phase three study (NCT00743743) [117] was being designed in order to determine the effects on cognitive and global functioning in patients with mild-to-moderate AD on standard therapy. Fifty patients (50–90 years old) had to be enrolled in the study. The treatment group had to receive 1 capsule daily for 52 weeks of Longevinex brand resveratrol supplement, containing 215 mg of resveratrol active ingredient, while the control group 1 capsule of placebo. However, this study was withdrawn prior to enrolment.

Another randomized, double-blind, placebo-controlled phase 3 study (NCT00678431) [118] recruited 27 subjects of both sexes (50–90 years old) with mild-to-moderate AD. The treatment group received liquid resveratrol (dose not reported) together with glucose and malate, using grape juice as the delivery system. The aim of this trial was to investigate the ability of resveratrol to slow the progression of AD. This endpoint was measured by the ADAS-Cog scale and Clinical Global Impression of Change (CGIC) scale at regular intervals up to 1 year after the study's beginning. Also, the adverse effects reported by patients were examined. Although this trial was completed in June 2011, results are not available at the moment.

Additionally, a randomized, double-blind, placebo-controlled phase 1 study (NCT01126229) [119] was aimed to assess the longer-term safety (3 months) and efficacy of resveratrol supplementation on cognitive function and physical performance in older adults. Thirty-two participants, of both sexes and aged 65–100 years, were enrolled. Subjects were randomly assigned with equal probability to receive either resveratrol (300 mg/day or 1000 mg/day) or placebo for 12 weeks. A follow-up evaluation was provided at 10 and 30 days following completion of the final post-treatment assessment. At the moment, the results on resveratrol safety have been published [120]; conversely, those about the effects on cognitive function and physical performance are still not available.

In the NCT01794351 [121] clinical trial (randomized, double-blind, placebo-controlled, cross-over study), the potentially cognitive enhancing effects of 500 mg *trans*-resveratrol in 50 healthy young humans (both sexes, 18–35 years old) were evaluated. In this study, participants received firstly placebo and then resveratrol, on separate days, with a 7–14 day wash-out period between visits and, in the second part of the study, first resveratrol and then placebo. The main outcome was to measure the number of participants with altered cognitive function which differed from the baseline, in a time range between 40 min and 6 h post-dose. The secondary outcome was to measure the number of participants with altered mood which differed from the baseline (time range 40 min–6 h post-dose). This study was completed in December 2012, but still results are not available.

Another larger double-blind, placebo-controlled phase four clinical trial (NCT01219244) [122] investigating whether dietary modification could provide positive effects on brain functions in elderly people with MCI is still recruiting participants. The researchers of this study planned to enrol 330 subjects (50–80 years old) with MCI. Participants will be randomly divided in 4 groups receiving placebo, or omega-3 supplementation, or resveratrol supplementation or they will undergo caloric restriction, for 6 months. The study plans also a second step in which the most effective dietary intervention will be combined with physical and cognitive training in order to highlighted the enhancing of memory functions. The effect of dietary modification on brain functions will be measured by ADAs-Cog scale. Moreover, functional and structural brain changes and plasma biomarkers will be evaluated prior to intervention and after 6 months of intervention.

The randomized double-blind placebo-controlled clinical trial NCT01766180 [123] has been designed to determine whether the intake of resveratrol (Resvida; resveratrol 150 mg/day), alone or in combination with Fruitflow-II (tomato extract; 150 mg/day), for a period of 3 months, is effective in improving memory. A cohort of 80 subjects (both sexes aged 50–80 years) with memory impairment will be enrolled. The effects of the medications on brain blood flow and fitness will be also evaluated to find out whether the possible improvement in memory is associated with the alterations in these parameters. Memory improvement will be measured by CANTAB (Cambridge Neuropsychological Test Automated Battery), maximal oxygen uptake and blood flow to the brain. At the moment, the present clinical trial is recruiting participants.

The clinical trial NCT02621554 [124] (randomized, double-blind, placebo-controlled phase 2/3 study) will investigate whether resveratrol could provide positive effects on memory and brain structures and functions in healthy elderly participants (both sexes $\geq$50 years old) with subjective memory complaints. Resveratrol (exact dose not reported) will be administered to the subjects for 6 months. Primary and secondary outcomes will be used to evaluate changes from baseline, after 6 and 12 months, with Verbal Learning Task Scores, MMSE score, structural and functional changes on the brain MRI images and plasma biomarkers. The present clinical trial is recruiting participants.

Additionally, a randomized double-blind clinical trial phase 1 (NCT02502253) [125] will evaluate the effects of a Bioactive Dietary Polyphenol Preparation (BDPP), a combination of three nutraceutical preparations (grape seed polyphenolic extract, resveratrol, and Concord grape juice) in patients with MCI and prediabetes. Forty-eight subjects of both sexes and aged 55–85 years will be enrolled. Participants will receive for 4 months BDPP preparation at low, moderate and high doses (the exact concentrations of BDPP are not reported in the website of clinicaltrial.gov). The main outcomes of this study will be to assess adverse events and serious adverse events, to confirm brain penetration of BDPP by measuring levels of its constituents in CBF, to evaluate the BDPP effect on mood with NPI and Cornell Scale for Depression in Dementia, and to assess the BDPP effect on cognition with a battery of memory, executive function, and attention measures. The present clinical trial is recruiting participants.

Finally, the study ACTRN12611001288910 [126] (placebo-controlled, double-blind, randomized, phase 1/2, crossover study) is aimed at evaluating the effect of resveratrol in red wine on cognitive function in older adults. Participants (20 healthy subjects ≥65 years old) will be randomized to receive either 100 mg of grape derived resveratrol in 100 mL of red wine and 100 mL of red wine, such that at the conclusion of the study all participants will have received both treatments. The main outcomes will be to assess the effects of a moderate daily amount of resveratrol-enriched red wine on cognitive performance in older adults using the Cognitive Demand Battery (CDB) and to establish whether the dose of resveratrol (100 mg) is significant enough to reach detectable concentrations in the body. At present, the recruitment has been completed.

5. Discussion

Our search retrieved five published clinical trials on curcumin and six on resveratrol, investigating their efficacy in preserving or restoring cognitive function. In the range of doses used and relatively to the duration of studies, curcumin and resveratrol appear to be generally safe and well tolerated.

Among the curcumin trials, three were performed in adult or old patients with AD of various degrees; among these, only one [98] was found to have positive effects on AD symptoms: it is worthwhile to point out that this study reported only three single cases. Two studies [99,100] enrolled healthy subjects and only in one of them [99] an improvement in cognitive function was observed; conversely, no effect was observed by Rainey-Smith et al. [100] in their one year long study.

Among the resveratrol studies, only one [115] enrolled patients with AD (mild-to-moderate); in this, a decrease of $A\beta_{40}$ and CSF plasma levels was observed but with no improvement in cognitive score. The other five studies enrolled young, healthy subjects or adult/old subjects with obesity or diabetes mellitus type 2. Results showed an increase in cerebral blood flow but cognitive function was not generally affected, except in one case [113]. Then, present data do not allow to draw conclusions on the efficacy of curcumin and resveratrol in neurodegenerative disorders.

Curcumin and resveratrol possess multitargeting biological effects, both in vitro and in vivo, such as inhibition of Aβ aggregation, reduction of oxidative stress, promotion of cell growth, inhibition of cholinesterase activity, inhibition of brain pro-inflammatory responses, prevention of neuronal cell death, enhancement of neuroprotective sirtuin-1 activity, etc., [8,130] that make them ideal candidates in the battle against neurodegenerative diseases. However, despite their attractive neuroprotective properties, the results obtained in clinical trials are generally disappointing: what is the reason for the discrepancy between pre-clinical and clinical data? Different points deserve to be taken into account in this regard.

First of all, the number of available studies is small and their experimental design is different. The number of subjects enrolled is generally small, too (<50 in eight out of eleven studies published); the duration of follow-up is <6 months in six out of 11 trials and sometimes less than one month, which is inadequate to detect potential changes in cognitive function. A further variable is represented by the dose, particularly as regards curcumin. Doses of curcumin used in the trials vary greatly: from 80 mg/day to 4 g/day. Of note, in patients with AD, Hishikawa et al. [98] observed an improvement of behavioral symptoms and quality of life with curcumin 100 mg/day. Analogously, in healthy subjects, Cox et al. [99] observed an improvement of cognitive functions with curcumin 80 mg/day (as Longvida® Optimized Curcumin). Instead, Baum et al. [96] administrating curcumin at 1 g/day and 4 g/day did not highlight any positive effect. These authors did not even find difference in curcumin plasma levels between 1 g/day and 4 g/day, suggesting that the use of curcumin at doses higher than one gram is not justified. Resveratrol doses used in the trials are generally in the range of between 250 mg/day and 500 mg/day.

Besides the dose, the clinical effect of a substance depends on its bioavailability, then on its formulation: this is a crucial point when talking about curcumin and resveratrol. In clinical trials, these substances are generally administered by oral route. Both curcumin and resveratrol have low water solubility and after oral administration, their absorption is very low (<1%), as reported in the clinical trial above described and in literature [131,132]. After absorption, the substances are metabolized mainly in glucuronides and sulfates while the plasma levels of parent compounds are very low [22]. Poor absorption, rapid metabolism within the human gastro-intestinal tract and rapid systemic elimination result in poor systemic bioavailability of curcumin and resveratrol: this has been the primary challenge to their clinical application [133–135]. To overcome these problems, different delivery systems, like adjuvants, nanoparticles, liposomes, micelles, phospholipid complexes and nanogels, have been investigated or are being developed as strategies to improve the bioavailability of the two polyphenols. Among the adjuvants, piperine, a known inhibitor of hepatic and intestinal glucuronidation, has been shown to strongly increase the bioavailability of curcumin and resveratrol when co-administered [136,137]. The solid lipid curcumin particle preparation, commercially available as Longvida®, has been reported to give increased bioavailability compared with a generic curcumin [138]. Theracurmin® is a nanoparticle-based curcumin preparation with a greater than 30-fold increase in bioavailability, compared with conventional curcumin [139]. The patented formulation Biocurcumax™ is reported to give a curcumin bioavailability of about 6.93-fold greater than normal curcumin owing to the synergism between the sesquiterpenoids present in turmeric and the curcuminoids [140]. In the formulation Longevinex®, resveratrol is supplemented with 5% quercetin and 5% rice bran phytate: these ingredients are micronized to increase the bioavailability. Resveratrol is sometimes administered in red wine to increase its bioavailability. In fact, the pharmacokinetics of resveratrol may dramatically change depending on the food matrix in which it is found: when it is part of wine uptake it is higher than the pure compound [134].

Noteworthy, some of the preparations mentioned above have been used in the clinical trials that gave positive results. For instance, Cox et al. [99] used the formulation Longvida® while Hishikawa et al. [98] administered turmeric as a source of curcumin. Studies have indicated that turmeric oil, present in turmeric, can enhance the bioavailability of curcumin. Moreover, some individual components of turmeric, including turmerin, turmerone, elemene, furanodiene, curdione, bisacurone, cyclocurcumin, calebin A, and germacrone possess biological activity that can potentiate the beneficial effects of curcumin [141]. In addition, Witte et al. [113] obtained a significant retention of memory by administering resveratrol in a formula with quercetin, while Wightman et al. [114] observed that piperine enhances the bioavailability of resveratrol and its effect on cerebral flow, even if the cognitive performance was not affected. We can then suppose that the use of novel formulations can allow to better highlight the possible clinical efficacy of curcumin and resveratrol.

Besides the problems above discussed, it has to be considered that Aβ-induced alterations occur in the earliest stages of AD. When symptoms occur there has already been a substantial loss of neurons, so it is only possible to counteract the symptoms; this is the reason for the limited efficacy of current pharmaceutical drugs and, probably, of the failure of curcumin and resveratrol. Then, it emerges in a compelling way the need for an early diagnosis of the disease that, in turn, requires the identification of suitable peripheral biomarkers, not only in the blood but also in other districts. In this context, the ongoing studies using curcumin in the early diagnosis of AD are of particular interest. This approach is based on the ability of curcumin to fluorescence and to bind Aβ both in the brain and in the retina [142,143]. Since the pathology in the retina can be detected before it could be detected in the brain, curcumin can represent a useful pre-clinical biomarker.

Furthermore, future studies aimed at highlighting the ability of new substances to prevent AD or to slow the progression of cognitive decline should be carried out in healthy older subjects and should have a long-lasting follow-up.

Finally, new drugs able to act in the early stages of AD are needed. Curcumin and resveratrol are pleiotropic substances that interfere with numerous pathophysiological mechanisms that precede the onset of AD, then they could be more likely effective at the earliest pre-clinical stages, before onset of symptoms and could act by slowing the disease progression.

As already stated, several clinical trials on curcumin and resveratrol are ongoing, most of them using curcumin and resveratrol formulations with high bioavailability; it is hoped that these trials provide more information on the possible efficacy of curcumin and resveratrol in preserving or restoring the cognitive function. Also, these, however, present some critical points, particularly as regards the standardization of products. For example, in the trial ACTRN12613000367741 [108], the treatment reported is "curcumin 20 g/day" but probably the dose is referred to the whole supplement (Longvida®) which contains 20% of curcumin, corresponding to 4 g of active substance. In the trial NCT02502253 [125], the treatment Bioactive Dietary Polyphenol Preparation (BDPP), a combination of grape seed polyphenolic extract [GSE], resveratrol, and Concord grape juice, is administered at low, moderate and high doses, but neither the doses nor the amount of resveratrol contained in the preparation is described. In order to obtain repeatable data it should be mandatory to use well standardized products: this should always be kept in mind in the search for natural products, particularly when they are used in the form of phytocomplexes.

6. Conclusions

AD is a multifactorial disorder that requires drugs capable of operating on multiple brain targets. Polyphenols, particularly curcumin and resveratrol, having pleiotropic protective effects appear to be ideal candidates to prevent or treat neurodegenerative disorders, however, their clinical efficacy and utility is still an open question. In order to exploit the protective properties of these compounds, some key points should be addressed.

Considering the scarce efficacy of current pharmacological treatments, the goal should be an early diagnosis of the pathology and intervention should be aimed at preventing or slowing down its progress. In this context, it appears of primary importance to identify suitable biomarkers, particularly blood biomarkers, easy to obtain and that can be repeated as necessary.

Curcumin and resveratrol, owing to their capability to interfere with a series of processes implicated in the early stages of pathology, when clinical symptoms have not yet appeared, could be useful in preventing neurodegeneration or slowing it down. However, it is of primary importance to establish the effective dose, improve the bioavailability of substances and use well standardized preparations, capable of ensuring plasma levels sufficient for the protective action. Considering that curcumin and resveratrol are generally marketed as food supplements and that for each substance exists a wide variety of preparations, the bioavailability of the different formulations should be assayed comparatively.

Finally, the potential preventive activity of curcumin and resveratrol should be evaluated in long-term exposure clinical trials, using specific designs, different from therapeutic effect trials. Such information is also requested by authorities like the FDA (Food and Drug Administration) and EFSA (European Food Safety Authority) to support health claims.

Acknowledgments: Silvia Di Giacomo has been supported by "Enrico ed Enrica Sovena" Foundation, Rome, Italy.

Abbreviations

The following abbreviations are used in this manuscript:

AD	Alzheimer disease
ADAS-Cog	Alzheimer's Disease Assessment Scale-Cognitive subscale
ADCS-ADL	Alzheimer's Disease Co-operative Study-Activities of Daily Living
AEs	Adverse Events
Aβ	Amyloid β
AUC	Area under the curve
BDPP	Bioactive Dietary Polyphenol Preparation
CANTAB	Cambridge Neuropsychological Test Automated Battery
CBF	Cerebral Blood Flow
CDB	Cognitive Demand Battery
CDR	Clinical Dementia Rating
CGIC	Clinical Global Impression of Change

CVR	Cerebral Vasodilator Responsiveness
DNMT1	DNA Methyltransferase
EFSA	European Food Safety Authority
FDA	Food and Drug Administration
FDG-PET	2-Deoxy-2-[fluorine-18]fluoro-D-glucose Positron Emission Tomography
FMD	Flow Mediated Dilatation
fMRI	functional Magnetic Resonance Imaging
HAT	Histone Acetyltransferases
HO-1	Heme oxygenase-1
iNOS	Inducible Nitric Oxide Synthase
MAPK	p38 Mitogen-activated protein kinase
MCI	Mild Cognitive Impairment
MMSE	Mini-Mental Status Examination
NF-kB	Nuclear factor kappa-light-chain-enhancer of activated B cells
NIRS	Near-Infrared Spectroscopy
NPI	Neuropsychiatric Inventory
NPI-Q	Neuropsychiatric Inventory-brief Questionnaire
PET	Positron Emission Tomography
RAI	Retinal Amyloid Index
RNS	Reactive Nitrogen Species
ROS	Reactive Oxygen Species
SAEs	Serious Adverse Events
SIRT-1	Sirtuin-1
STAT1	Signal Transducer and Activator of Transcription 1
STAT3	Signal Transducer and Activator of Transcription 3
TNF-α	Tumour Necrosis Factor α

References

1. Spagnuolo, C.; Napolitano, M.; Tedesco, I.; Moccia, S.; Milito, A.; Russo, G.L. Neuroprotective role of natural polyphenols. *Curr. Top. Med. Chem.* **2016**, *16*, 1943–1950. [CrossRef] [PubMed]
2. Zhang, Y.J.; Gan, R.Y.; Li, S.; Zhou, Y.; Li, A.N.; Xu, D.P.; Li, H.B. Antioxidant phytochemicals for the prevention and treatment of chronic diseases. *Molecules* **2015**, *20*, 21138–21156. [CrossRef] [PubMed]
3. Alzheimer's Disease International. The Global Voice on Dementia. Available online: https://www.alz.co.uk/research/WorldAlzheimerReport2015.pdf (accessed on 22 August 2016).
4. World Health Organization. Available online: http://www.who.int/medicines/areas/priority_medicines/BP6_11Alzheimer.pdf (accessed on 22 August 2016).
5. Dorszewska, J.; Prendecki, M.; Oczkowska, A.; Dezor, M.; Kozubski, W. Molecular basis of familial and sporadic Alzheimer's disease. *Curr. Alzheimer Res.* **2016**, *13*, 952–963. [CrossRef] [PubMed]
6. Apetz, N.; Munch, G.; Govindaraghavan, S.; Gyengesi, E. Natural compounds and plant extracts as therapeutics against chronic inflammation in Alzheimer's disease—A translational perspective. *CNS Neurol. Disord. Drug Targets* **2014**, *13*, 1175–1191. [CrossRef] [PubMed]
7. Kumar, A.; Singh, A.; Ekavali. A review on Alzheimer's disease pathophysiology and its management: An update. *Pharmacol. Rep.* **2015**, *67*, 195–203. [CrossRef] [PubMed]
8. Goozee, K.G.; Shah, T.M.; Sohrabi, H.R.; Rainey-Smith, S.R.; Brown, B.; Verdile, G.; Martins, R.N. Examining the potential clinical value of curcumin in the prevention and diagnosis of Alzheimer's disease. *Br. J. Nutr.* **2016**, *115*, 449–465. [CrossRef] [PubMed]
9. Libro, R.; Giacoppo, S.; Soundara Rajan, T.; Bramanti, P.; Mazzon, E. Natural phytochemicals in the treatment and prevention of dementia: An overview. *Molecules* **2016**, *21*, 518. [CrossRef] [PubMed]
10. Reddy, P.H.; Tripathi, R.; Troung, Q.; Tirumala, K.; Reddy, T.P.; Anekonda, V.; Shirendeb, U.P.; Calkins, M.J.; Reddy, A.P.; Mao, P.; et al. Abnormal mitochondrial dynamics and synaptic degeneration as early events in Alzheimer's disease: Implications to mitochondria-targeted antioxidant therapeutics. *Biochim. Biophys. Acta* **2012**, *1822*, 639–649. [CrossRef] [PubMed]
11. Noda, M. Dysfunction of glutamate receptors in microglia may cause neurodegeneration. *Curr. Alzheimer Res.* **2016**, *13*, 381–386. [CrossRef] [PubMed]

12. Goedert, M.; Klug, A.; Crowther, R.A. Tau protein, the paired helical filament and Alzheimer disease. *J. Alzheimers Dis.* **2006**, *9*, 195–207. [PubMed]
13. Di Domenico, F.; Pupo, G.; Giraldo, E.; Badìa, M.C.; Monllor, P.; Lloret, A.; Schininà, M.E.; Giorgi, A.; Cini, C.; Tramutola, A.; et al. Oxidative signature of cerebrospinal fluid from mild cognitive impairment and Alzheimer disease patients. *Free Radic. Biol. Med.* **2016**, *91*, 1–9. [CrossRef] [PubMed]
14. Sliwinska, A.; Kwiatkowski, D.; Czarny, P.; Toma, M.; Wigner, P.; Drzewoski, J.; Fabianowska-Majewska, K.; Szemraj, J.; Maes, M.; Galecki, P.; et al. The levels of 7,8-dihydrodeoxyguanosine (8-oxoG) and 8-oxoguanine DNA glycosylase 1 (OGG1)—A potential diagnostic biomarkers of Alzheimer's disease. *J. Neurol. Sci.* **2016**, *368*, 155–159. [CrossRef] [PubMed]
15. Faller, P.; Hureau, C.; Berthoumieu, O. Role of metal ions in the self-assembly of the Alzheimer's amyloid-β peptide. *Inorg. Chem.* **2013**, *52*, 12193–12206. [CrossRef] [PubMed]
16. Gella, A.; Durany, N. Oxidative stress in Alzheimer disease. *Cell Adh. Migr.* **2009**, *3*, 88–93. [CrossRef] [PubMed]
17. McGeer, P.L.; McGeer, E.G. Local neuroinflammation and the progression of Alzheimer's disease. *J. Neurovirol.* **2002**, *8*, 529–538. [CrossRef] [PubMed]
18. Steiner, N.; Balez, R.; Karunaweera, N.; Lind, J.M.; Munch, G.; Ooi, L. Neuroprotection of Neuro2a cells and the cytokine suppressive and anti-inflammatory mode of action of resveratrol in activated RAW264.7 macrophages and C8-B4 microglia. *Neurochem. Int.* **2015**, *95*, 46–54. [CrossRef] [PubMed]
19. Daniilidou, M.; Koutroumani, M.; Tsolaki, M. Epigenetic mechanisms in Alzheimer's disease. *Curr. Med. Chem.* **2011**, *18*, 1751–1756. [CrossRef] [PubMed]
20. Mastroeni, D.; Grover, A.; Delvaux, E.; Whiteside, C.; Coleman, P.D.; Rogers, J. Epigenetic mechanisms in Alzheimer's disease. *Neurobiol. Aging* **2011**, *32*, 1161–1180. [CrossRef] [PubMed]
21. Smith, A.R.; Smith, R.G.; Condliffe, D.; Hannon, E.; Schalkwyk, L.; Mill, J.; Lunnon, K. Increased DNA methylation near TREM2 is consistently seen in the superior temporal gyrus in Alzheimer's disease brain. *Neurobiol. Aging* **2016**, *47*, 35–40. [CrossRef] [PubMed]
22. Shindikar, A.; Singh, A.; Nobre, M.; Kirolikar, S. Curcumin and resveratrol as promosing natural remedies with nanomedicine approach for the effective treatment of triple negative breast cancer. *J. Oncol.* **2016**, *2016*, 9750785. [CrossRef] [PubMed]
23. Du, Q.; Hu, B.; An, H.M.; Shen, K.P.; Xu, L.; Deng, S.; Wei, M.M. Synergistic anticancer effects of curcumin and resveratrol in Hepa1-6 hepatocellular carcinoma cells. *Oncol. Rep.* **2013**, *29*, 1851–1858. [PubMed]
24. Masuelli, L.; di Stefano, E.; Fantini, M.; Mattera, R.; Benvenuto, M.; Marzocchella, L.; Sacchetti, P.; Focaccetti, C.; Bernardini, R.; Tresoldi, I.; et al. Resveratrol potentiates the in vitro and in vivo anti-tumoral effects of curcumin in head and neck carcinomas. *Oncotarget* **2014**, *5*, 10745–10762. [CrossRef] [PubMed]
25. Aggarwal, B.B.; Sundaram, C.; Malani, N.; Ichikawa, H. Curcumin: The Indian solid gold. *Adv. Exp. Med. Biol.* **2007**, *595*, 1–75. [PubMed]
26. Gupta, S.C.; Sung, B.; Kim, J.H.; Prasad, S.; Li, S.; Aggarwal, B.B. Multitargeting by turmeric, the golden spice: From kitchen to clinic. *Mol. Nutr. Food Res.* **2013**, *57*, 1510–1528. [CrossRef] [PubMed]
27. Rajakrishnan, V.; Viswanathan, P.; Rajasekharan, K.N.; Menon, V.P. Neuroprotective role of curcumin from Curcuma longa on ethanol-induced brain damage. *Phytother. Res.* **1999**, *13*, 571–574. [CrossRef]
28. Shytle, R.D.; Tan, J.; Bickford, P.C.; Rezai-Zadeh, K.; Hou, L.; Zeng, J.; Sanberg, P.R.; Sanberg, C.D.; Alberte, R.S.; Fink, R.C.; et al. Optimized turmeric extract reduces β-amyloid and phosphorylated tau protein burden in Alzheimer's transgenic mice. *Curr. Alzheimer Res.* **2012**, *9*, 500–506. [CrossRef] [PubMed]
29. Ganguli, M.; Chandra, V.; Kamboh, M.I.; Johnston, J.M.; Dodge, H.H.; Thelma, B.K.; Juyal, R.C.; Pandav, R.; Belle, S.H.; DeKosky, S.T. Apolipoprotein E polymorphism and Alzheimer disease: The Indo-US cross-national dementia study. *Arch. Neurol.* **2000**, *57*, 824–830. [CrossRef] [PubMed]
30. Chandra, V.; Pandav, R.; Dodge, H.H.; Johnston, J.M.; Belle, S.H.; DeKosky, S.T.; Ganguli, M. Incidence of Alzheimer's disease in a rural community in India: the Indo-US study. *Neurology* **2001**, *57*, 985–989. [CrossRef] [PubMed]
31. Shaji, S.; Bose, S.; Verghese, A. Prevalence of dementia in an urban population in Kerala, India. *Br. J. Psychiatry* **2005**, *186*, 136–140. [CrossRef] [PubMed]
32. Ng, T.P.; Chiam, P.C.; Lee, T.; Chua, H.C.; Lim, L.; Kua, E.H. Curry consumption and cognitive function in the elderly. *Am. J. Epidemiol.* **2006**, *164*, 898–906. [CrossRef] [PubMed]

33. Cvejic, J.M.; Djekic, S.V.; Petrovic, A.V.; Atanackovic, M.T.; Jovic, S.M.; Brceski, I.D.; Gojkovic-Bukarica, L.C. Determination of *trans*- and *cis*-Resveratrol in Serbian Commercial Wines. *J. Chromatogr. Sci.* **2010**, *48*, 229–234. [CrossRef] [PubMed]
34. Shi, J.; He, M.; Cao, J.; Wang, H.; Ding, J.; Jiao, Y.; Li, R.; He, J.; Wang, D.; Wang, Y. The comparative analysis of the potential relationship between resveratrol and stilbene synthase gene family in the development stages of grapes (*Vitis quinquangularis* and *Vitis vinifera*). *Plant Physiol. Biochem.* **2014**, *74*, 24–32. [CrossRef] [PubMed]
35. Moreno, M.; Castro, E.; Falqué, E. Evolution of *trans*- and *cis*- resveratrol content in red grapes (*Vitis vinifera* L. cv Menciá, Albarello and Merenzao) during ripening. *Eur. Food Res. Technol.* **2008**, *227*, 667–674. [CrossRef]
36. Trela, B.C.; Waterhouse, A.L. Resveratrol: Isomeric molar absorptivities and stability. *J. Agric. Food Chem.* **1996**, *44*, 1253–1257. [CrossRef]
37. Smoliga, J.M.; Baur, J.A.; Hausenblas, H.A. Resveratrol and health—A comprehensive review of human clinical trials. *Mol. Nutr. Food Res.* **2011**, *55*, 1129–1141. [CrossRef] [PubMed]
38. Luchsinger, J.A.; Noble, J.M.; Scarmeas, N. Diet and Alzheimer's disease. *Curr. Neurol. Neurosci. Rep.* **2007**, *7*, 366–372. [CrossRef] [PubMed]
39. Orgogozo, J.M.; Dartigues, J.F.; Lafont, S.; Letenneur, L.; Commenges, D.; Salamon, R.; Renaud, S.; Breteler, M.B. Wine consumption and dementia in the elderly: A prospective community study in the Bordeaux area. *Rev. Neurol.* **1997**, *153*, 185–192. [PubMed]
40. Ono, K.; Hasegawa, K.; Naiki, H.; Yamada, M. Curcumin has potent anti-amyloidogenic effects for Alzheimer's β-amyloid fibrils in vitro. *J. Neurosci. Res.* **2004**, *75*, 742–750. [CrossRef] [PubMed]
41. Lim, G.P.; Chu, T.; Yang, F.; Beech, W.; Frautschy, S.A.; Cole, G.M. The curry spice curcumin reduces oxidative damage and amyloid pathology in an Alzheimer transgenic mouse. *J. Neurosci.* **2001**, *21*, 8370–8377. [PubMed]
42. Fu, Z.; Aucoin, D.; Ahmed, M.; Ziliox, M.; van Nostrand, W.E.; Smith, S.O. Capping of Aβ42 oligomers by small molecule inhibitors. *Biochemistry* **2014**, *53*, 7893–7903. [CrossRef] [PubMed]
43. Mithu, V.S.; Sarkar, B.; Bhowmik, D.; Das, A.K.; Chandrakesan, M.; Maiti, S.; Madhu, P.K. Curcumin alters the salt bridge-containing turn region in amyloid β(1-42) aggregates. *J. Biol. Chem.* **2014**, *289*, 11122–11131. [CrossRef] [PubMed]
44. Frautschy, S.A.; Hu, W.; Kim, P.; Miller, S.A.; Chu, T.; Harris-White, M.E.; Cole, G.M. Phenolic anti-inflammatory antioxidant reversal of Aβ-induced cognitive deficits and neuropathology. *Neurobiol. Aging* **2001**, *22*, 993–1005. [CrossRef]
45. Ahmed, T.; Enam, S.A.; Gilani, A.H. Curcuminoids enhance memory in an amyloid-infused rat model of Alzheimer's disease. *Neuroscience* **2010**, *169*, 1296–1306. [CrossRef] [PubMed]
46. Belviranlı, M.; Okudan, N.; Atalık, K.E.; Öz, M. Curcumin improves spatial memory and decreases oxidative damage in aged female rats. *Biogerontology* **2013**, *14*, 187–196. [CrossRef] [PubMed]
47. Marambaud, P.; Zhao, H.; Davies, P. Resveratrol promotes clearance of Alzheimer's disease amyloid-β peptides. *J. Biol. Chem.* **2005**, *280*, 37377–37382. [CrossRef] [PubMed]
48. Bastianetto, S.; Ménard, C.; Quirion, R. Neuroprotective action of resveratrol. *Biochim. Biophys. Acta* **2015**, *1852*, 1195–1201. [CrossRef] [PubMed]
49. Richard, T.; Poupard, P.; Nassra, M.; Papastamoulis, Y.; Iglesias, M.L.; Krisa, S.; Waffo-Teguo, P.; Merillon, J.M.; Monti, J.P. Protective effect of epsilon-viniferin on betaamyloid peptide aggregation investigated by electrospray ionization mass spectrometry. *Bioorg. Med. Chem.* **2011**, *19*, 3152–3155. [CrossRef] [PubMed]
50. Granzotto, A.; Zatta, P. Resveratrol acts not through anti-aggregative pathways but mainly via its scavenging properties against Aβ and Aβ-metal complexes toxicity. *PLoS ONE* **2011**, *6*, e21565. [CrossRef] [PubMed]
51. Kim, J.; Lee, H.J.; Lee, K.W. Naturally occurring phytochemicals for the prevention of Alzheimer's disease. *J. Neurochem.* **2010**, *112*, 1415–1430. [CrossRef] [PubMed]
52. Wahlster, L.; Arimon, M.; Nasser-Ghodsi, N.; Post, K.L.; Serrano-Pozo, A.; Uemura, K.; Berezovska, O. Presenilin-1 adopts pathogenic conformation in normal aging and in sporadic Alzheimer's disease. *Acta Neuropathol.* **2013**, *125*, 187–199. [CrossRef] [PubMed]
53. Wei, Q.Y.; Chen, W.F.; Zhou, B.; Yang, L.; Liu, Z.L. Inhibition of lipid peroxidation and protein oxidation in rat liver mitochondria by curcumin and its analogues. *Biochim. Biophys. Acta* **2006**, *1760*, 70–77. [CrossRef] [PubMed]

54. Agnihotri, N.; Mishra, P.C. Scavenging mechanism of curcumin toward the hydroxyl radical: A theoretical study of reactions producing ferulic acid and vanillin. *J. Phys. Chem. A* **2011**, *115*, 14221–14232. [CrossRef] [PubMed]
55. Baum, L.; Ng, A. Curcumin interaction with copper and iron suggests one possible mechanism of action in Alzheimer's disease animal models. *J. Alzheimers Dis.* **2004**, *6*, 367–377. [PubMed]
56. Banerjee, R. Effect of curcumin on the metal ion induced fibrillization of amyloid-β peptide. *Spectrochim. Acta A Mol. Biomol. Spectrosc.* **2014**, *117*, 798–800. [CrossRef] [PubMed]
57. Nishinaka, T.; Ichijo, Y.; Ito, M.; Kimura, M.; Katsuyama, M.; Iwata, K.; Miura, T.; Terada, T.; Yabe-Nishimura, C. Curcumin activates human glutathione *S*-transferase P1 expression through antioxidant response element. *Toxicol. Lett.* **2007**, *170*, 238–247. [CrossRef] [PubMed]
58. Ishrat, T.; Hoda, M.N.; Khan, M.B.; Yousuf, S.; Ahmad, M.; Khan, M.M.; Ahmad, A.; Islam, F. Amelioration of cognitive deficits and neurodegeneration by curcumin in rat model of sporadic dementia of Alzheimer's type (SDAT). *Eur. Neuropsychopharmacol.* **2009**, *19*, 636–647. [CrossRef] [PubMed]
59. Motterlini, R.; Foresti, R.; Bassi, R.; Green, C.J. Curcumin, an antioxidant and anti-inflammatory agent, induces heme oxygenase-1 and protects endothelial cells against oxidative stress. *Free Radic. Biol. Med.* **2000**, *28*, 1303–1312. [CrossRef]
60. González-Reyes, S.; Guzmán-Beltrán, S.; Medina-Campos, O.N.; Pedraza-Chaverri, J. Curcumin pretreatment induces Nrf2 and an antioxidant response and prevents hemin-induced toxicity in primary cultures of cerebellar granule neurons of rats. *Oxid. Med. Cell Longev.* **2013**, *2013*, 801418. [CrossRef] [PubMed]
61. Begum, A.N.; Jones, M.R.; Lim, G.P.; Morihara, T.; Kim, P.; Heath, D.D.; Rock, C.L.; Pruitt, M.A.; Yang, F.; Hudspeth, B.; et al. Curcumin structure-function, bioavailability, and efficacy in models of neuroinflammation and Alzheimer's disease. *J. Pharmacol. Exp. Ther.* **2008**, *326*, 196–208. [CrossRef] [PubMed]
62. Zhuang, H.; Kim, Y.S.; Koehler, R.C.; Dore, S. Potential mechanism by which resveratrol, a red wine constituent, protects neurons. *Ann. N. Y. Acad. Sci.* **2003**, *993*, 276–286. [CrossRef] [PubMed]
63. Candelario-Jalil, E.; de Oliveira, A.C.; Graf, S.; Bhatia, H.S.; Hull, M.; Munoz, E.; Fiebich, B.L. Resveratrol potently reduces prostaglandin E_2production and free radical formation in lipopolysaccharide-activated primary rat microglia. *J. Neuroinflam.* **2007**, *4*, 25. [CrossRef] [PubMed]
64. Jang, J.H.; Surh, Y.J. Protective effect of resveratrol on β-amyloid- induced oxidative PC12 cell death. *Free Radic. Biol. Med.* **2003**, *34*, 1100–1110. [CrossRef]
65. Kwon, K.J.; Kim, H.J.; Shin, C.Y.; Han, S.H. Melatonin potentiates the neuroprotective properties of resveratrol against betaamyloid-induced neurodegeneration by modulating AMP activated protein kinase pathways. *J. Clin. Neurol.* **2010**, *6*, 127–137. [CrossRef] [PubMed]
66. Koukoulitsa, C.; Villalonga-Barber, C.; Csonka, R.; Alexi, X.; Leonis, G.; Dellis, D.; Hamelink, E.; Belda, O.; Steele, B.R.; Micha-Screttas, M.; et al. Biological and computational evaluation of resveratrol inhibitors against Alzheimer's disease. *J. Enzyme Inhib. Med. Chem.* **2016**, *31*, 67–77. [CrossRef] [PubMed]
67. Cao, Z.; Li, Y. Potent induction of cellular antioxidants and phase 2 enzymes by resveratrol in cardiomyocytes: Protection against oxidative and electrophilic injury. *Eur. J. Pharmacol.* **2004**, *489*, 39–48. [CrossRef] [PubMed]
68. Kwon, K.J.; Kim, J.N.; Kim, M.K.; Lee, J.; Ignarro, L.J.; Kim, H.J.; Shin, C.Y.; Han, S.H. Melatonin synergistically increases resveratrolinduced heme oxygenase-1 expression through the inhibition of ubiquitin-dependent proteasome pathway: A possible role in neuroprotection. *J. Pineal Res.* **2011**, *50*, 110–123. [PubMed]
69. Sharma, M.; Gupta, Y.K. Chronic treatment with trans-resveratrol prevents intracerebroventricular streptozotocin induced cognitive impairment and oxidative stress in rats. *Life Sci.* **2002**, *71*, 2489–2498. [CrossRef]
70. Kumar, A.; Naidu, P.S.; Seghal, N.; Padi, S.S. Neuroprotective effects of resveratrol against intracerebroventricular colchicine-induced cognitive impairment and oxidative stress in rats. *Pharmacology* **2007**, *79*, 17–26. [CrossRef] [PubMed]
71. Sadigh-Eteghad, S.; Majdi, A.; Mahmoudi, J.; Golzari, S.E.; Talebi, M. Astrocytic and microglial nicotinic acetylcholine receptors: An overlooked issue in Alzheimer's disease. *J. Neural. Transm.* **2016**. [CrossRef] [PubMed]

72. Nanji, A.A.; Jokelainen, K.; Tipoe, G.L.; Rahemtulla, A.; Thomas, P.; Dannenberg, A.J. Curcumin prevents alcohol-induced liver disease in rats by inhibiting the expression of NF-κB-dependent genes. *Am. J. Physiol. Gastrointest. Liver Physiol.* **2003**, *284*, G321–G327. [CrossRef] [PubMed]
73. Bengmark, S. Curcumin, an atoxic antioxidant and natural NF-κB, cyclooxygenase-2, lipooxygenase, and inducible nitric oxide synthase inhibitor: A shield against acute and chronic diseases. *J. Parenter. Enter. Nutr.* **2006**, *30*, 45–51. [CrossRef]
74. Sandur, S.K.; Ichikawa, H.; Pandey, M.K.; Kunnumakkara, A.B.; Sung, B.; Sethi, G.; Aggarwal, B.B. Role of pro-oxidants and antioxidants in the anti-inflammatory and apoptotic effects of curcumin (diferuloylmethane). *Free Radic. Biol. Med.* **2007**, *43*, 568–580. [CrossRef] [PubMed]
75. Karunaweera, N.; Raju, R.; Gyengesi, E.; Münch, G. Plant polyphenols as inhibitors of NF-κB induced cytokine production—A potential antiinflammatory treatment for Alzheimer's disease? *Front. Mol. Neurosci.* **2015**, *8*, 24. [CrossRef] [PubMed]
76. Millington, C.; Sonego, S.; Karunaweera, N.; Rangel, A.; Aldrich-Wright, J.R.; Campbell, I.L.; Gyengesi, E.; Münch, G. Chronic neuroinflammation in Alzheimer's disease: New perspectives on animal models and promising candidate drugs. *BioMed Res. Int.* **2014**, *2014*, 309129. [CrossRef] [PubMed]
77. Venigalla, M.; Sonego, S.; Gyengesi, E.; Sharman, M.J.; Münch, G. Novel promising therapeutics against chronic neuroinflammation and neurodegeneration in Alzheimer's disease. *Neurochem. Int.* **2016**, *95*, 63–74. [CrossRef] [PubMed]
78. Wang, Q.; Xu, J.; Rottinghaus, G.E.; Simonyi, A.; Lubahn, D.; Sun, G.Y.; Sun, A.Y. Resveratrol protects against global cerebral ischemic injury in gerbils. *Brain Res.* **2002**, *958*, 439–447. [CrossRef]
79. Bi, X.L.; Yang, J.Y.; Dong, Y.X.; Wang, J.M.; Cui, Y.H.; Ikeshima, T.; Zhao, Y.Q.; Wu, C.F. Resveratrol inhibits nitric oxide and TNF-α production by lipopolysaccharide-activated microglia. *Int. Immunopharmacol.* **2005**, *5*, 185–193. [CrossRef] [PubMed]
80. Cheng, X.; Wang, Q.; Li, N.; Zhao, H. Effects of resveratrol on hippocampal astrocytes and expression of TNF-α in Alzheimer's disease model rate. *J. Hyg. Res.* **2015**, *44*, 610–614.
81. Rahman, I.; Biswas, S.K.; Kirkham, P.A. Regulation of inflammation and redox signaling by dietary polyphenols. *Biochem. Pharmacol.* **2006**, *72*, 1439–1452. [CrossRef] [PubMed]
82. Huang, T.C.; Lu, K.T.; Wo, Y.Y.; Wu, Y.J.; Yang, Y.L. Resveratrol protects rats from Aβ-induced neurotoxicity by the reduction of iNOS expression and lipid peroxidation. *PLoS ONE* **2011**, *6*, e29102. [CrossRef] [PubMed]
83. Yao, Y.; Li, J.; Niu, Y.; Yu, J.Q.; Yan, L.; Miao, Z.H.; Zhao, X.X.; Li, Y.J.; Yao, W.X.; Zheng, P.; et al. Resveratrol inhibits oligomeric Aβ-induced microglial activation via NADPH oxidase. *Mol. Med. Rep.* **2015**, *12*, 6133–6139. [PubMed]
84. Capiralla, H.; Vingtdeux, V.; Zhao, H.; Sankowski, R.; Al-Abed, Y.; Davies, P.; Marambaud, P. Resveratrol mitigates lipopolysaccharide- and Aβ-mediated microglial inflammation by inhibiting the TLR4/NF-κB/STAT signaling cascade. *J. Neurochem.* **2012**, *120*, 461–472. [CrossRef] [PubMed]
85. Sezgin, Z.; Dincer, Y. Alzheimer's disease and epigenetic diet. *Neurochem. Int.* **2014**, *78*, 105–116. [CrossRef] [PubMed]
86. Boyanapalli, S.S.; Tony Kong, A.N. "Curcumin, the king of spices": Epigenetic regulatory mechanisms in the prevention of cancer, neurological, and inflammatory diseases. *Curr. Pharmacol. Rep.* **2015**, *1*, 129–139. [CrossRef] [PubMed]
87. Hardy, M.T.; Tollefsbol, T.O. Epigenetic diet: Impact on the epigenome and cancer. *Epigenomics* **2011**, *3*, 503–518. [CrossRef] [PubMed]
88. Feng, J.; Zhou, Y.; Campbell, S.L.; Le, T.; Li, E.; Sweatt, J.D.; Silva, A.J.; Fan, G. Dnmt1 and Dnmt3a maintain DNA methylation and regulate synaptic function in adult forebrain neurons. *Nat. Neurosci.* **2010**, *13*, 423–430. [CrossRef] [PubMed]
89. Fan, G.; Beard, C.; Chen, R.Z.; Csankovszki, G.; Sun, Y.; Siniaia, M.; Biniszkiewicz, D.; Bates, B.; Lee, P.P.; Kuhn, R.; et al. DNA hypomethylation perturbs the function and survival of CNS neurons in postnatal animals. *J. Neurosci.* **2001**, *21*, 788–797. [PubMed]
90. Iskandar, B.J.; Rizk, E.; Meier, B.; Hariharan, N.; Bottiglieri, T.; Finnell, R.H.; Jarrard, D.F.; Banerjee, R.V.; Skene, J.H.; Nelson, A.; et al. Folate regulation of axonal regeneration in the rodent central nervous system through DNA methylation. *J. Clin. Investig.* **2010**, *120*, 1603–1616. [CrossRef] [PubMed]
91. Huber, K.; Superti-Furga, G. After the grape rush: Sirtuins as epigenetic drug targets in neurodegenerative disorders. *Bioorg. Med. Chem.* **2011**, *19*, 3616–3624. [CrossRef] [PubMed]

92. Porquet, D.; Grinan-Ferre, C.; Ferrer, I.; Camins, A.; Sanfeliu, C.; del Valle, J.; Pallàs, M. Neuroprotective role of *trans*-resveratrol in a murine model of familial Alzheimer's disease. *J. Alzheimers Dis.* **2014**, *42*, 1209–1220. [PubMed]
93. National Institutes of Health, Clinical Trials.gov. Available online: https://clinicaltrials.gov/ (accessed on 15 June 2016).
94. Australian New Zealand Clinical Trials Registry. Available online: http://anzctr.org.au (accessed on 15 June 2016).
95. Lamport, D.J.; Pal, D.; Moutsiana, C.; Field, D.T.; Williams, C.M.; Spencer, J.P.; Butler, L.T. The effect of flavanol-rich cocoa on cerebral perfusion in healthy older adults during conscious resting state: A placebo controlled, crossover, acute trial. *Psychopharmacology* **2015**, *232*, 3227–3234. [CrossRef] [PubMed]
96. Baum, L.; Lam, C.W.; Cheung, S.K.; Kwok, T.; Lui, V.; Tsoh, J.; Lam, L.; Leung, V.; Hui, E.; Ng, C.; et al. Six-month randomized, placebo-controlled, double-blind, pilot clinical trial of curcumin in patients with Alzheimer disease. *J. Clin. Psychopharmacol.* **2008**, *28*, 110–113. [CrossRef] [PubMed]
97. Ringman, J.M.; Frautschy, S.A.; Teng, E.; Begum, A.N.; Bardens, J.; Beigi, M.; Gylys, K.H.; Badmaev, V.; Heath, D.D.; Apostolova, L.G.; et al. Oral curcumin for Alzheimer's disease: Tolerability and efficacy in a 24-week randomized, double blind, placebo-controlled study. *Alzheimers Res. Ther.* **2012**, *4*, 43. [CrossRef] [PubMed]
98. Hishikawa, N.; Takahashi, Y.; Amakusa, Y.; Tanno, Y.; Tuji, Y.; Niwa, H.; Murakami, N.; Krishna, U.K. Effects of turmeric on Alzheimer's disease with behavioral and psychological symptoms of dementia. *AYU* **2012**, *33*, 499–504. [CrossRef] [PubMed]
99. Cox, K.H.; Pipingas, A.; Scholey, A.B. Investigation of the effects of solid lipid curcumin on cognition and mood in a healthy older population. *J. Psychopharmacol.* **2015**, *29*, 642–651. [CrossRef] [PubMed]
100. Rainey-Smith, S.R.; Brown, B.M.; Sohrabi, H.R.; Shah, T.; Goozee, K.G.; Gupta, V.B.; Martins, R.N. Curcumin and cognition: A randomised, placebo-controlled, double-blind study of community-dwelling older adults. *Br. J. Nutr.* **2016**, *115*, 2106–2113. [CrossRef] [PubMed]
101. National Institutes of Health, Clinical Trials.gov. Early Intervention in Mild Cognitive Impairment (MCI) With Curcumin + Bioperine. Available online: https://clinicaltrials.gov/ct2/show/NCT00595582 (accessed on 15 June 2016).
102. National Institutes of Health, Clinical Trials.gov. Efficacy and Safety of Curcumin Formulation in Alzheimer's Disease. Available online: https://clinicaltrials.gov/ct2/show/NCT01001637 (accessed on 15 June 2016).
103. National Institutes of Health, Clinical Trials.gov. 18-Month Study of Curcumin (Curcumin). Available online: https://clinicaltrials.gov/ct2/show/NCT01383161 (accessed on 15 June 2016).
104. National Institutes of Health, Clinical Trials.gov. Curcumin and Yoga Therapy for Those at Risk for Alzheimer's Disease. Available online: https://clinicaltrials.gov/ct2/show/NCT01811381 (accessed on 15 June 2016).
105. Australian New Zealand Clinical Trials Registry. Investigation of the Effects of Longvida Curcumin on Cognitive Function, Mood and Biomarkers of Health. Available online: https://www.anzctr.org.au/Trial/Registration/TrialReview.aspx?id=370499 (accessed on 15 June 2016).
106. Australian New Zealand Clinical Trials Registry. McCusker KARVIAH: Curcumin in Alzheimer's Disease Prevention. Available online: https://www.anzctr.org.au/Trial/Registration/TrialReview.aspx?ACTRN=12613000681752 (accessed on 15 June 2016).
107. Australian New Zealand Clinical Trials Registry. The Epigenetic Effect of Curcumin as Measured in the Blood and Seen within Lifestyle, for the Prevention of Alzheimer's Disease. Available online: https://www.anzctr.org.au/Trial/Registration/TrialReview.aspx?id=366926 (accessed on 15 June 2016).
108. Australian New Zealand Clinical Trials Registry. This Study Will Evaluate if an Eye Examination Can Identify Changes in the Structure of the Retina Which May Help in the Early Detection of Alzheimer's Disease. Available online: https://www.anzctr.org.au/Trial/Registration/TrialReview.aspx?id=363949 (accessed on 15 June 2016).
109. Australian New Zealand Clinical Trials Registry. Imaging of Retinal Amyloid Plaques in Alzheimer's Disease—Longitudinal Study. Available online: https://www.anzctr.org.au/Trial/Registration/TrialReview.aspx?id=368267 (accessed on 15 June 2016).
110. Australian New Zealand Clinical Trials Registry. Imaging of Retinal Amyloid Plaques in Alzheimer's Disease—Middle Aged Controls Study. Available online: https://www.anzctr.org.au/Trial/Registration/TrialReview.aspx?id=368764 (accessed on 15 June 2016).

111. Kennedy, D.; Wightman, E.L.; Reay, J.L.; Lietz, G.; Okello, E.J.; Wilde, A.; Haskell, C.F. Effects of resveratrol on cerebral blood flow variables and cognitive performance in humans: A double-blind, placebo-controlled, crossover investigation. *Am. J. Clin. Nutr.* **2010**, *91*, 1590–1597. [CrossRef] [PubMed]
112. Wong, R.H.; Berry, N.M.; Coates, A.M.; Buckley, J.D.; Bryan, J.; Kunz, I.; Howe, P.R. Chronic resveratrol consumption improves brachial flow-mediated dilatation in healthy obese adults. *J. Hypertens.* **2013**, *31*, 1819–1827. [CrossRef] [PubMed]
113. Witte, A.V.; Kerti, L.; Margulies, D.S.; Flöel, A. Effects of resveratrol on memory performance, hippocampal functional connectivity, and glucose metabolism in healthy older adults. *J. Neurosci.* **2014**, *34*, 7862–7870. [CrossRef] [PubMed]
114. Wightman, E.L.; Reay, JL.; Haskell, CF.; Williamson, G.; Dew, T.P.; Kennedy, D.O. Effects of resveratrol alone or in combination with piperine on cerebral blood flow parameters and cognitive performance in human subjects: A randomised, double-blind, placebo-controlled, cross-over investigation. *Br. J. Nutr.* **2014**, *112*, 203–213. [CrossRef] [PubMed]
115. Turner, R.S.; Thomas, R.G.; Craft, S.; van Dyck, C.H.; Mintzer, J.; Reynolds, B.A.; Brewer, J.B.; Rissman, R.A.; Raman, R.; Aisen, P.S. Alzheimer's disease cooperative study. A randomized, double-blind, placebo-controlled trial of resveratrol for Alzheimer disease. *Neurology* **2015**, *85*, 1383–1391. [CrossRef] [PubMed]
116. Wong, R.H.; Nealon, R.S.; Scholey, A.; Howe, P.R. Low dose resveratrol improves cerebrovascular function in type 2 diabetes mellitus. *Nutr. Metab. Cardiovasc. Dis.* **2016**, *26*, 393–399. [CrossRef] [PubMed]
117. National Institutes of Health, Clinical Trials.gov. Pilot Study of the Effects of Resveratrol Supplement in Mild-to-moderate Alzheimer's Disease. Available online: https://clinicaltrials.gov/ct2/show/NCT00743743 (accessed on 15 June 2016).
118. National Institutes of Health, Clinical Trials.gov. Randomized Trial of a Nutritional Supplement in Alzheimer's Disease. Available online: https://clinicaltrials.gov/ct2/show/NCT00678431 (accessed on 15 June 2016).
119. National Institutes of Health, Clinical Trials.gov. Resveratrol for Improved Performance in the Elderly (RIPE). Available online: https://clinicaltrials.gov/ct2/show/NCT01126229 (accessed on 15 June 2016).
120. Anton, S.D.; Embry, C.; Marsiske, M.; Lu, X.; Doss, H.; Leeuwenburgh, C.; Manini, T.M. Safety and metabolic outcomes of resveratrol supplementation in older adults: Results of a twelve-week, placebo-controlled pilot study. *Exp. Gerontol.* **2014**, *57*, 181–187. [CrossRef] [PubMed]
121. National Institutes of Health, Clinical Trials.gov. Cognitive Effects of 500 mg Trans-resveratrol. Available online: https://clinicaltrials.gov/ct2/show/NCT01794351 (accessed on 15 June 2016).
122. National Institutes of Health, Clinical Trials.gov. Effects of Dietary Interventions on the Brain in Mild Cognitive Impairment (MCI). Available online: https://clinicaltrials.gov/ct2/show/NCT01219244 (accessed on 15 June 2016).
123. National Institutes of Health, Clinical Trials.gov. Cerebrovascular and Cognitive Improvement by Resveratrol (resVida) and Fruitflow-II (CCIRF-II) (CCIRF-II). Available online: https://clinicaltrials.gov/ct2/show/NCT01766180 (accessed on 15 June 2016).
124. National Institutes of Health, Clinical Trials.gov. Impact of Resveratrol on Brain Function and Structure. Available online: https://clinicaltrials.gov/ct2/show/NCT02621554 (accessed on 15 June 2016).
125. National Institutes of Health, Clinical Trials.gov. BDPP Treatment for Mild Cognitive Impairment (MCI) and Prediabetes (BDPP). Available online: https://clinicaltrials.gov/ct2/show/NCT02502253 (accessed on 15 June 2016).
126. Australian New Zealand Clinical Trials Registry. The Effect of Resveratrol in Red Wine on Cognitive Function in Older Adults: Preliminary Study. Available online: https://www.anzctr.org.au/Trial/Registration/TrialReview.aspx?id=347694 (accessed on 15 June 2016).
127. Lovibond, P.F.; Lovibond, S.H. The structure of negative emotional states: Comparison of the Depression Anxiety Stress Scales (DASS) with the Beck Depression and Anxiety Inventories. *Behav. Res. Ther.* **1995**, *3*, 335–343. [CrossRef]
128. Nasreddine, Z.S.; Phillips, N.A.; Bédirian, V.; Charbonneau, S.; Whitehead, V.; Collin, I.; Cummings, J.L.; Chertkow, H. The Montreal Cognitive Assessment, MoCA: A brief screening tool for mild cognitive impairment. *J. Am. Geriatr. Soc.* **2005**, *53*, 695–699. [CrossRef] [PubMed]
129. National Institutes of Health, Clinical Trials.gov. Early Detection of Mild Cognitive Impairment in Individual Patients. Available online: https://clinicaltrials.gov/ct2/show/study/NCT00243451 (accessed

on 15 June 2016).

130. Ahmed, T.; Javed, S.; Javed, S.; Tariq, A.; Šamec, D.; Tejada, S.; Nabavi, S.F.; Braidy, N.; Nabavi, S.M. Resveratrol and Alzheimer's disease: Mechanistic insights. *Mol. Neurobiol.* **2016**. [CrossRef] [PubMed]
131. Cheng, A.L.; Hsu, C.H.; Lin, J.K.; Hsu, M.M.; Ho, Y.F.; Shen, T.S.; Ko, J.Y.; Lin, J.T.; Lin, B.R.; Ming-Shiang, W.; et al. Phase I clinical trial of curcumin, a chemopreventive agent, in patients with high-risk or pre-malignant lesions. *Anticancer Res.* **2001**, *21*, 2895–2900. [PubMed]
132. Cottart, C.H.; Nivet-Antoine, V.; Beaudeux, J.L. Review of recent data on the metabolism, biological effects, and toxicity of resveratrol in humans. *Mol. Nutr. Food Res.* **2014**, *58*, 7–21. [CrossRef] [PubMed]
133. Kanai, M. Therapeutic applications of curcumin for patients with pancreatic cancer. *World J. Gastroenterol.* **2014**, *20*, 9384–9391. [PubMed]
134. Erdogan, C.S.; Vang, O. Challenges in analyzing the biological effects of resveratrol. *Nutrients* **2016**, *8*, 353. [CrossRef] [PubMed]
135. Morbidelli, L. Polyphenol-based nutraceuticals for the control of angiogenesis: Analysis of the critical issues for human use. *Pharmacol. Res.* **2016**, *111*, 384–393. [CrossRef] [PubMed]
136. Prasad, S.; Tyagi, A.K.; Aggarwal, B.B. Recent developments in delivery, bioavailability, absorption and metabolism of curcumin: the Golden pigment from golden spice. *Cancer Res. Treat.* **2014**, *46*, 2–18. [CrossRef] [PubMed]
137. Johnson, J.J.; Nihal, M.; Siddiqui, I.A.; Scarlett, C.O.; Bailey, H.H.; Mukhtar, H.; Ahmad, N. Enhancing the bioavailability of resveratrol by combining it with piperine. *Mol. Nutr. Food Res.* **2011**, *55*, 1169–1176. [CrossRef] [PubMed]
138. Nahar, P.P.; Slitt, A.L.; Seeram, N.P. Anti-inflammatory effects of novel standardized solid lipid curcumin formulations. *J. Med. Food* **2015**, *18*, 786–792. [CrossRef] [PubMed]
139. Sasaki, H.; Sunagawa, Y.; Takahashi, K.; Imaizumi, A.; Fukuda, H.; Hashimoto, T.; Wada, H.; Katanasaka, Y.; Kakeya, H.; Fujita, M.; et al. Innovative preparation of curcumin for improved oral bioavailability. *Biol. Pharm. Bull.* **2011**, *34*, 660–665. [CrossRef] [PubMed]
140. Antony, B.; Merina, B.; Iyer, V.S.; Judy, N.; Lennertz, K.; Joyal, S. A pilot cross-over study to evaluate human oral bioavailability of BCM-95®CG (Biocurcumax™), a novel bioenhanced preparation of curcumin. *Indian J. Pharm. Sci.* **2008**, *70*, 445–449. [CrossRef] [PubMed]
141. Aggarwal, B.B.; Yuan, W.; Li, S.; Gupta, S.C. Curcumin-free turmeric exhibits anti-inflammatory and anticancer activities: Identification of novel components of turmeric. *Mol. Nutr. Food Res.* **2013**, *57*, 1529–1542. [CrossRef] [PubMed]
142. Ryu, E.K.; Choe, Y.S.; Lee, K.H.; Choi, Y.; Kim, BT. Curcumin and dehydrozingerone derivatives: Synthesis, radiolabeling, and evaluation for β-amyloid plaque imaging. *J. Med. Chem.* **2006**, *49*, 6111–6119. [CrossRef] [PubMed]
143. Koronyo-Hamaoui, M.; Koronyo, Y.; Ljubimov, A.V.; Miller, C.A.; Ko, M.K.; Black, K.L.; Schwartz, M.; Farkas, D.L. Identification of amyloid plaques in retinas from Alzheimer's patients and noninvasive in vivo optical imaging of retinal plaques in a mouse model. *Neuroimage* **2011**, *54*, S204–S217. [CrossRef] [PubMed]

12

Protective Effects of Costunolide against Hydrogen Peroxide-Induced Injury in PC12 Cells

Chong-Un Cheong [1,†], Ching-Sheng Yeh [2,3,4,5,†], Yi-Wen Hsieh [6], Ying-Ray Lee [7], Mei-Ying Lin [8], Chung-Yi Chen [2,*] and Chien-Hsing Lee [9,*]

1 Department of Intensive Care Medicine, Chi Mei Medical Center, Liouying, Tainan City 73657, Taiwan; jhnchong@me.com
2 Department of Nutrition and Health Science, School of Medical and Health Sciences, Fooyin University, Kaohsiung City 83102, Taiwan; janson.yeh@msa.hinet.net
3 Bio-Medical Technology Developmental Center, Fooyin University, Kaohsiung City 83102, Taiwan
4 Department of Medical Technology, School of Medical and Health Sciences, Fooyin University, Kaohsiung City 83102, Taiwan
5 Department of Medical Research, Fooyin University Hospital, Ping-Tung County 92847, Taiwan
6 Department of Mackay Memorial Hospital Taitung Branch, Taitung County 95054, Taiwan; yisnolly@gmail.com
7 Department of Medical Research, Chiayi Christian Hospital, Chiayi City 60002, Taiwan; yingray.lee@gmail.com
8 Cancer Center, Kaohsiung Medical University Hospital, Kaohsiung City 80708, Taiwan; eileen26854@yahoo.com.tw
9 Department of Nursing, Min-Hwei Junior College of Health Care Management, Tainan City 73658, Taiwan
* Correspondence: xx377@fy.edu.tw (C.-Y.C.); chlee0818@gmail.com (C.-H.L.)

† These authors contributed equally to this work.

Academic Editor: Thomas J. Schmidt

Abstract: Oxidative stress-mediated cellular injury has been considered as a major cause of neurodegenerative diseases including Alzheimer's and Parkinson's diseases. The scavenging of reactive oxygen species (ROS) mediated by antioxidants may be a potential strategy for retarding the diseases' progression. Costunolide (CS) is a well-known sesquiterpene lactone, used as a popular herbal remedy, which possesses anti-inflammatory and antioxidant activity. This study aimed to investigate the protective role of CS against the cytotoxicity induced by hydrogen peroxide (H_2O_2) and to elucidate potential protective mechanisms in PC12 cells. The results showed that the treatment of PC12 cells with CS prior to H_2O_2 exposure effectively increased the cell viability. Furthermore, it decreased the intracellular ROS, stabilized the mitochondria membrane potential (MMP), and reduced apoptosis-related protein such as caspase 3. In addition, CS treatment attenuated the cell injury by H_2O_2 through the inhibition of phosphorylation of p38 and the extracellular signal-regulated kinase (ERK). These results demonstrated that CS is promising as a potential therapeutic candidate for neurodegenerative diseases resulting from oxidative damage and further research on this topic should be encouraged.

Keywords: reactive oxygen species; costunolide; PC12 cells; mitochondria membrane potential

---

1. Introduction

Reactive oxygen species (ROS), a substance resulting from neuronal injury during oxidative stress, regulates many cellular activities under physiological conditions [1]. Oxidative stress- mediated cellular injury has long been associated with a variety of neurodegenerative diseases such as Alzheimer's disease, Parkinson's disease, stroke, and amyotrophic lateral sclerosis [2–5]. Furthermore, H_2O_2 is thought to be the major precursor of ROS and has been utilized extensively as an inducer of oxidative damage to interpret mechanisms and the neuroprotective potential of therapeutics [6].

Several evidences have showed that H_2O_2 induces cytotoxicity in rat pheochromocytoma (PC12), which has neuron-like characteristics and provides a useful model system in analyzing the neurological apoptosis and the prevention mechanisms of antioxidants [7–9]. Moreover, H_2O_2-induced apoptosis has been linked to various key alterations including in anti-apoptosis proteins, pro-apoptosis proteins and caspases. Therapeutic strategies focusing on prevention of the ROS mediated by antioxidants seem to have potential for delaying the diseases' progression [10]. Many synthetic antioxidants have been demonstrated to be strong radical scavengers, but they are also carcinogenic and cause liver damage [11]. Therefore, much attention has recently been focused on the isolation and identification of antioxidants from natural sources with neuroprotective potential [12,13].

Costunolide (CS) is a sesquiterpene lactone found in the leaves of *Laurus nobilis* (Lauraceae), which has been reported to have anti-inflammatory [14], neuronal dopaminergic cells protection [15], anti-viral and anti-fungal properties [16,17], as well as cytotoxic effects on various human cancer cells [18] and antioxidant activity [19]. The chemical structure of CS is shown in Figure 1. However, its neuroprotective activity has yet to be explored. In this study, we used H_2O_2-induced oxidative damage in PC12 cells as an in vitro model to determine the neuroprotective activity of CS and to further investigate the mechanism.

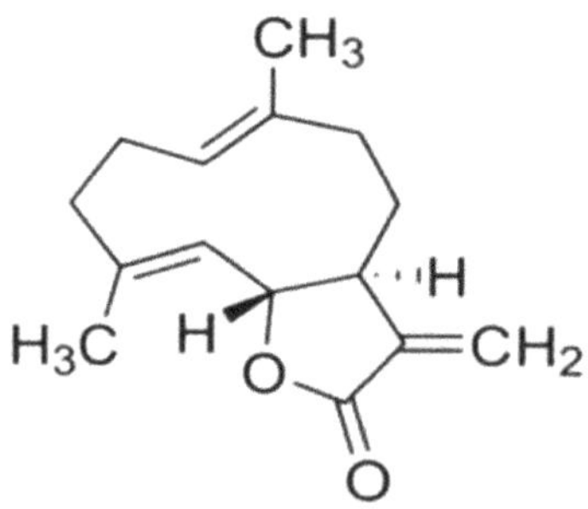

Figure 1. Chemical structure of costunolide (CS).

2. Results and Discussion

2.1. *Effect of Costunolide on Viability of H_2O_2-Induced PC12 Cells*

Overproduction of ROS causes damages to the cellular structures of neurons including lipids and membranes, proteins, and DNA [20]. The oxidative stress-induced ROS is involved in the pathophysiology of major neurodegenerative diseases such as Parkinson's and Alzheimer's diseases [20–22]. Several reports suggest therapeutic strategies focused on searching for the potential targets involved in the neuroprotection of natural compounds that can scavenge free radicals and protect cells from oxidative damage [12,13]. Previous studies have revealed that CS possesses antioxidant activities [19]. However, whether CS can exert protective effects against oxidative cytotoxicity in neuronal models as a result of its antioxidant properties has not been established in the literature.

A pilot study revealed that H_2O_2 ranging from 0.1 to 1.5 mM leads to cell death in a dose dependent manner and 0.75 mM H_2O_2 induced cell injury in a moderate manner (Figure 2A). These morphological alterations are reported illustrated in Figure 2B. The aim of the study was to investigate the effects of antioxidants over a short time frame (0–6 h). Therefore this concentration (0.75 mM H_2O_2) was used for all further experiments. The high concentration of H_2O_2 exposure of PC12 cells is consistent with investigations of the neuroprotective effects of macranthoin G [9] and the flavonoid extracts [23].

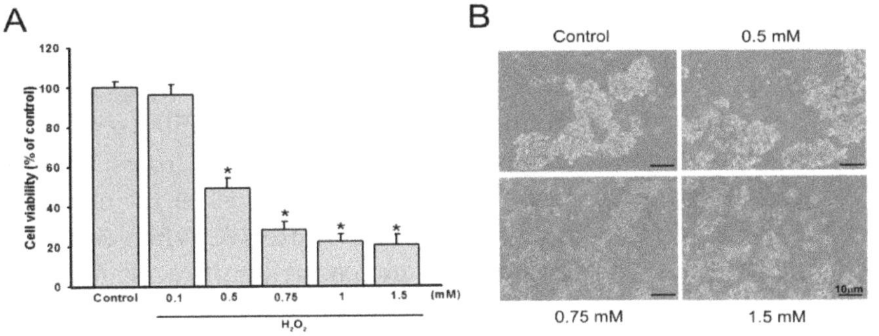

Figure 2. Effects of H_2O_2 on PC12 cell viability and cell morphology. (**A**) Effect of H_2O_2 on viability of PC12 cells (exposure to 4 h). A MTT assay showed that H_2O_2 decreased cell viability in a concentration-dependent manner; (**B**) treatments with different concentrations induced cell morphological alterations. Data were summarized from three independent experiments. * $p < 0.05$ vs. control group.

To characterize the effects of CS on cell viability in the H_2O_2-stressed cultured PC12 cells, the cells were incubated with CS and 0.75 mM H_2O_2. The H_2O_2-induced cell death of cells was determined by MTT assays. As shown in Figure 3A, PC12 cells exposed to CS (0–200 μM) for 4 h did not exhibit any significant viability or proliferation alterations. However, incubation with 0.75 mM H_2O_2 for 4 h resulted in a cell viability rate of 26.9% compared to the control (Figure 3B). In contrast, pretreatment of the cells with CS (10, 30, 50, or 100 μM) for 1 h could remarkably restore cell survival to 34.0%, 55.33%, 90.8%, and 95.87%, respectively. The potency of 100 μM vitamin E was similar to that of 50 μM CS (data not shown). Moreover, the H_2O_2-induced neuronal injury was accompanied by changes in cell morphology as observed in the loss of the characteristic round form and grouping shaped in PC12 cells. According to the respective calculations, it was shown that the protection rates of CS were reported in Figure 3C. Results suggested that CS could be considered as a neuroprotective agent against H_2O_2-induced oxidative stress.

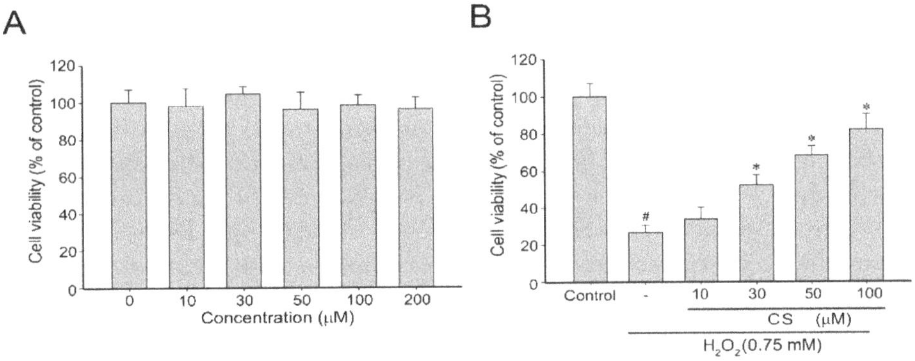

C

Group	Dose (μM)	Cell Viability (%)	Protection Rate (%)
control group	-	100 ± 6.5	-
model group (0.75 mMH_2O_2)	-	29.3 ± 6.0 #	-
CS	30	52.7 + 3.0 *	25.2 + 6.2
	100	79.2 ± 2.6 *	50.2 ± 5.4

Figure 3. Cytotoxicity and cytoprotective activity of costunolide (CS). (**A**) PC12 cells were pretreated with various concentrations of CS for 4 h; (**B**) Cell viability of PC12 cells pretreated with CS (10, 30, 50 and 100 μM) 1 h before exposure to H_2O_2 (0.75 mM) 4 h was measured by the MTT assay. Data are presented as mean ± SD (n = 3) and (**C**) The protection rates of CS are shown. Values with the same superscript letters are not significantly different from each other. # $p < 0.01$ compared with the control group; * $p < 0.05$, compared with the model group.

2.2. Effect of CS on H_2O_2-Induced ROS Production and Mitochondria Membrane Potential (MMP) in PC12 Cells

Oxidative stress-induced ROS production contributes to cell death by oxidation of many important proteins, leading to mitochondrial dysfunction and cell death [24,25]. To provide further evidence that CS could prevent H_2O_2-induced ROS generation and oxidative stress, levels of ROS production in the cells were determined using the fluorescence probe DCFH-DA for measuring the fluorescent compound dichlorofluorescein (DCF) [26]. As shown in Figure 4A, when cells were only exposed to 0.75 mM H_2O_2 for 6 h, the DCF fluorescence intensity increased significantly (305.18% of control group). Pretreatment with CS suppressed the fluorescence intensity in the H_2O_2-induced PC12 cells, suggesting that CS exerts its antioxidant effect in the intracellular compartment. A recent study indicated that the CS possessed protective effects on ethanol-induced oxidative gastrointestinal mucosal injury through restoration of oxidative stress markers, such as superoxide dismutase (SOD) and malondialdehyde (MDA) [27]. These results confirm that CS has antioxidant activity against ROS.

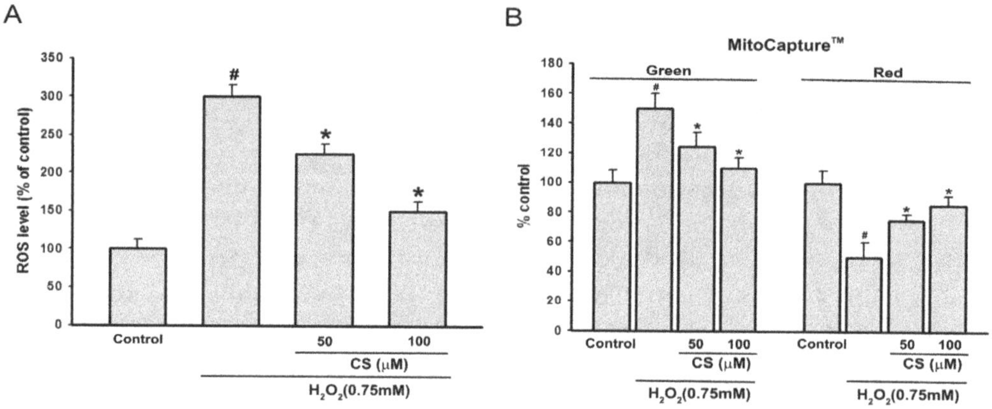

Figure 4. Effect of costunolide (CS) on H_2O_2-induced intracellular accumulation of ROS and mitochondria membrane potential (MMP). Intracellular ROS levels and MMP were measured using the MitoCapture™ Kit. PC12 cells were pretreated with various concentrations of CS for 30 min before exposure to 0.75 mM H_2O_2 for 6 h. (**A**) Histogram showing the ROS level in PC12 cells after treatment with H_2O_2 in presence or absence of CS compared to untreated groups; (**B**) Histogram showing the number of cells with a low potential in PC12 cells after treatment with H_2O_2 in presence or absence of CS compared to untreated groups. Cells were stained with MitoCapture™ solution, demonstrating both a reduced number of healthy cells (red signal) and increased number of cells with disrupted mitochondrial potential (green signal) in the presence of CS. Data are presented as mean ± SD ($n = 3$). Values with the same superscript letters are not significantly different from each other at # $p < 0.01$ compared with the control group; * $p < 0.05$, compared with the model group.

Excessive ROS production would damage mitochondrial membrane integrity and affect the energy production in mitochondria, resulting in mitochondrial dysfunction [28,29]. Furthermore, mitochondrial dysfunction includes a decrease in mitochondria membrane potential (MMP), activation of caspase-3, and apoptosis [30]. Therefore, we studied the effect of CS on MMP induced by H_2O_2 using the MitoCapture™ Apoptosis Detection Kit. The MitoCapture™ fluorescent dye was used as a marker for apoptosis. In healthy cells, the reagent congregates in the mitochondria and is detected as a red fluorescence signal. Conversely, in apoptotic cells, the dye remains in the cell cytosol (due to the disrupted mitochondrial membrane potential) and can be monitored as a green fluorescent signal [31]. Exposure of PC12 cells to H_2O_2 (0.75 mM) for 6 h induced a significant loss of MMP (Figure 4B), green fluorescence was increased by 45% ± 8%, while red fluorescence was decreased by 51% ± 6% (in both cases $n = 30$ and $p < 0.001$ compared with controls). Pretreatment with 50 μM CS significantly enhanced the reduction in MMP induced by H_2O_2, demonstrating that CS might change the occurrence of mitochondrial dysfunction after oxidative stress.

2.3. *Effect of CS on H_2O_2-Induced Apoptosis in PC12 Cells*

ROS have been demonstrated to induce damage biological molecules resulting in apoptotic or necrotic cell death [32]. Caspase-3 has been reported to be a key executioner caspase involved in neuronal apoptosis which modulates the mitochondria-dependent pathway [31]. To determine whether the cytoprotection by CS was due to the inhibition of apoptosis, the PC12 cells were treated with H_2O_2 and various concentrations of CS. As shown in Figure 5A, H_2O_2 treatment caused a remarkable increase of caspase-3 activity. However, adding 50 and 100 μM CS before H_2O_2 treatment decreased the caspase-3 activity to 205.68% and 158.63%, respectively. It can therefore be concluded that CS was effective in decreasing H_2O_2-induced apoptotic cell death. This supports the conclusion that CS inhibits H_2O_2-induced apoptosis through the regulation of intracellular ROS levels and mitochondria-dependent caspase-3 pathway.

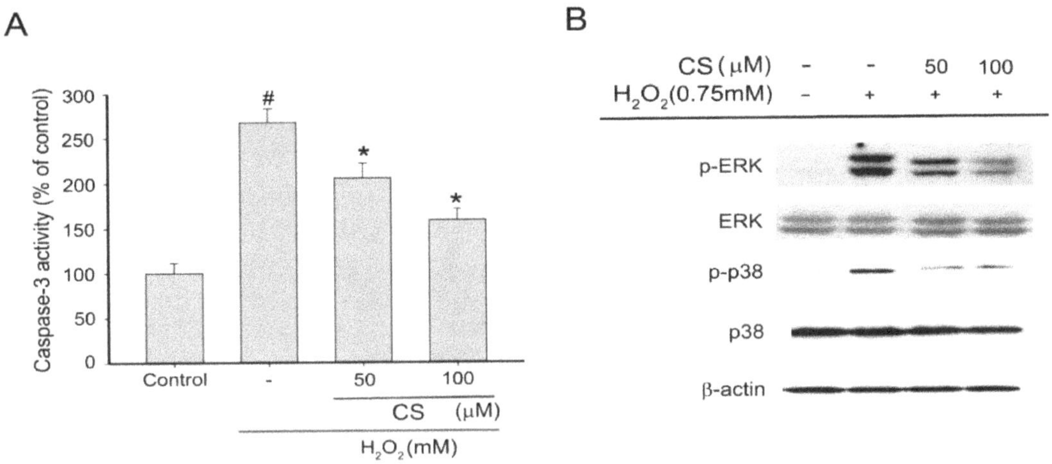

Figure 5. Effect of costunolide (CS) on H_2O_2-induced apoptosis in PC12 cells. PC12 cells were pretreated with various concentrations of MCG for 30 min before exposure to 0.75 mM H_2O_2 for 6 h. (**A**) The effect of CS on caspase-3 activity in H_2O_2-induced PC12 cells. Cells were pretreated with various concentrations of CS for 30 min before exposure to 0.75 mM H_2O_2 for 6 h. Caspase-3 activity was determined using a commercial kit according to the manufacturer's instruction. Values with the same color bars with the same superscript letters are not significantly different from each other at # $p < 0.01$ compared with the control group; * $p < 0.05$, compared with the model group; (**B**) Following the same treatment, the levels of phospho- or total mitogen activated protein kinases (MAPKs) (ERK and p38) were identified by their antibodies. Results are representative of three experiments.

2.4. *Effect of CS on MAPK Phosphorylation in H_2O_2-Induced PC12 Cells*

The mitogen-activated protein kinases (MAPK) signaling pathway plays an important role in cell proliferation, differentiation, and apoptosis [33,34]. They are also involved in ROS-mediated oxidative stress. ROS activates MAPKs in PC12 cells leading to apoptosis through activation of various downstream signal related events, such as MMP dissipation and activation of caspase-3 [35–38]. To further explore the effect of CS on the modulation of upstream signaling events against H_2O_2-stimulated oxidative stress, we examined MAPKs pathway by the immunoblot analysis. As shown in Figure 5B, pretreatment of cells with 50 and 100 μM CS significantly inhibited the H_2O_2-induced activation of phosphorylation of p38 MAPK and ERK. Consistent with the previous results, CS markedly inhibited LPS-induced activation of p38 MAPK and ERK [39]. A number of reports have shown that NF-κB/Rel activity is mediated by MAPKs [40]. Thus, our results provided a possible mechanism responsible for the neuroprotective effect of CS on NF-κB/Rel activity. Taken together, the inhibitory effects of CS on H_2O_2-induced apoptosis in PC12 cells was not only due to ROS scavenging, but also to the specific modulation of phosphorylation of p38 and ERK.

In addition, the neuroprotective effect of CS was also observed in dopamine-induced apoptosis in SH-SY5Y cells through reduction of α-synuclen [15] which increases the rate of production of ROS [41]. These results confirmed that CS is a cytoprotective agent for neurodegenerative diseases caused by ROS.

3. Materials and Methods

3.1. Chemicals and Reagents

Costunolide (CS), dimethylsulfoxide (DMSO), 1,1-diphenyl-2-picrylhydrazyl (DPPH), and 3-(4,5-dimethylthiazol-2-yl)-2,5-diphenyltetrazolium bromide (MTT) were obtained from Sigma (St. Louis, MO, USA). Dulbecco's modified Eagle's medium (DMEM) was purchased from Hyclone (Logan, UT, USA). Fetal bovine serum (FBS) and a penicillin/streptomycin mixture were purchased from Gibco (Grand Island, NY, USA). Vitamin E, catechin hydrate, Reactive Oxygen Species Assay Kit (S0033), cell lysis buffer for western blots and immunoprecipitation (IP) (P0013), 6× SDS-PAGE Sample Loading Buffer (P0015F) were obtained from Cell Signaling Technology (Danvers, MA, USA).

3.2. Cell Culture

PC12 cells were obtained from the American Type Culture Collection (ATCC), Rockville, MD, USA). PC12 cells were cultured in RPMI 1640 supplemented with 5% heat-inactivated FBS, 10% HS, 100 U/mL of penicillin, and 100 μg/mL of streptomycin. Cells were incubated at 37 °C in a humidified atmosphere of 95% air and 5% CO_2.

3.3. Cell Viability Assay

Cytoprotective activity of CS on H_2O_2-induced cell injury was investigated by an MTT assay. The PC12 cells were seeded into 96 well plates at a density of 5×10^4 cells/well for 16 h and then pretreated with vehicle alone or different concentrations of CS for 30 min before exposure to 0.75 mM H_2O_2 for 6 h. After removing the supernatant of each well, a total of 10 μL of MTT solution (5 mg/mL in phosphate-buffered saline (PBS)) and 90 μL of FBS-free medium were added to each well at the time of incubation for 4 h at 37 °C. The dark blue formazan crystals formed inside the intact mitochondria were solubilized with 100 μL of MTT stop solution (containing 10% sodium dodecyl sulfate (SDS) and 0.01 M hydrochloric acid). The amount of MTT formazan was determined based on the adsorption at 550 nm in a microplate reader (SpectraMax 250, Molecular Devices Inc., Sunnyvale, CA, USA). The optical density of formazan formed in control cells was taken as 100% viability. The protection rate of tested compounds was calculated using the following equation/protection rate (%) = (cell viability of drug group − cell viability of model group)/(cell viability of control group − cell viability of model group) × 100%.

3.4. Measurement of ROS

Generation of intracellular ROS was detected using a ROS-sensitive fluorescent probe (DCFH-DA). DCFH-DA is oxidized to highly fluorescent dichlorofluorescein (DCF) in the presence of ROS, which is readily detected by a flow cytometry [25]. A total of 1×10^5 PC12 cells was plated per well in 6 well plates with 2 mL culture medium for 16 h for stabilization and exposed to CS for 30 min before exposure to 0.75 mM H_2O_2 for 6 h. The cells were detached by gentle pipetting and washed with PBS. Cells were treated with 20 μM DHFH-DA for 30 min in the dark at room temperature. After DCFH-DA was removed, the cells were rinsed by PBS and collected in 15 mL centrifuge tubes by gentle centrifugation. Then, the supernatants were aspirated and cell pellets re-suspended in 1 mL PBS. Cells were finally transferred to flow cytometry tubes and intracellular ROS was measured via flow cytometry (Becton-Dickinson, Franklin Lakes, NJ, USA) at an excitation wavelength of 498 nm and an emission wavelength of 522 nm. The mean fluorescent intensity (MFI) of 10,000 cells was analyzed using three replicates for each experimental condition.

3.5. Measurement of Mitochondrial Transmembrane Potential

Mitochondrial transmembrane potential was evaluated with a MitoCapture™ Mitochondrial Apoptosis Detection kit (MBL, Nagoya, Japan), according to the manufacturer's instructions. CS were subjected to assays at 4 h. Images were taken under a fluorescence microscope using a bandpass filter to detect FITC and rhodamine. The cells with many aggregates giving off a bright red fluorescence represented those with a intact mitochondrial transmembrane potential and were enumerated.

3.6. Measurement of Caspase-3 Activity

Caspase-3 activity was measured using a commercial kit (Beyotime, Haimen, China) according to manufacturer's instruction. Briefly, a total of 1×10^6 cells was plated per well in 6 well plates with 2 mL culture medium for 16 h and exposed to CS for 30 min before exposure to 0.75 mM H_2O_2 for 6 h. Cells were harvested, washed twice with cold PBS and resuspended in lysis buffer on ice for 4 min. Next, cell lysates were centrifuged at 10,000× g at 4 °C for 10 min. Caspase-3 activity was measured by using reaction buffer and optical density was determined based on the adsorption at 405 nm using reaction buffer and optical density was determined based on the adsorption at 405 nm using an Infinite M200 Pro spectrophotometer (Tecan, Männedorf, Switzerland).

3.7. Data Analysis

All tests were carried out in triplicate (n = 3). The data are expressed as the mean ± standard derivation (SD). One-way analysis of variance (ANOVA) was used to determine the significant differences between the groups followed by a Dunnett's t-test for multiple comparisons. A probability <0.05 was considered as significant. All analyses were performed using SPSS for Windows 7, version 19.0 (IBM Corp., New York, NY, USA).

4. Conclusions

The neuroprotective effect of CS against H_2O_2-induced apoptosis in PC12 cells was investigated. It was found that CS can decrease H_2O_2-induced oxidative stress in PC12 cells by decreasing the ROS level and elevating MMP as well as restoring the mitochondria-dependent caspase-3 pathway. Furthermore, CS possibly affects upstream regulatory elements, such as p38, and ERK to attenuate the oxidative stress injury induced by H_2O_2 in PC12 cells. CS has been proved to possess aqueous solubility, good intestinal absorption and blood-brain barrier penetration [42]. These results demonstrate the potential of CS, providing a basis for further studies on its application to combat neurologic diseases, despite the fact that CS can be quite cytotoxic against other cells so its use to combat neurological disorders would probably be quite limited.

Acknowledgments: This study was supported by a Chi-Mei Medical Center Liouying Research Grant (CLFHR10228) and National Science Council of Taiwan (MOST 104-2320-B-242-001-MY3).

Author Contributions: C.-S.Y. and C.-H.L. conceived and designed the experiments; Y.-W.H. and C.-S.Y. performed the experiments; C.-S.Y. and C.-H.L. analyzed the data; C.-U.C., Y.-R.L. and C.-Y.C. contributed reagents/materials/analysis tools; M.-Y.L. and C.-H.L. wrote the paper.

Abbreviations

ROS	Reactive oxygen species
CS	Costunolide
H_2O_2	Hydrogen peroxide
MMP	Mitochondria membrane potential
ERK	Extracellular signal-regulated kinase

References

1. Zuo, L.; Zhou, T.; Pannell, B.K.; Ziegler, A.C.; Best, T.M. Biological and physiological role of reactive oxygen species-the good, the bad and the ugly. *Acta Physiol. (Oxf.)* **2015**, *214*, 329–348. [CrossRef] [PubMed]
2. Niranjan, R. The role of inflammatory and oxidative stress mechanisms in the pathogenesis of Parkinson's disease: Focus on astrocytes. *Mol. Neurobiol.* **2014**, *49*, 28–38. [CrossRef] [PubMed]
3. Sugawara, T.; Chan, P.H. Reactive oxygen radicals and pathogenesis of neuronal death after cerebral ischemia. *Antioxid. Redox Signal.* **2003**, *5*, 597–607. [CrossRef] [PubMed]
4. Ince, P.G.; Shaw, P.J.; Candy, J.M.; Mantle, D.; Tandon, L.; Ehmann, W.D.; Markesbery, W.R. Iron, selenium and glutathione peroxidase activity are elevated in sporadic motor neuron disease. *Neurosci. Lett.* **1994**, *182*, 87–90. [CrossRef]
5. Brieger, K.; Schiavone, S.; Miller, F.J., Jr.; Krause, K.H. Reactive oxygen species: From health to disease. *Swiss. Med. Wkly.* **2012**, *142*, w13659. [CrossRef] [PubMed]
6. Yu, Y.; Du, J.R.; Wang, C.Y.; Qian, Z.M. Protection against hydrogen peroxide-induced injury by Z-ligustilide in PC12 cells. *Exp. Brain Res.* **2008**, *184*, 307–312. [CrossRef] [PubMed]
7. Xiao, H.; Lv, F.; Xu, W.; Zhang, L.; Jing, P.; Cao, X. Deprenyl prevents MPP(+)-induced oxidative damage in PC12 cells by the upregulation of Nrf2-mediated NQO1 expression through the activation of PI3K/Akt and Erk. *Toxicology* **2011**, *290*, 286–294. [CrossRef] [PubMed]
8. Chen, B.; Yue, R.; Yang, Y.; Zeng, H.; Chang, W.; Gao, N.; Yuan, X.; Zhang, W.; Shan, L. Protective effects of (*E*)-2-(1-hydroxyl-4-oxocyclohexyl) ethyl caffeine against hydrogen peroxide-induced injury in PC12 cells. *Neurochem. Res.* **2015**, *40*, 531–541. [CrossRef] [PubMed]
9. Hu, W.; Wang, G.; Li, P.; Wang, Y.; Si, C.L.; He, J.; Long, W.; Bai, Y.; Feng, Z.; Wang, X. Neuroprotective effects of macranthoin G from *Eucommia ulmoides* against hydrogen peroxide-induced apoptosis in PC12 cells via inhibiting NF-kappaB activation. *Chem. Biol. Interact.* **2014**, *224C*, 108–116. [CrossRef] [PubMed]
10. Finkel, T.; Holbrook, N.J. Oxidants, oxidative stress and the biology of ageing. *Nature* **2000**, *408*, 239–247. [CrossRef] [PubMed]
11. Valentao, P.; Fernandes, E.; Carvalho, F.; Andrade, P.B.; Seabra, R.M.; Bastos, M.L. Antioxidative properties of cardoon (*Cynara cardunculus* L.) infusion against superoxide radical, hydroxyl radical, and hypochlorous acid. *J. Agric. Food Chem.* **2002**, *50*, 4989–4993. [CrossRef] [PubMed]
12. Wang, S.; Jin, D.Q.; Xie, C.; Wang, H.; Wang, M.; Xu, J.; Guo, Y. Isolation, characterization, and neuroprotective activities of sesquiterpenes from *Petasites japonicus*. *Food Chem.* **2013**, *141*, 2075–2082. [CrossRef] [PubMed]
13. Mansouri, M.T.; Farbood, Y.; Sameri, M.J.; Sarkaki, A.; Naghizadeh, B.; Rafeirad, M. Neuroprotective effects of oral gallic acid against oxidative stress induced by 6-hydroxydopamine in rats. *Food Chem.* **2013**, *138*, 1028–1033. [CrossRef] [PubMed]
14. Park, H.J.; Jung, W.T.; Basnet, P.; Kadota, S.; Namba, T. Syringin 4-*O*-beta-glucoside, a new phenylpropanoid glycoside, and costunolide, a nitric oxide synthase inhibitor, from the stem bark of *Magnolia sieboldii*. *J. Nat. Prod.* **1996**, *59*, 1128–1130. [CrossRef] [PubMed]
15. Ham, A.; Lee, S.J.; Shin, J.; Kim, K.H.; Mar, W. Regulatory effects of costunolide on dopamine metabolism-associated genes inhibit dopamine-induced apoptosis in human dopaminergic SH-SY5Y cells. *Neurosci. Lett.* **2012**, *507*, 101–105. [CrossRef] [PubMed]
16. Chen, H.C.; Chou, C.K.; Lee, S.D.; Wang, J.C.; Yeh, S.F. Active compounds from *Saussurea lappa* Clarks that suppress hepatitis B virus surface antigen gene expression in human hepatoma cells. *Antivir. Res.* **1995**, *27*, 99–109. [CrossRef]
17. Wedge, D.E.; Galindo, J.C.; Macias, F.A. Fungicidal activity of natural and synthetic sesquiterpene lactone analogs. *Phytochemistry* **2000**, *53*, 747–757. [CrossRef]
18. Park, S.H.; Choi, S.U.; Lee, C.O.; Yoo, S.E.; Yoon, S.K.; Kim, Y.K.; Ryu, S.Y. Costunolide, a sesquiterpene from the stem bark of *Magnolia sieboldii*, inhibits the RAS-farnesyl-proteintransferase. *Planta Med.* **2001**, *67*, 358–359. [CrossRef] [PubMed]
19. Eliza, J.; Daisy, P.; Ignacimuthu, S. Antioxidant activity of costunolide and eremanthin isolated from *Costus speciosus* (Koen ex. Retz) Sm. *Chem. Biol. Interact.* **2010**, *188*, 467–472. [CrossRef] [PubMed]
20. Valko, M.; Leibfritz, D.; Moncol, J.; Cronin, M.T.; Mazur, M.; Telser, J. Free radicals and antioxidants in normal physiological functions and human disease. *Int. J. Biochem. Cell Biol.* **2007**, *39*, 44–84. [CrossRef] [PubMed]

21. Dasuri, K.; Zhang, L.; Keller, J.N. Oxidative stress, neurodegeneration, and the balance of protein degradation and protein synthesis. *Free Radic. Biol. Med.* **2013**, *62*, 170–185. [CrossRef] [PubMed]
22. Zuo, L.; Hemmelgarn, B.T.; Chuang, C.C.; Best, T.M. The Role of Oxidative Stress-Induced Epigenetic Alterations in Amyloid-beta Production in Alzheimer's Disease. *Oxid. Med. Cell. Longev.* **2015**, *2015*, 604658. [CrossRef] [PubMed]
23. Horakova, L.; Licht, A.; Sandig, G.; Jakstadt, M.; Durackova, Z.; Grune, T. Standardized extracts of flavonoids increase the viability of PC12 cells treated with hydrogen peroxide: Effects on oxidative injury. *Arch. Toxicol.* **2003**, *77*, 22–29. [PubMed]
24. Avery, S.V. Molecular targets of oxidative stress. *Biochem. J.* **2011**, *434*, 201–210. [CrossRef] [PubMed]
25. Luo, P.; Chen, T.; Zhao, Y.; Xu, H.; Huo, K.; Zhao, M.; Yang, Y.; Fei, Z. Protective effect of Homer 1a against hydrogen peroxide-induced oxidative stress in PC12 cells. *Free Radic. Res.* **2012**, *46*, 766–776. [CrossRef] [PubMed]
26. Zuo, L.; Shiah, A.; Roberts, W.J.; Chien, M.T.; Wagner, P.D.; Hogan, M.C. Low Po(2) conditions induce reactive oxygen species formation during contractions in single skeletal muscle fibers. *Am. J. Physiol. Regul. Integr. Comp. Physiol.* **2013**, *304*, R1009–R1016. [CrossRef] [PubMed]
27. Zheng, H.; Chen, Y.; Zhang, J.; Wang, L.; Jin, Z.; Huang, H.; Man, S.; Gao, W. Evaluation of protective effects of costunolide and dehydrocostuslactone on ethanol-induced gastric ulcer in mice based on multi-pathway regulation. *Chem. Biol. Interact.* **2016**, *250*, 68–77. [CrossRef] [PubMed]
28. Li, S.Y.; Jia, Y.H.; Sun, W.G.; Tang, Y.; An, G.S.; Ni, J.H.; Jia, H.T. Stabilization of mitochondrial function by tetramethylpyrazine protects against kainate-induced oxidative lesions in the rat hippocampus. *Free Radic. Biol. Med.* **2010**, *48*, 597–608. [CrossRef] [PubMed]
29. Karbowski, M.; Neutzner, A. Neurodegeneration as a consequence of failed mitochondrial maintenance. *Acta Neuropathol.* **2012**, *123*, 157–171. [CrossRef] [PubMed]
30. Kim, K.Y.; Cho, H.J.; Yu, S.N.; Kim, S.H.; Yu, H.S.; Park, Y.M.; Mirkheshti, N.; Kim, S.Y.; Song, C.S.; Chatterjee, B.; et al. Interplay of reactive oxygen species, intracellular Ca^{2+} and mitochondrial homeostasis in the apoptosis of prostate cancer cells by deoxypodophyllotoxin. *J. Cell. Biochem.* **2013**, *114*, 1124–1134. [CrossRef] [PubMed]
31. Cheah, Y.H.; Nordin, F.J.; Tee, T.T.; Azimahtol, H.L.; Abdullah, N.R.; Ismail, Z. Antiproliferative property and apoptotic effect of xanthorrhizol on MDA-MB-231 breast cancer cells. *Anticancer Res.* **2008**, *28*, 3677–3689. [PubMed]
32. Li, C.; Li, X.; Suzuki, A.K.; Zhang, Y.; Fujitani, Y.; Nagaoka, K.; Watanabe, G.; Taya, K. Effects of exposure to nanoparticle-rich diesel exhaust on pregnancy in rats. *J. Reprod. Dev.* **2013**, *59*, 145–150. [CrossRef] [PubMed]
33. Zarubin, T.; Han, J. Activation and signaling of the p38 MAP kinase pathway. *Cell Res.* **2005**, *15*, 11–18. [CrossRef] [PubMed]
34. Qi, M.; Elion, E.A. MAP kinase pathways. *J. Cell Sci.* **2005**, *118*, 3569–3572. [CrossRef] [PubMed]
35. Ge, R.; Ma, W.H.; Li, Y.L.; Li, Q.S. Apoptosis induced neurotoxicity of Di-*n*-butyl-di-(4- chlorobenzohydroxamato) Tin (IV) via mitochondria-mediated pathway in PC12 cells. *Toxicol. In Vitro* **2013**, *27*, 92–102. [CrossRef] [PubMed]
36. Wu, F.; Wang, Z.; Gu, J.H.; Ge, J.B.; Liang, Z.Q.; Qin, Z.H. p38(MAPK)/p53-Mediated Bax induction contributes to neurons degeneration in rotenone-induced cellular and rat models of Parkinson's disease. *Neurochem. Int.* **2013**, *63*, 133–140. [CrossRef] [PubMed]
37. Khodagholi, F.; Tusi, S.K.; Alamdary, S.Z.; Amini, M.; Ansari, N. 3-Thiomethyl-5,6-(dimethoxyphenyl)-1,2,4-triazine improves neurite outgrowth and modulates MAPK phosphorylation and HSPs expression in H_2O_2-exposed PC12 cells. *Toxicol. In Vitro* **2012**, *26*, 907–914. [CrossRef] [PubMed]
38. Hwang, S.L.; Yen, G.C. Modulation of Akt, JNK, and p38 activation is involved in citrus flavonoid-mediated cytoprotection of PC12 cells challenged by hydrogen peroxide. *J. Agric. Food Chem.* **2009**, *57*, 2576–2582. [CrossRef] [PubMed]
39. Kang, J.S.; Yoon, Y.D.; Lee, K.H.; Park, S.K.; Kim, H.M. Costunolide inhibits interleukin-1beta expression by down-regulation of AP-1 and MAPK activity in LPS-stimulated RAW 264.7 cells. *Biochem. Biophys. Res. Commun.* **2004**, *313*, 171–177. [CrossRef] [PubMed]
40. Hagemann, C.; Blank, J.L. The ups and downs of MEK kinase interactions. *Cell Signal.* **2001**, *13*, 863–875. [CrossRef]

41. Angelova, P.R.; Horrocks, M.H.; Klenerman, D.; Gandhi, S.; Abramov, A.Y.; Shchepinov, M.S. Lipid peroxidation is essential for alpha-synuclein-induced cell death. *J. Neurochem.* **2015**, *133*, 582–589. [CrossRef] [PubMed]
42. Pitchai, D.; Roy, A.; Banu, S. In vitro and in silico evaluation of NF-kappaB targeted costunolide action on estrogen receptor-negative breast cancer cells-a comparison with normal breast cells. *Phytother. Res.* **2014**, *28*, 1499–1505. [CrossRef] [PubMed]

Permissions

All chapters in this book were first published by MDPI; hereby published with permission under the Creative Commons Attribution License or equivalent. Every chapter published in this book has been scrutinized by our experts. Their significance has been extensively debated. The topics covered herein carry significant findings which will fuel the growth of the discipline. They may even be implemented as practical applications or may be referred to as a beginning point for another development.

The contributors of this book come from diverse backgrounds, making this book a truly international effort. This book will bring forth new frontiers with its revolutionizing research information and detailed analysis of the nascent developments around the world.

We would like to thank all the contributing authors for lending their expertise to make the book truly unique. They have played a crucial role in the development of this book. Without their invaluable contributions this book wouldn't have been possible. They have made vital efforts to compile up to date information on the varied aspects of this subject to make this book a valuable addition to the collection of many professionals and students.

This book was conceptualized with the vision of imparting up-to-date information and advanced data in this field. To ensure the same, a matchless editorial board was set up. Every individual on the board went through rigorous rounds of assessment to prove their worth. After which they invested a large part of their time researching and compiling the most relevant data for our readers.

The editorial board has been involved in producing this book since its inception. They have spent rigorous hours researching and exploring the diverse topics which have resulted in the successful publishing of this book. They have passed on their knowledge of decades through this book. To expedite this challenging task, the publisher supported the team at every step. A small team of assistant editors was also appointed to further simplify the editing procedure and attain best results for the readers.

Apart from the editorial board, the designing team has also invested a significant amount of their time in understanding the subject and creating the most relevant covers. They scrutinized every image to scout for the most suitable representation of the subject and create an appropriate cover for the book.

The publishing team has been an ardent support to the editorial, designing and production team. Their endless efforts to recruit the best for this project, has resulted in the accomplishment of this book. They are a veteran in the field of academics and their pool of knowledge is as vast as their experience in printing. Their expertise and guidance has proved useful at every step. Their uncompromising quality standards have made this book an exceptional effort. Their encouragement from time to time has been an inspiration for everyone.

The publisher and the editorial board hope that this book will prove to be a valuable piece of knowledge for researchers, students, practitioners and scholars across the globe.

List of Contributors

Christian Galasso, Ida Orefice, Paola Pellone, Roberta Miele, Adrianna Ianora, Christophe Brunet and Clementina Sansone
Department of Marine Biotechnology, Stazione Zoologica Anton Dohrn, Villa Comunale, 80121 Naples, Italy

Paola Cirino
Department of Research Infrastructures for Marine Biological Resources, Stazione Zoologica Anton Dohrn, Villa Comunale, 80121 Naples, Italy

Johant Lakey-Beitia
Center for Biodiversity and Drug Discovery, Instituto de Investigaciones Científicas y Servicios de Alta Tecnología (INDICASAT AIP), Clayton, City of Knowledge 0843-01103, Panama

Jagadeesh Kumar D.
Department of Biotechnology, Sir M. Visvesvaraya Institute of Technology, Bangalore 562157, India

Muralidhar L. Hegde
Department of Radiation Oncology, Houston Methodist Research Institute, Houston, TX 77030, USA
Center for Neuroregeneration, Department of Neurosurgery, Houston Methodist, Houston, Texas 77030, USA
Weill Medical College of Cornell University, New York, NY 10065, USA

K.S. Rao
Center for Neuroscience, Instituto de Investigaciones Científicas y Servicios de Alta Tecnología (INDICASAT AIP), Clayton, City of Knowledge 0843-01103, Panama

Maria Grazia Morgese, Lucia Morgano, Paolo Tucci, Luigia Trabace and Stefania Schiavone
Department of Clinical and Experimental Medicine, University of Foggia, Foggia 71121, Italy

Emanuela Mhillaj and Maria Bove
Department of Physiology and Pharmacology, "Sapienza" University of Rome, Rome 00185, Italy

Matteo Francavilla
STAR Agroenergy Research Group, University of Foggia, Via Gramsci, 89-91, Foggia 71121, Italy
Institute of Marine Science, National Research Council, via Pola 4, Lesina 71010, Italy

Dorothea Kaufmann, Ahmad Tahrani, Florian Herrmann and Michael Wink
Institute of Pharmacy and Molecular Biotechnology, Department of Biology, Ruprecht Karls University Heidelberg, Heidelberg 69120, Germany

Anudeep Kaur Dogra
Centre for Pharmacognosy and Phytotherapy, The School of Pharmacy, University of London, 29-39 Brunswick Square, London WC1N 1AX, UK

Changmin Kim, Woojin Kim and Yangseok Kim
Department of Physiology, College of Korean Medicine, Kyung Hee University, 26 Kyunghee-daero, Dongdamoon-gu, Seoul 02447, Korea

Sun Kwang Kim
Department of Physiology, College of Korean Medicine, Kyung Hee University, 26 Kyunghee-daero, Dongdamoon-gu, Seoul 02447, Korea
Department of Science in Korean Medicine, Graduate School, Kyung Hee University, 26 Kyunghee-daero, Dongdamoon-gu, Seoul 02447, Korea

Ji Hwan Lee
Department of Science in Korean Medicine, Graduate School, Kyung Hee University, 26 Kyunghee-daero, Dongdamoon-gu, Seoul 02447, Korea

Dongxing Li
Department of Anesthesiology, Renji Hospital, School of Medicine, Shanghai Jiaotong University, 573 Xujiahui Rd., Dapiqiao, Huangpu Qu, Shanghai 200025, China

Kyungjin Lee
Department of Herbology, College of Korean Medicine, Kyung Hee University, 26 Kyunghee-daero, Dongdamoon-gu, Seoul 02447, Korea

Jianming Wu, Haixia Chen, Hua Li, Yong Tang, Shousong Cao and Dalian Qin
Department of Pharmacology, School of Pharmacy, Sichuan Medical University, Luzhou 86646-000, Sichuan, China

Le Yang
Chengdu Analytical Applications Center, Shimadzu (China) Co. Ltd., Chengdu 86610-063, Sichuan, China

Santa Cirmi, Nadia Ferlazzo and Michele Navarra
Department of Chemical, Biological, Pharmaceutical and Environmental Sciences, University of Messina, viale Annunziata, Messina I-98168, Italy

Giovanni E. Lombardo
Department of Health Sciences, University "Magna Graecia" of Catanzaro, Catanzaro I-88100, Italy

Elvira Ventura-Spagnolo
Department of Biotechnology and Legal Medicine, University of Palermo, Palermo I-90127, Italy

Sebastiano Gangemi
Department of Clinical and Experimental Medicine, University of Messina, Messina I-98125, Italy
Institute of Applied Sciences and Intelligent Systems (ISASI), National Research Council (CNR), Pozzuoli I-80078, Italy

Gioacchino Calapai
Department of Biomedical and Dental Sciences and Morphofunctional Imaging, University of Messina, Messina I-98125, Italy

Atsushi Sawamoto, Satoshi Okuyama, Kana Yamamoto, Mitsunari Nakajima and Yoshiko Furukawa
Department of Pharmaceutical Pharmacology, College of Pharmaceutical Sciences, Matsuyama University, 4-2 Bunkyo-cho, Matsuyama, Ehime 790-8578, Japan

Yoshiaki Amakura and Morio Yoshimura
Department of Pharmacognosy, College of Pharmaceutical Sciences, Matsuyama University, 4-2 Bunkyo-cho, Matsuyama, Ehime 790-8578, Japan

Rita Citraro, Antonio Leo, Eugenio Donato Di Paola, Ermenegildo Santangelo, Rossana Aiello, Emilio Russo and Giovambattista De Sarro
Department of Science of Health, School of Medicine and Surgery, University of Catanzaro, Catanzaro I-88100, Italy

Pellegrino Lippiello
Department of Pharmacy, University of Naples Federico II, Naples I-80131, Italy

Rosaliana Libro, Sabrina Giacoppo, Thangavelu Soundara Rajan, Placido Bramanti and Emanuela Mazzon
IRCCS Centro Neurolesi "Bonino-Pulejo", Via Provinciale Palermo, Contrada Casazza, 98124 Messina, Italy

Gabriela Mazzanti and Silvia Di Giacomo
Department of Physiology and Pharmacology, Sapienza—University of Rome, P.le Aldo Moro 5, 00185 Rome, Italy

Chong-Un Cheong
Department of Intensive Care Medicine, Chi Mei Medical Center, Liouying, Tainan City 73657, Taiwan

Chung-Yi Chen
Department of Nutrition and Health Science, School of Medical and Health Sciences, Fooyin University, Kaohsiung City 83102, Taiwan

Ching-Sheng Yeh
Department of Nutrition and Health Science, School of Medical and Health Sciences, Fooyin University, Kaohsiung City 83102, Taiwan
Bio-Medical Technology Developmental Center, Fooyin University, Kaohsiung City 83102, Taiwan
Department of Medical Technology, School of Medical and Health Sciences, Fooyin University, Kaohsiung City 83102, Taiwan
Department of Medical Research, Fooyin University Hospital, Ping-Tung County 92847, Taiwan

Yi-Wen Hsieh
Department of Mackay Memorial Hospital Taitung Branch, Taitung County 95054, Taiwan

Ying-Ray Lee
Department of Medical Research, Chiayi Christian Hospital, Chiayi City 60002, Taiwan

Mei-Ying Lin
Cancer Center, Kaohsiung Medical University Hospital, Kaohsiung City 80708, Taiwan

Chien-Hsing Lee
Department of Nursing, Min-Hwei Junior College of Health Care Management, Tainan City 73658, Taiwan

Gihyun Lee
Department of Physiology, College of Korean Medicine, Kyung Hee University, 26 Kyunghee-daero, Dongdaemoon-gu, Seoul 02447, Korea
Department of Research and Development, National Development Institute of Korean Medicine, 94 Hwarang-ro, Gyeongsan-si, Gyeongsangbuk-do 38540, Korea

Index

P

R

S

T

U

www.ingramcontent.com/pod-product-compliance
Lightning Source LLC
LaVergne TN
LVHW060543210926
848485LV00005B/1245
* 9 7 8 1 6 3 9 2 7 7 4 7 6 *